2010
YEAR BOOK OF
ANESTHESIOLOGY AND PAIN MANAGEMENT™

The 2010 Year Book Series

Year Book of Anesthesiology and Pain Management™: Drs Chestnut, Abram, Black, Gravlee, Lien, Mathru and Roizen

Year Book of Cardiology®: Drs Gersh, Cheitlin, Elliott, Gold, Graham, and Sundt

Year Book of Critical Care Medicine®: Drs Dellinger, Parrillo, Balk, Dorman, Dries, and Zanotti-Cavazzoni

Year Book of Dermatology and Dermatologic Surgery™: Dr Del Rosso

Year Book of Diagnostic Radiology®: Drs Osborn, Abbara, Birdwell, Elster, Manaster, Oestreich, Offiah, Rosado de Christenson, and Walker

Year Book of Emergency Medicine®: Drs Hamilton, Bruno, Handly, Mullin, Quintana, and Ramoska

Year Book of Endocrinology®: Drs Schott, Apovian, Clarke, Eugster, Ludlam, Meikle, Ovalle, Schinner, Schteingart, and Toth

Year Book of Gastroenterology™: Drs Talley, Dempsey, Harnois, Lange, Pearson, Picco, Rombeau, and Scolapio

Year Book of Hand and Upper Limb Surgery®: Drs Yao and Steinmann

Year Book of Medicine®: Drs Barker, Berney, Garrick, Gersh, Khardori, LeRoith, Talley, and Thigpen

Year Book of Neonatal and Perinatal Medicine®: Drs Fanaroff, Benitz, Neu, and Papile

Year Book of Neurology and Neurosurgery®: Drs Klimo and Rabinstein

Year Book of Obstetrics, Gynecology, and Women's Health®: Drs Dungan and Shulman

Year Book of Oncology®: Drs Thigpen, Arceci, Bauer, Byhardt, Gordon, and Lawton

Year Book of Ophthalmology®: Drs Rapuano, Cohen, Eagle, Flanders, Hammersmith, Myers, Nelson, Penne, Sergott, Shields, Tipperman, and Vander

Year Book of Orthopedics®: Drs Morrey, Beauchamp, Huddleston, Swiontkowski, and Trigg

Year Book of Otolaryngology-Head and Neck Surgery®: Drs Sindwani, Balough, Franco, Gapany, and Mitchell

Year Book of Pathology and Laboratory Medicine®: Drs Raab, Parwani, Bejarano, and Bissell

Year Book of Pediatrics®: Dr Stockman

Year Book of Plastic and Aesthetic Surgery™: Drs Miller, Gosain, Gurtner, Gutowski, Ruberg, Salisbury, and Smith

Year Book of Psychiatry and Applied Mental Health®: Drs Talbott, Ballenger, Buckley, Frances, Krupnick, and Mack

Year Book of Pulmonary Disease®: Drs Barker, Jones, Maurer, Raza, Tanoue, and Willsie

Year Book of Sports Medicine®: Drs Shephard, Cantu, Feldman, Jankowski, Khan, Nieman, Pierrynowski, and Rowland

Year Book of Surgery®: Drs Copeland, Behrns, Daly, Eberlein, Fahey, Huber, Jones, Mozingo, and Pruett

Year Book of Urology®: Drs Andriole and Coplen

Year Book of Vascular Surgery®: Drs Moneta, Gillespie, Starnes, and Watkins

2010

The Year Book of ANESTHESIOLOGY AND PAIN MANAGEMENT™

Editor-in-Chief

David H. Chestnut, MD

Associate Editors

Stephen E. Abram, MD
Susan Black, MD
Glenn P. Gravlee, MD
Cynthia A. Lien, MD
Mali Mathru, MD, FCCP
Michael F. Roizen, MD

ELSEVIER
MOSBY

ELSEVIER
MOSBY

Vice President, Continuity: John A. Schrefer
Developmental Editor: Yonah Korngold
Production Manager: Donna M. Skelton
Electronic Article Manager: Travis L. Ross
Illustrations and Permissions Coordinator: Linda Jones

2010 EDITION

Composition by TNQ Books and Journals Pvt Ltd, India

Editorial Office:
Elsevier
1600 John F. Kennedy Boulevard
Suite 1800
Philadelphia, PA 19103-2899

International Standard Serial Number: 1073-5437
International Standard Book Number: 978-0-323-06824-6

Editorial Board

Table of Contents

Journals Represented

Journals represented in this YEAR BOOK are listed below.

Acta Anaesthesiologica Scandinavica
Acta Obstetricia et Gynecologica Scandinavica
Acta Paediatrica
American Heart Journal
American Journal of Epidemiology
American Journal of Obstetrics and Gynecology
American Journal of Preventive Medicine
American Journal of Surgery
American Surgeon
Anaesthesia
Anaesthesia and Intensive Care
Anesthesia & Analgesia
Anesthesiology
Annals of Internal Medicine
Annals of Plastic Surgery
Annals of Surgery
Annals of Thoracic Surgery
Archives of Disease in Childhood
Archives of Internal Medicine
Archives of Physical Medicine and Rehabilitation
Arthritis & Rheumatism
Brain Research
British Journal of Anaesthesia
British Journal of Ophthalmology
British Journal of Surgery
British Medical Association
Canadian Family Physician
Canadian Journal of Anaesthesia
Cancer Epidemiology, Biomarkers & Prevention
Cell Cycle
Chest
Child Development
Circulation
Clinical Orthopaedics and Related Research
Critical Care Medicine
Diabetes Care
Digestive Diseases and Sciences
European Journal of Pain
European Journal of Obstetrics & Gynecology and Reproductive Biology
European Journal of Vascular and Endovascular Surgery
Headache
Hepatology
Hypertension
Intensive Care Medicine
International Journal of Behavioral Nutrition and Physical Activity
International Journal of Cancer
International Journal of Clinical Practice

International Journal of Gynecology & Obstetrics
International Journal of Obstetric Anesthesia
Journal of Bone and Joint Surgery American
Journal of Cardiothoracic and Vascular Anesthesia
Journal of Clinical Anesthesia
Journal of Clinical Investigation
Journal of Clinical Neuroscience
Journal of Epidemiology & Community Health
Journal of Neurosurgery
Journal of Neurosurgery Spine
Journal of Pain
Journal of Pain and Symptom Management
Journal of the American College of Cardiology
Journal of the American Dietetic Association
Journal of the American Geriatrics Society
Journal of the American Medical Association
Journal of the American Society of Echocardiography
Journal of Thoracic and Cardiovascular Surgery
Kidney International
Lancet
Medical Care
Medicine and Science in Sports and Exercise
Nature
Neurology
Neurosurgery
New England Journal of Medicine
Obstetrics & Gynecology
Pain
Proceedings of the National Academy of Sciences of the United States of America
Regional Anesthesia and Pain Medicine
Scandinavian Journal of Rheumatology
Science
Sleep
Sleep & Breathing
Spine
Spine Journal
Stroke
Surgery
Surgical Neurology
Thorax
World Journal of Surgery

Standard Abbreviations

The following terms are abbreviated in this edition: acquired immunodeficiency syndrome (AIDS), cardiopulmonary resuscitation (CPR), central nervous system (CNS), cerebrospinal fluid (CSF), computed tomography (CT), deoxyribonucleic acid (DNA), electrocardiography (ECG), health maintenance organization (HMO), human immunodeficiency virus (HIV), intensive care unit (ICU), intramuscular (IM), intravenous (IV), magnetic resonance (MR) imaging (MRI), ribonucleic acid (RNA), ultrasound (US), and ultraviolet (UV).

Note

The Year Book of Anesthesiology and Pain Management™ is a literature survey service providing abstracts of articles published in the professional literature. Every effort is made to ensure the accuracy of the information presented in these pages. Neither the editors nor the publisher of the Year Book of Anesthesiology and Pain Management™ can be responsible for errors in the original materials. The editors' comments are their own opinions. Mention of specific products within this publication does not constitute endorsement.

To facilitate the use of the Year Book of Anesthesiology and Pain Management™ as a reference tool, all illustrations and tables included in this publication are now identified as they appear in the original article. This change is meant to help the reader recognize that any illustration or table appearing in the Year Book of Anesthesiology and Pain Management™ may be only one of many in the original article. For this reason, figure and table numbers will often appear to be out of sequence within the Year Book of Anesthesiology and Pain Management™.

Introduction

It is an honor and a privilege for me to continue my service as Editor-in-Chief of the 2010 Year Book of Anesthesiology and Pain Management. I am happy that our distinguished editorial board remains intact for 2010.

I recently reviewed the selections for this edition and, as in past editions of the Year Book of Anesthesiology and Pain Management, the anesthesiology subspecialties (eg, cardiothoracic anesthesia, critical care medicine, neuroanesthesia, obstetric anesthesia, pain medicine, pediatric anesthesia, regional anesthesia) are well represented. Once again, sepsis and acute lung injury are the subjects of a number of the critical care medicine selections. The obstetric anesthesia chapter includes several selections that address the relationship between intrapartum neuraxial analgesia and obstetric outcome. Several selections address the implications of the increasing cesarean delivery rate for both mothers and neonates. And the obstetric anesthesia chapter also includes several selections that assess the efficacy of various vasopressor regimens for the prophylaxis and/or treatment of maternal hypotension during cesarean delivery. Postoperative analgesia continues to be a subject of high interest, and the pediatric anesthesia chapter includes a selection that assesses the use of continuous peripheral nerve blockade for postoperative analgesia in children.

This edition also includes a number of interesting selections that are not related to a specific subspecialty of anesthesiology. Skilled airway management remains the "bread and butter" for anesthesia providers, and several selections provide helpful information on airway management in both adults and children. A number of selections address issues related to neuromuscular blockade, including the use of sugammadex for reversal of rocuronium-induced neuromuscular blockade. Other selections discuss intraoperative awareness in both adults and children. And of special interest are the selections that address the effects of diet, exercise, and smoking cessation on aging and risk reduction.

In my current position, I divide my time between the clinical practice of anesthesiology and my administrative role as director of medical education for a large integrated health system and associate dean for a regional campus of a large school of medicine and public health. As a result, I spend a significant amount of time with medical students. I am happy to tell those students that I enjoy the practice of medicine today more than ever before! The practice of anesthesiology—and the opportunity to spend time with patients during some of their most significant and stressful life events—is surely a great and special privilege, as well as an awesome responsibility.

One of the joys of editing the Year Book is the opportunity to integrate lifelong learning with my daily clinical practice. I hope that you are enjoying your practice as much as I enjoy mine. Likewise, I hope that you will enjoy reading these selections and accompanying comments as much as my editorial colleagues and I have enjoyed preparing them for you.

David H. Chestnut, MD

1 Studies of Outcomes, Risks, Costs, and Benefits

Residual Neuromuscular Blockade and Critical Respiratory Events in the Postanesthesia Care Unit

Murphy GS, Szokol JW, Marymont JH, et al (Evanston Northwestern Healthcare, IL)

Anesth Analg 107:130-137, 2008

Background.—Incomplete recovery of neuromuscular function may impair pulmonary and upper airway function and contribute to adverse respiratory events in the postanesthesia care unit (PACU). The aim of this investigation was to assess and quantify the severity of neuromuscular blockade in patients with signs or symptoms of critical respiratory events (CREs) in the PACU.

Methods.—We collected data over a 1-yr period. PACU nurses identified patients with evidence of a predefined CRE during the first 15 min of PACU admission. Train-of-four (TOF) ratios were immediately quantified in these patients using acceleromyography (cases). TOF data were also collected in a control group that consisted of patients undergoing a general anesthetic during the same period who were matched with the cases by age, sex, and surgical procedure.

Results.—A total of 7459 patients received a general anesthetic during the 1-yr period, of whom 61 developed a CRE. Forty-two of these cases were matched with controls and constituted the study group for statistical analysis. The most common CREs among matched cases were severe hypoxemia (22 of 42 patients; 52.4%) and upper airway obstruction (15 of 42 patients; 35.7%). There were no significant differences between the cases and matched controls in any measured preoperative or intraoperative variables. Mean ($\pm$SD) TOF ratios were 0.62 ($\pm$0.20) in the cases, with 73.8% of the cases having TOF ratios <0.70. In contrast, TOF values in the controls were 0.98 ($\pm$0.07) (a difference of −0.36 with a 95% confidence interval of −0.43 to −0.30, $P < 0.0001$), and no control patients were observed to have TOF values <0.70 (the 95% confidence interval of the difference was 59%–85%, $P < 0.0001$).

Conclusions.—A high incidence of severe residual blockade was observed in patients with CREs, which was absent in control patients without CREs. These findings suggest that incomplete neuromuscular recovery is an important contributing factor in the development of adverse respiratory events in the PACU.

▶ In spite of the use of intermediate-acting neuromuscular blocking agents, patients continue to arrive in the postanesthesia care unit with unacceptable levels of neuromuscular blockade.[1-4] Without quantitative monitoring (a train-of-four monitor that displays the train-of-four ratio), patients are likely to continue to arrive in the postanesthesia care unit with inadequate recovery of muscle strength. Adequate recovery of strength is increasingly defined as a train-of-four ratio ≥0.9. Lesser degrees of recovery in volunteer trials are associated with malaise and visual disturbances,[5] decreased hypoxic ventilatory drive,[6] decreased coordination of the musculature associated with swallowing, and increased incidence of aspiration.[7]

In spite of the substantial documented incidence of residual postoperative neuromuscular block and the findings in several volunteer trials, there had been, until this study, only 2 prospective trials of the consequences of residual neuromuscular block.[8,9] Berg found an increased incidence of postoperative pulmonary complications, such as a new requirement for oxygen or pneumonia, in patients with train-of-four ratios <0.7 on arrival to the postanesthesia care unit following maintenance of neuromuscular block with pancuronium. Other factors associated with development of pulmonary complications included advance age, abdominal surgery, and a long duration of surgery. The more recent study by Murphy confirms the finding of the earlier trial, that postoperative residual neuromuscular block has clinical effects. It also demonstrates that patients with a train-of-four ratio <0.9 are at increased risk for critical respiratory events in the postanesthesia care unit. Critical respiratory events are defined as upper airway obstruction, hypoxemia, signs of pending respiratory failure, inability to breathe deeply when asked to do so, a feeling as if it is difficult to breathe, swallow, or speak and suspicion of pulmonary aspiration. In the almost 7500 patients studied, the incidence of critical respiratory events was 0.8%. The most commonly observed critical respiratory events were hypoxemia and airway obstruction. In the critical respiratory event group only 9.5% of patients had train-of-four ratios ≥0.9; 16.7% had train-of-four ratios ≥0.7 and <0.9, and most patients (73.8%) had train-of-four ratios <0.7. In contrast, in the matched control group no patients had train-of-four ratios <0.7 and the majority (90.5%) had train-of-four ratios ≥0.9.

While the incidence of critical respiratory events is low (<1%), it is not negligible. In a moderately sized hospital providing 10 000 anesthetics/year with general anesthesia and muscle relaxation, one can anticipate that there will be approximately 80 of these events each year. Until clinicians are routinely using monitors of neuromuscular block that measure and display train-of-four values, occurrence of critical respiratory events needs to be anticipated and postanesthesia care unit staff trained to look for and appropriately manage these events in order to minimize their potential for long-term effects.

C. A. Lien, MD

References

1. Murphy GS, Szokol JW, Marymount JH, et al. Intraoperative acceleromyographic monitoring reduces the risk of residual neuromuscular blockade and adverse respiratory events in the postanestehsia care unit. *Anesthesiology.* 2008;109:389-398.
2. Cammu G, DeWhitte J, De Veylder J, et al. Postoperative residual paralysis in outpatients versus inpatients. *Anesth Analg.* 2006;102:426-429.
3. Hayes AH, Mirakhur RK, Breslin DS, Reid JE, McCourt KC. Postoperative residual block after intermediate-acting neuromuscular blocking drugs. *Anaesthesia.* 2001;98:1333-1337.
4. Baillard C, Gehan G, Reboul-Marty J, Larmignat P, Samama CM, Cupa M. Residual curarization in the recovery room after vecuronium. *Br J Anaesth.* 2000;84:394-395.
5. Kopman AF, Yee PS, Neuman GG. Relationship of the train-of-four fade ratio to clinical signs and symptoms of residual paralysis in awake volunteers. *Anesthesiology.* 1997;86:765-771.
6. Erikkson LI, Sato M, Severinghaus JW. Effect of a vecuronium-induced partial neuromuscular block on hypoxic ventilator response. *Anesthesiology.* 1993;78:693-699.
7. Eriksson LI, Sundman E, Olsson R, et al. Functional assessment of the pharynx at rest and during swallowing in partially paralyzed humans: Simultaneous videomanometry and mechanomyography of awake human volunteers. *Anesthesiology.* 1997;78:693-699.
8. Berg H, Viby-Mogensen J, Roed J, et al. Residual neuromuscular block is a risk factor for postoperative pulmonary complications. a prospective, randomized and blinded study of postoperative pulmonary complications after atracurium, vecuronium, and pancuronium. *Acta Anaesthesiol Scand.* 1997;41:1095-1103.
9. Murphy GS, Szokol JW, Marymont JH, et al. Intraoperative acceleromyographic monitoring reduces the risk of residual neuromuscular blockade and adverse respiratory events in the postanesthesia care unit. *Anesthesiology.* 2008;109:389-398.

Complications associated with postoperative antibiotic prophylaxis after breast surgery

Throckmorton AD, Hoskin T, Boostrom SY, et al (Mayo Clinic, Rochester, MN; et al)

Am J Surg 198:553-556, 2009

Background.—Evidence supports single-dose preoperative antibiotic (ABX) prophylaxis for breast surgery; however, limited data exist regarding the incidence and type of antibiotic complications postoperatively.

Methods.—Breast/axillary surgeries between July 2004 and June 2006 were reviewed. Complications were analyzed by antibiotic group: preoperative prophylaxis, postoperative prophylaxis, and therapeutic intent. The Fisher exact test was used to compare complication rates.

Results.—A total of 389 patients underwent breast/axillary surgeries during the study period. A total of 363 (93%) patients received ABX:

353 (91%) received a single preoperative dose, 91 (23%) received postoperative ABX prophylaxis, and 76 (201%) received ABX for therapeutic intent. Among patients receiving ABX, 15 (4%) had an ABX-related complication. The ABX-related complication rate was significantly higher among those receiving postoperative prophylaxis (5.5%; 5 of 91) compared with those receiving preoperative ABX alone (0%; 0 of 214) (P =.002).

Conclusions.—Drug-related complications were uncommon with preoperative ABX prophylaxis. Considering the potential complications of ABX after breast surgery, the use of postoperative prophylaxis should be reexamined.

▶ Postoperative infection rates have recently become an area of intense interest as efforts are being made to minimize both length of hospital stay and complications associated with surgery. Protocols exist in each operating room to dictate how a surgical area should be prepped, what type of drapes should be used, and how surgeons should scrub for surgery and anesthesiologists should place invasive monitors. Prepping solutions that must be used—whether for physicians or patients—vary from one hospital to the next and are constantly being changed as new solutions that are potentially more effective become available. Even the solutions with which we clean our operating rooms change from time to time.

In an effort to minimize postoperative infections, anesthesiologists are monitored in terms of whether or not they administer prophylactic antibiotics within an hour before surgical incision. Later administration is not effective.[1-4] While studies indicate that infection rates are decreased with administration of one dose of preoperative antibiotics,[5–7] prolonged administration may increase risk of infection with resistant organisms.[5] As most patients undergoing surgical procedures receive prophylactic antibiotics, the risks associated with the exposure to these medications need to be established.

In this relatively small retrospective analysis of operations done from 2004-2006, no patient of the 214 who received only a single dose of antibiotics preoperatively developed any complication potentially associated with its administration. Just over 5% of patients who received antibiotics for postoperative prophylaxis had a complication attributed to antibiotic therapy.

Interestingly, while this was a study of complications associated with antibiotic therapy, and not a study of efficacy, 2 patients receiving postoperative antibiotic prophylaxis developed infections requiring treatment. Five of seventy-three patients receiving postoperative antibiotic prophylaxis developed complications related to antibiotic therapy, a percentage not dissimilar from the number of patients requiring treatment of an infection postoperatively who had not received antibiotic prophylaxis.

Certainly, more work needs to be done aligning requirement for administration of prophylactic antibiotics to all patients requiring it within an hour of surgical incision with what is best for patients. There seems to be little indication for postoperative antibiotic prophylaxis and considerable risk associated with their administration in patients who have had breast surgery.

C. A. Lien, MD

References

1. Burke JF. The effective period of preventive antibiotic action in experimental incisions and dermal lesions. *Surgery.* 1961;50:161-168.
2. Polk HC Jr, Lopez-Mayor JF. Postoperative wound infection: a prospective study of determinant factors and prevention. *Surgery.* 1969;66:97-103.
3. Classen DC, Evans RS, Pestotnik SL, Horn SD, Menlove RL, Burke JP. The timing of prophylactic administration of antibiotics and the risk of surgical-wound infection. *N Engl J Med.* 1992;326:281-286.
4. Polk HC Jr, Trachtenberg L, Finn MP. Antibiotic activity in surgical incisions: the basis for prophylaxis in selected operations. *JAMA.* 1980;244:1353-1354.
5. Harbarth S, Samore MH, Lichtenberg D, Carmeli Y. Prolonged antibiotic prophylaxis after cardiovascular surgery and its effect on surgical site infections and antimicrobial resistance. *Circulation.* 2000;101:2916-2921.
6. Su HY, Ding DC, Chen DC, Lu MF, Liu JY, Chang FY. Prospective randomized comparison of single-dose versus 1-day cefazolin for prophylaxis in gynecologic surgery. *Acta Obstet Gynecol Scand.* 2005;84:384-389.
7. Throckmorton AD, Boughey JC, Boostrom SY, et al. Postoperative antibiotics and infection rates in breast surgery patients. *Ann Surg Oncol.* 2009;16:2464-2469.

Nocturia and snoring: predictive symptoms for obstructive sleep apnea

Romero E, Krakow B, Haynes P, et al (Sleep and Human Health Inst, Albuquerque, NM)

Sleep Breath Epub ahead of print, 2009

Purpose.—Current screening for obstructive sleep apnea (OSA) emphasizes self-reported snoring and other breathing symptoms. Nocturia, a symptom with a precise pathophysiological link to sleep apnea, has not been assessed as a screening tool for this common disorder of sleep respiration. In a large sample of adults presenting to area sleep centers, we aimed to determine the predictive power of nocturia for OSA and compare findings with other markers of OSA commonly used to screen for this disease.

Methods.—This was a retrospective chart review. A consecutive sample of 1,007 adult patients seeking treatment at two sleep centers in New Mexico completed detailed medical and sleep history questionnaires and completed diagnostic polysomnography testing. The sensitivity, specificity, positive predictive value (PPV), and negative predictive value (NPV) of nocturia, snoring, high body mass index, sex, and age for OSA were determined. Hierarchical linear regression determined unique variance contribution to the apnea-hypopnea index, the objective measure of sleep apnea severity.

Results.—The results are as follows: sensitivities-snoring, 82.6% and nocturia, 84.8%; specificities-snoring, 43.0% and nocturia, 22.4%; PPVs-snoring, 84.7% and nocturia, 80.6%; and NPVs-snoring, 39.6%

and nocturia, 27.9%. With hierarchical linear regression, patient-reported nocturia frequency predicted apnea-hypopnea index (OSA severity) above and beyond body mass index, sex, age, and self-reported snoring ($P < 0.0001$).

Conclusions.—Nocturia appears comparable to snoring as a screening tool for OSA in patients presenting to a sleep medical center. Research in urology and primary care clinics is needed to definitively clarify the use of nocturia as a screening instrument for obstructive sleep apnea.

▶ This article on nocturia, snoring, and predictive symptoms for obstructive sleep apnea was an eye opener for me. I always thought of nocturia as something relating to benign prosthetic hypertrophy, but apparently nocturia also proves to be a very useful screen for obstructive sleep apnea. In fact, one that is almost as good as snoring. It is also a risk for nocturnal falls and mild to severe equality of life impairment. Apparently nocturia occurs because of the negative intrathoracic pressure swings that occur with obstructive breathing resulting in release of atrial natriuretic peptide and increased urine production during sleep. So in preoperative clinic when one is screening for obstructive sleep apnea in addition to looking at waist size and neck size, maybe we should be asking also about nocturia frequency.

M. F. Roizen, MD

The effect of teenage maternal obesity on perinatal outcomes

Haeri S, Guichard I, Baker AM, et al (Univ of North Carolina School of Medicine, Chapel Hill)

Obstet Gynecol 113:300-304, 2009

Objective.—To estimate the effect of obesity on perinatal outcomes among inner-city teenage pregnant women.

Methods.—In this retrospective cohort study, we reviewed all nulliparous teenaged (aged 18 years and younger) deliveries at the Washington Hospital Center between 2000 and 2004. Overweight and obese teenagers (body mass index at or above 25.0 kg/m) were compared with normal-weight (body mass index less than 25.0 kg/m) teenagers. Frequencies and odds ratios for adverse maternal-fetal outcomes were calculated.

Results.—Of the 10,322 deliveries that occurred during the study period, 712 (7%) were to teenagers. Among the 458 nulliparous teenaged mothers, 274 (60%) were normal weight and 184 (40%) were overweight/obese. Compared with normal-weight teens ($n = 274$), obese teens ($n = 78$) were at higher risk for cesarean delivery (adjusted odds ration [OR] 4.3, 95% confidence interval [CI] 2.4-7.6) and gestational diabetes (adjusted OR 4.2, 95% CI 1.5-12.1). Overweight teens ($n = 106$) had lower risk for preterm birth at less than 37 and less than 34 weeks of gestation (adjusted OR 0.28, 95% CI 0.10-0.77 and adjusted OR 0.11, 95% CI 0.01-0.80, respectively).

Conclusion.—Overweight and obese teenage mothers are at increased risk for adverse perinatal outcomes. Research on optimal weight for pregnant teens and weight control interventions is needed.
Level of Evidence.—II.

▶ The article says it all. It seems that we probably really don't have an ability to influence this that is whether the women gets obese or not while pregnant (although hopefully our book "You Having a Baby" might have an effect), and those of you involved in teaching early birthing classes might be able to have an effect. But it does imply what all of us probably know: if a woman comes into the delivery room who is obese, there is a much greater chance for C section and perinatal problems.

From another standpoint, if you or your spouse becomes pregnant, remember the mantra eating for 1.1—that is, the right amount of food during pregnancy is not an eating for 2 mantra that belongs in the proverbial diaper genie never to be heard of, seen, or touched again. The pregnant woman really wants to eat about 10% more than she normally ate for the proper nutrition for the child.

M. F. Roizen, MD

At concentrations that inhibit mTOR, resveratrol suppresses cellular senescence

Demidenko ZN, Blagosklonny MV (Oncotarget, Albany, NY)
Cell Cycle 8:1901-1904, 2009

Here we demonstrated that, at cytostatic, near-toxic concentrations, resveratrol inhibited S6 phosphorylation and prevented the senescence morphology in human cells. Using a sensitive functional assay, we found that resveratrol partially prevented loss of the proliferative potential associated with cellular senescence. Resveratrol was less effective than rapamycin, because aging-suppression by resveratrol was limited by its toxicity at high concentrations. We discuss whether concentrations of resveratrol that inhibit mTOR (target of rapamycin) and suppress cellular senescence are clinically achievable and whether partial inhibition of mTOR by resveratrol might be sufficient to affect organismal aging.

▶ This is another article where resveratrol, which appears to affect part of the "DAF 16-sweet 16-gene" complex appears to decrease senescence. Everyone knows that resveratrol is found in red wine, and you will probably learn that it is also in knotweed and a bunch of other things. Unfortunately, none of the resveratrol available in the United States is made in a way that keeps it in its active configuration so that it seems not worth taking it in pill form yet, but if data like this are confirmed in humans, you can bet your bottom dollar that active resveratrol or other drugs that turn on this "sweet 16" pathway will be available for our use before too long.

M. F. Roizen, MD

Lifestyle intervention in obese children with non-alcoholic fatty liver disease: 2-year follow-up study

Reinehr T, Schmidt C, Toschke AM, et al (Univ of Witten-Herdecke, Datteln, Germany)
Arch Dis Child 94:437-442, 2009

Objective.—Non-alcoholic fatty liver disease (NAFLD) is the most common cause of liver disease in obese youth. Lifestyle intervention was demonstrated to improve NAFLD but follow-up studies after end of intervention are lacking. Furthermore the necessary degree of overweight reduction for improvement of NAFLD remains unknown.

Methods.—We examined standard deviation score of body mass index (SDS-BMI) and transaminases in 152 obese children with NAFLD diagnosed by ultrasound at baseline, at the end of a 1-year intervention and 2 years after baseline. Within-subject changes of these parameters were compared by participation in the intervention based on physical activity, nutrition education and behaviour therapy.

Results.—In contrast to 43 children without lifestyle intervention, participation in lifestyle intervention (n = 109) was associated with a significant decrease of transaminases and overweight 1 and 2 years after baseline (1 year: alanine transaminase (ALT) −10 U/l (−14 to −6); aspartate transaminase (AST) −5 U/l (−7 to −3); SDS-BMI −0.23 (−0.30 to −0.16); 2 years: ALT −9 U/l (−12 to −6); AST −6 U/l (−7 to −4); SDS-BMI −0.30 (−0.37 to −0.22); data as mean changes and 95% confidence interval compared to baseline). Any degree of overweight reduction was associated with a significant decrease of NAFLD prevalence. The greatest decrease of NAFLD prevalence (1 year: −89% (95% CI −72% to −100%); 2 years: −94% (95% CI −83% to −100%)) was observed in children with the greatest overweight reduction (SDS-BMI decrease >0.5).

Conclusions.—Multidisciplinary lifestyle intervention is effective to improve NAFLD even in the 1-year follow-up after the end of intervention. A minimal reduction of overweight led to an improvement of NAFLD.

Trial Registration Number.—NCT00435734.

▶ What is really disturbing in the United States is that where non-alcoholic steatorrheic hepatitis was present in 1% of United States citizens in 1990 and 10% in 1999, as many as 35% of individuals exhibited it in 2004-2005. The good thing is that lifestyle interventions in children with this potentially lethal disease can be treated simply by overweight reduction. I say simply, but nothing is really that simple when it comes to overweight.

M. F. Roizen, MD

Sick at work–a risk factor for long-term sickness absence at a later date?

Hansen CD, Andersen JH (Herning Hosp, Denmark)

J Epidemiol Community Health 63:397-402, 2009

Background.—Little is known about the long-term consequences of sickness presence (ie, going to work despite ill-health), although one study suggests an association with coronary heart disease. This study examined the effect of sickness presence on future long-term sickness absence.

Methods.—Information from a random sample of 11 838 members of the Danish core workforce was collected from questionnaires, containing questions about work, family and attitudes towards sickness absence. Information on prospective sickness absence spells of at least 2 weeks was derived from an official register during a follow-up period of 1.5 years.

Results.—Sickness presence is associated with long-term sickness absence of at least 2 weeks' duration as well as with spells lasting at least 2 months. Participants who had gone to work ill more than six times in the year prior to baseline had a 74% higher risk of becoming sick-listed for more than 2 months, even when controlling for a wide range of potential confounders as well as baseline health status and previous long-term sickness absence. The association was consistent for most subgroups of employees reporting various symptoms, but either disappeared or became insignificant when analysing subgroups of employees with specific chronic diseases.

Conclusions.—Going to work ill repeatedly is associated with long-term sickness absence at a later date. For this reason, researchers and policy-makers should consider this phenomenon more carefully when planning future studies of sickness absence or when laying out new policies.

▶ This is an unusual study, and one that I had never seen elsewhere relating to people who come to work sick and work that way. What the data indicate is that such people, in addition to being less productive at work, clearly, when they are sick, also have an increased sickness and disability later in life.

M. F. Roizen, MD

Aspirin for the Prevention of Cardiovascular Events in Patients With Peripheral Artery Disease: A Meta-analysis of Randomized Trials

Berger JS, Krantz MJ, Kittelson JM, et al (Univ of Pennsylvania, Philadelphia; Univ of Colorado Denver School of Medicine; Colorado School of Public Health, Denver; et al)

JAMA 301:1909-1919, 2009

Context.—Randomized trials have shown that aspirin decreases the risk of cardiovascular events in patients with symptomatic coronary and cerebrovascular disease. Despite guideline recommendations for secondary prevention in peripheral artery disease (PAD), the effect of aspirin in this population is not well established.

Objective.—To investigate the effect of aspirin on cardiovascular event rates in patients with PAD.

Data Sources and Study Selection.—MEDLINE, the Cochrane Central Register of Controlled Trials, EMBASE, Science Citation Index (1966 to December 2008), and unpublished studies from the supplemental index of the Antithrombotic Trialists' Collaboration. Eligible studies were prospective, randomized controlled trials of aspirin therapy, with or without dipyridamole that reported cardiovascular event rates. Eighteen trials involving 5269 individuals were identified.

Data Extraction.—Studies were reviewed to determine the number of participants, mean follow-up, and the primary end point of cardiovascular events (nonfatal myocardial infarction [MI], nonfatal stroke, and cardiovascular death). Data on the secondary end points of all-cause mortality, major bleeding, and the individual components of the primary outcome measure were also abstracted. For the primary end point, the analysis had 88% power to detect a 25% reduction and 70% power to detect a 20% reduction in cardiovascular events in the aspirin group compared with the control group.

Data Synthesis.—Among 5269 participants, cardiovascular events were experienced by 251 (8.9%) of 2823 patients taking aspirin (alone or with dipyridamole) and by 269 (11.0%) of 2446 in the control group (pooled relative risk [RR], 0.88; 95% confidence interval [CI], 0.76-1.04). Aspirin therapy was associated with a reduction in the secondary outcome of nonfatal stroke (52 of 2823 vs 76 of 2446; RR, 0.66; 95% CI, 0.47-0.94) but was not associated with significant reductions in all-cause or cardiovascular mortality, MI, or major bleeding. In the subset of 3019 participants taking aspirin alone vs control, aspirin was associated with a nonsignificant reduction in cardiovascular events (125 of 1516 vs 144 of 1503; RR, 0.75; 95% CI, 0.48-1.18), a significant reduction in nonfatal stroke (32 of 1516 vs 51 of 1503; RR, 0.64; 95% CI, 0.42-0.99), but no statistically significant reductions in all-cause or cardiovascular mortality, MI, or major bleeding.

Conclusions.—In patients with PAD, treatment with aspirin alone or with dipyridamole resulted in a statistically nonsignificant decrease in the primary end point of cardiovascular events and a significant reduction in nonfatal stroke. Results for the primary end point may reflect limited statistical power. Additional randomized controlled trials of aspirin therapy are needed to establish the net benefit and bleeding risks in PAD.

▶ Despite a lack of a primary end point, aspirin use in patients with peripheral artery disease clearly decreased the risk of stroke. It is clear to me that we should continue aspirin in the perioperative period if it is at all possible, as such patients with peripheral vascular disease are at high risk of stroke and heart attack, and probably not just in the long term, but also probably perioperatively.

M. F. Roizen, MD

Good Semen Quality and Life Expectancy: A Cohort Study of 43,277 Men

Jensen TK, Jacobsen R, Christensen K, et al (Univ of Southern Denmark, Odense; et al)

Am J Epidemiol 170:559-565, 2009

Fertility status may predict later mortality, but no studies have examined the effect of semen quality on subsequent mortality. Men referred to the Copenhagen Sperm Analysis Laboratory by general practitioners and urologists from 1963 to 2001 were, through a unique personal identification number, linked to the Danish central registers that hold information on all cases of cancer, causes of death, and number of children in the Danish population. The men were followed until December 31, 2001, death, or censoring, whichever occurred first, and the total mortality and cause-specific mortality of the cohort were compared with those of all age-standardized Danish men or according to semen characteristics. Among 43,277 men without azospermia referred for infertility problems, mortality decreased as the sperm concentration increased up to a threshold of 40 million/mL. As the percentages of motile and morphologically normal spermatozoa and semen volume increased, mortality decreased in a dose-response manner ($P_{trend} < 0.05$). The decrease in mortality among men with good semen quality was due to a decrease in a wide range of diseases and was found among men both with and without children; therefore, the decrease in mortality could not be attributed solely to lifestyle and/or social factors. Semen quality may therefore be a fundamental biomarker of overall male health.

▶ This is an amazing study in that irrespective of everything else it appears that good sperm quality correlates directly with longevity. Maybe that is the best biomarker of aging in men—sperm quality and sperm production. Have you had your sperm tested yet?

M. F. Roizen, MD

Exposure to Smoking Imagery in the Movies and Experimenting with Cigarettes among Mexican Heritage Youth

Wilkinson AV, Spitz MR, Prokhorov AV, et al (The Univ of Texas M.D. Anderson Cancer Ctr, Houston; et al)

Cancer Epidemiol Biomarkers Prev 18:3435-3443, 2009

There is growing evidence that an adolescent's decision to try cigarettes is influenced by level of exposure to movies in which smoking is portrayed. Less is known about how ethnicity affects this process. We examined whether acculturation and/or country of birth influence the relationship between exposure to smoking imagery in the movies and experimenting with cigarettes among Mexican origin youth. We prospectively followed 1,328 Mexican origin adolescents ages 11 to 13 years at baseline. We assessed which of 50 movies (randomly selected from a pool of 250 popular contemporary movies released from 1999 to 2004 and content analyzed for smoking) adolescents had seen. Smoking behavior was assessed at baseline and at 6-month intervals over 24 months. Ten percent of the adolescents had experimented at baseline; 17% tried subsequently. Multivariate analyses revealed, as exposure to smoking imagery in the movies increased, the chances of having ever experimented [adjusted odds ratio (AOR) = 1.27; 95% confidence interval (CI), 1.10-1.48] and of being a new experimenter (AOR = 1.19; 95% CI, 1.01-1.40) increased, equivalent to a 4.2% increased risk of ever and a 3.0% increased risk of new experimenting for each additional quartile of movie exposure. This effect was moderated by country of birth. For Mexican-born youth, exposure to smoking imagery in the movies was the strongest independent predictor of new experimentation (AOR = 1.52; 95% CI, 1.14-2.05). For U.S.-born youth, we observed a ceiling effect: the percent of experimenters increased with increasing exposure, and then flattened. Among Mexican-born youth, exposure to smoking imagery in the movies may be an important part of the acculturation process associated with smoking initiation.

▶ Perhaps what was most interesting in this article is that increased watching of smoking in movies increases experimentation and likelihood of cigarette smoking. Mexican born youth may have as much as 40% of their smoking habit triggered by movies, and movie smoking may trigger more than 20% of the smoking risk in non-Mexican heritage United States born youth. The good news is that there are only about 400 movies or so with smoking seen by non-Mexican heritage youth, and that non-Mexican heritage youth reach a plateau or maximum in their tendency to smoke from watching movies. The bad news is that there seems to be no plateau in movie triggered tendency to smoke in Mexican heritage youth in America, who on average watch 600 movies with smoking by age 18. We should really ban cigarettes in movies, and I applaud Disney for not having any smoking in any movie they produce.

M. F. Roizen, MD

Metabolic Syndrome and Insulin Resistance in Division 1 Collegiate Football Players

Borchers JR, Clem KL, Habash DL, et al (Ohio State Univ, Columbus)
Med Sci Sports Exerc 41:2105-2110, 2009

Purpose.—To estimate the prevalence of metabolic syndrome and insulin resistance in a cohort of Division 1 collegiate football players.

Methods.—Ninety football players were evaluated in a cross-sectional study to estimate the prevalence of metabolic syndrome, insulin resistance, and associated risk factors. Obesity was defined as a body fat ≥25% determined by BOD POD measurements. The National Cholesterol Education Program Adult Treatment Panel III criteria were used to estimate prevalence of metabolic syndrome. Quantitative insulin sensitivity check index calculations were performed to estimate prevalence of insulin resistance. Linear regression techniques were used to determine association between body fat percentage and other measured continuous parameters. Fisher exact test was used to determine association between nominal variables, and one-way ANOVA compared the three groups defined by position.

Results.—Summary measures showed a small prevalence of abnormal individual measurements. There was an association between body fat percentage and most evaluated parameters ($P < 0.05$). The prevalence of obesity, insulin resistance, and metabolic syndrome was 21%, 21%, and 9%, respectively. Obesity is closely associated with metabolic syndrome ($P < 0.0001$) and insulin resistance ($P < 0.0001$) in this population. All subjects with metabolic syndrome were obese, and the odds for insulin resistance in the obese group are 10.6 times the odds for the nonobese group. Linemen ($n = 29$) had 19 of the 19 obese subjects, 13 of the 19 subjects with insulin resistance, and all subjects with metabolic syndrome.

Conclusions.—There is a strong association between obesity and both metabolic syndrome and insulin resistance in Division 1 collegiate football players. Linemen are at significant risk for metabolic syndrome and insulin resistance compared with other positions. This may be predictive of future health problems in Division 1 collegiate football players, especially linemen.

▶ Well, guess which football players have all the metabolic syndrome, all the insulin resistance, and almost all of the obesity in football? That's right, it's the linemen. The prevalence of obesity, insulin resistance, and metabolic syndrome was 21%, all due to linemen. Twenty-one percent had insulin resistance and 9% of the total group had metabolic syndrome, and this is in college athletes. It is bad enough that collegiate football is associated with concussions and brain dysfunction from concussions, but now metabolic syndrome and insulin resistance too? More time is needed in the weight room, guys.

M. F. Roizen, MD

Effects of Exercise Modality on Insulin Resistance and Functional Limitation in Older Adults: A Randomized Controlled Trial

Davidson LE, Hudson R, Kilpatrick K, et al (Queen's Univ, Ontario, Canada)

Arch Intern Med 169:122-131, 2009

Background.—Authorities advocate that resistance and aerobic exercise are essential for reducing risk factors for chronic disease and disability in older adults. However, the incremental effects of combined resistance and aerobic exercise compared with either modality alone on risk factors for disease and disability is generally unknown.

Methods.—Participants were 136 sedentary, abdominally obese older men and women recruited from September 30, 2002, through November 15, 2006, at Queen's University. Participants were randomized to 1 of the following 4 groups for 6 months: resistance exercise, aerobic exercise, resistance and aerobic exercise (combined exercise), or nonexercise control. Primary outcomes were analyzed by an intent-to-treat model and included changes in insulin resistance by hyperinsulinemic-euglycemic clamp and functional limitation using the average change in 4 tests combined (average z score).

Results.—After controlling for age, sex, and baseline value, insulin resistance improved compared with controls in the aerobic exercise and the combined exercise groups but not in the resistance exercise group. Improvement (mean [SE]) in the combined exercise group was greater than in the resistance exercise group (9.2 [1.3] vs 1.8 [1.3] mg/mL/μIU per kilogram of skeletal muscle per minute ×100 [$P < .001$]) but not in the aerobic exercise group (9.2 [1.3] vs 6.5 [1.3] mg/mL/μIU per kilogram of skeletal muscle per minute ×100 [$P = .46$]). Functional limitation improved significantly in all groups compared with the control group. Improvement in the combined exercise group was greater than in the aerobic exercise group (0.5 [0.1] vs −0.0 [0.1]; standard units, z score [$P = .003$]) but not in the resistance exercise group. Improvement in the resistance exercise group was not different from the aerobic exercise group.

Conclusion.—The combination of resistance and aerobic exercise was the optimal exercise strategy for simultaneous reduction in insulin resistance and functional limitation in previously sedentary, abdominally obese older adults.

Trial Registration.—clinicaltrials.gov Identifier: NCT00520858.

▶ Clearly, aerobic exercise seems to be better for diabetics, and the ability of resistance exercise to add functional mobility and strength to the decrease in insulin resistance seems be an important reason to first do walking and other things that lead to aerobic exercise, and then to do resistance exercise. But don't forget the resistance.

M. F. Roizen, MD

Egg Consumption and Risk of Type 2 Diabetes in Men and Women

Djoussé L, Gaziano JM, Buring JE, et al (Brigham and Women's Hosp, Boston, MA)

Diabetes Care 32:295-300, 2009

Objective.—Whereas limited and inconsistent findings have been reported on the relation between dietary cholesterol or egg consumption and fasting glucose, no previous study has examined the association between egg consumption and type 2 diabetes. This project sought to examine the relation between egg intake and the risk of type 2 diabetes in two large prospective cohorts.

Research Design and Methods.—In this prospective study, we used data from two completed randomized trials: 20,703 men from the Physicians' Health Study I (1982–2007) and 36,295 women from the Women's Health Study (1992–2007). Egg consumption was ascertained using questionnaires, and we used the Cox proportional hazard model to estimate relative risks of type 2 diabetes.

Results.—During mean follow-up of 20.0 years in men and 11.7 years in women, 1,921 men and 2,112 women developed type 2 diabetes. Compared with no egg consumption, multivariable adjusted hazard ratios for type 2 diabetes were 1.09 (95% CI 0.87–1.37), 1.09 (0.88–1.34), 1.18 (0.95–1.45), 1.46 (1.14–1.86), and 1.58 (1.25–2.01) for consumption of <1, 1, 2–4, 5–6, and ≥7 eggs/week, respectively, in men (P for trend <0.0001). Corresponding multivariable hazard ratios for women were 1.06 (0.92–1.22), 0.97 (0.83–1.12), 1.19 (1.03–1.38), 1.18 (0.88–1.58), and 1.77 (1.28–2.43), respectively (*P* for trend <0.0001).

Conclusions.—These data suggest that high levels of egg consumption (daily) are associated with an increased risk of type 2 diabetes in men and women. Confirmation of these findings in other populations is warranted.

► My mom always fed me eggs, but now at least I have kept down to egg whites and one full egg per week. But eggs are in a lot of foods and used in a lot of ways. This study didn't look at egg whites, only at whole egg, so we will have to hope that egg whites don't have the same effect as eggs in promoting Type 2 diabetes.

M. F. Roizen, MD

Rapamycin fed late in life extends lifespan in genetically heterogenous mice

Harrison DE, Strong R, Sharp ZD, et al (The Jackson Laboratory, Bar Harbor, ME; The Univ of Texas Health Science Ctr at San Antonio; et al)

Nature 460:392-395, 2009

Inhibition of the TOR signalling pathway by genetic or pharmacological intervention extends lifespan in invertebrates, including yeast, nematodes and fruit flies. However, whether inhibition of mTOR signalling can extend lifespan in a mammalian species was unknown. Here we report that rapamycin, an inhibitor of the mTOR pathway, extends median and maximal lifespan of both male and female mice when fed beginning at 600 days of age. On the basis of age at 90% mortality, rapamycin led to an increase of 14% for females and 9% for males. The effect was seen at three independent test sites in genetically heterogeneous mice, chosen to avoid genotype-specific effects on disease susceptibility. Disease patterns of rapamycin-treated mice did not differ from those of control mice. In a separate study, rapamycin fed to mice beginning at 270 days of age also increased survival in both males and females, based on an interim analysis conducted near the median survival point. Rapamycin may extend lifespan by postponing death from cancer, by retarding mechanisms of ageing, or both. To our knowledge, these are the first results to demonstrate a role for mTOR signalling in the regulation of mammalian lifespan, as well as pharmacological extension of lifespan in both genders. These findings have implications for further development of interventions targeting mTOR for the treatment and prevention of age-related diseases.

▶ This study shows that disturbing the "DAF 16"—"sweet 16"-gene complex slows age related diseases. In this study, starting to feed rats rapamycin, which inhibited the mTOR signalling pathway, increased lifespan by between 9% and 14%. This again led support to the concept that agents affecting the DAF 16 complex may in fact allow us to go through 3 residencies in our working lifespan (see article #2 in this series).

M. F. Roizen, MD

Breast Cancer after Use of Estrogen plus Progestin in Postmenopausal Women

Chlebowski RT, for the WHI Investigators (Los Angeles Biomedical Res Inst at Harbor–UCLA Med Ctr, Torrance, CA; et al)
N Engl J Med 360:573-587, 2009

Background.—Following the release of the 2002 report of the Women's Health Initiative (WHI) trial of estrogen plus progestin, the use of menopausal hormone therapy in the United States decreased substantially. Subsequently, the incidence of breast cancer also dropped, suggesting a cause-and-effect relation between hormone treatment and breast cancer. However, the cause of this decrease remains controversial.

Methods.—We analyzed the results of the WHI randomized clinical trial — in which one study group received 0.625 mg of conjugated equine estrogens plus 2.5 mg of medroxyprogesterone acetate daily and another group received placebo — and examined temporal trends in breast-cancer diagnoses in the WHI observational-study cohort. Risk factors for breast cancer, frequency of mammography, and time-specific incidence of breast cancer were assessed in relation to combined hormone use.

Results.—In the clinical trial, there were fewer breast-cancer diagnoses in the group receiving estrogen plus progestin than in the placebo group in the initial 2 years of the study, but the number of diagnoses increased over the course of the 5.6-year intervention period. The elevated risk decreased rapidly after both groups stopped taking the study pills, despite a similar frequency of mammography. In the observational study, the incidence of breast cancer was initially about two times as high in the group receiving menopausal hormones as in the placebo group, but this difference in incidence decreased rapidly in about 2 years, coinciding with year-to-year reductions in combined hormone use. During this period, differences in the frequency of mammography between the two groups were unchanged.

Conclusions.—The increased risk of breast cancer associated with the use of estrogen plus progestin declined markedly soon after discontinuation of combined hormone therapy and was unrelated to changes in frequency of mammography.

► What is amazing to me in this study, which is the follow-up study to the Women's Health Initiative, is that in no place do they talk about the use of aspirin in such patients as a routine. Aspirin has been shown in multiple trials to decrease breast cancer incidence, and probably could solve this problem as well as the increased clotting problem that estrogens plus the conjugated progestins are associated with. It would be great to have a trial of low dose estradiol plus micronized progestin plus aspirin versus placebo. My guess is you would see less heart attacks, less strokes, less memory loss, and maybe no increase or even a decrease in breast cancer. Why they aren't mentioning aspirin is hidden from my understanding, and makes one wonder if we will ever see such a study. I guess only journal editors may be able to force this on the investigators.

M. F. Roizen, MD

A systematic review of the evidence supporting a causal link between dietary factors and coronary heart disease

Mente A, de Koning L, Shannon HS, et al (Hamilton General Hosp, Ontario, Canada)

Arch Intern Med 169:659-669, 2009

Background.—Although a wealth of literature links dietary factors and coronary heart disease (CHD), the strength of the evidence supporting valid associations has not been evaluated systematically in a single investigation.

Methods.—We conducted a systematic search of MEDLINE for prospective cohort studies or randomized trials investigating dietary exposures in relation to CHD. We used the Bradford Hill guidelines to derive a causation score based on 4 criteria (strength, consistency, temporality, and coherence) for each dietary exposure in cohort studies and examined for consistency with the findings of randomized trials.

Results.—Strong evidence supports valid associations (4 criteria satisfied) of protective factors, including intake of vegetables, nuts, and "Mediterranean" and high-quality dietary patterns with CHD, and associations of harmful factors, including intake of trans-fatty acids and foods with a high glycemic index or load. Among studies of higher methodologic quality, there was also strong evidence for monounsaturated fatty acids and "prudent" and "western" dietary patterns. Moderate evidence (3 criteria) of associations exists for intake of fish, marine omega-3 fatty acids, folate, whole grains, dietary vitamins E and C, beta carotene, alcohol, fruit, and fiber. Insufficient evidence (≤2 criteria) of association is present for intake of supplementary vitamin E and ascorbic acid (vitamin C); saturated and polyunsaturated fatty acids; total fat; alpha-linolenic acid; meat; eggs; and milk. Among the dietary exposures with strong evidence of causation from cohort studies, only a Mediterranean dietary pattern is related to CHD in randomized trials.

Conclusions.—The evidence supports a valid association of a limited number of dietary factors and dietary patterns with CHD. Future evaluation of dietary patterns, including their nutrient and food components, in cohort studies and randomized trials is recommended.

▶ It seems pretty simple: more fruits, vegetables, only 100% whole grain, and a little alcohol seem to be the keys. It ain't rocket science, but, when you hit age 90, it will make you smarter than the average rocket scientist.

M. F. Roizen, MD

Trends in Hypertension Prevalence, Awareness, Treatment, and Control Rates in United States Adults Between 1988–1994 and 1999–2004

Cutler JA, Sorlie PD, Wolz M, et al (Natl Heart, Lung, and Blood Inst, Bethesda, MD; et al)

Hypertension 52:818-827, 2008

This study assesses trends in hypertension prevalence, blood pressure distributions and mean levels, and hypertension awareness, treatment, and control among US adults, age ≥18 years, between the third National Health and Nutrition Examination Survey (1988–1994) and the 1999–2004 National Health and Nutrition Examination Survey, a period of ≈10 years. The age-standardized prevalence rate increased from 24.4% to 28.9% ($P < 0.001$), with the largest increases among non-Hispanic women. Depending on gender and race/ethnicity, from one fifth to four fifths of the increase could be accounted for by increasing body mass index. Among hypertensive persons, there were modest increases in awareness ($P = 0.04$), from 68.5% to 71.8%. The rate for men increased from

61.6% to 69.3% ($P = 0.001$), whereas the rate for women did not change significantly. Rates remained higher for women than for men, although the difference narrowed considerably. Improvements in treatment and control rates were larger: 53.1% to 61.4% and 26.1% to 35.1%, respectively (both $P < 0.001$). The greatest increases occurred among non-Hispanic white men and non-Hispanic black persons, especially men. Mexican American persons showed improvement in treatment and control rates, but these rates remained the lowest among race/ethnic subgroups (47.4% and 24.3%, respectively). Among all of the race/ethnic groups, women continued to have somewhat better awareness, treatment, and control, except for control rates among non-Hispanic white persons, which became higher in men. Differences between non-Hispanic black and white persons in awareness, treatment, and control were small. These divergent trends may translate into disparate trends in cardiovascular disease morbidity and mortality.

▶ This is one of the most disturbing articles this year. Clearly, 40 years after the Veteran's studies showing how important hypertension is, how easy control of it could be with what are now very generic medicines, and how important that was to survival and to quality of life, still less than 70% of people are aware of their hypertension, and only 31% get even what I would call barely acceptable control. How this can happen in this day and age with IT systems and knowing how vital this is to our overall costs of care is mind boggling to me. One benefit of anesthesia and close monitoring of blood pressure should be to acknowledge the presence of hypertension if we spot it, and push on the patients through email and other systems to get control. Clearly, we can send out copies of the Veteran's study or even copies of 1 or 2 of the key figures in that study (ie, key graphs of the study) that would give patients the visualization that without treatment over a 5 year period, the average 50-year-old male with moderate hypertension in that study was dead (terminating morbid events includes deaths and total disability) 33% of the time within 5 years, whereas treatment reduced that to 6%. And, this was with inexpensive medicines that are all clearly generic by now. I think we have an obligation to do that to patients we spot as hypertensive or who are probably hypertensive in the peri-operative period.

M. F. Roizen, MD

Effect of varying levels of disease management on smoking cessation: a randomized trial

Ellerbeck EF, Mahnken JD, Cupertino AP, et al (Univ of Kansas Med Ctr)
Ann Intern Med 150:437-446, 2009

Background.—Cigarette smoking is a chronic, relapsing illness that is inadequately addressed in primary care practice.

Objective.—To compare cessation rates among smokers who receive pharmacotherapy alone or combined with either moderate- or high-intensity disease management that includes counseling and provider feedback.

Design.—Randomized clinical trial from June 2004 to December 2007.

Setting.—50 rural primary care practices.

Participants.—750 persons who smoke more than 10 cigarettes per day.

Intervention.—Pharmacotherapy alone (n = 250), pharmacotherapy supplemented with up to 2 counseling calls (moderate-intensity disease management) (n = 249), or pharmacotherapy supplemented with up to 6 counseling calls (high-intensity disease management) (n = 251). Interventions were offered every 6 months for 2 years. All participants were offered free pharmacotherapy. Moderate-intensity and high-intensity disease management recipients had postcounseling progress reports faxed to their physicians.

Measurements.—Self-reported, point-prevalence smoking abstinence at 24 months (primary outcome) and overall (0 to 24 months) analyses of smoking abstinence, utilization of pharmacotherapy, and discussions about smoking with physicians (secondary outcomes). Research assistants who were blinded to treatment assignment conducted outcome assessments.

Results.—Pharmacotherapy utilization was similar across treatment groups, with 473 of 741 (63.8%), 302 of 739 (40.9%), 175 of 732 (23.9%), and 179 of 726 (24.7%) participants requesting pharmacotherapy during the first, second, third, and fourth 6-month treatment cycles, respectively. Of participants who saw a physician during any given treatment cycle, 37.5% to 59.5% reported that they had discussed smoking cessation with their physician; this did not differ across the treatment groups. Abstinence rates increased throughout the study, and overall (0 to 24 months) analyses demonstrated higher abstinence among the high-intensity disease management group than the moderate-intensity disease management group (odds ratio [OR], 1.43 [95% CI, 1.00 to 2.03]) and among the combined disease management groups than the pharmacotherapy-alone group (OR, 1.47 [CI, 1.08 to 2.00]). Self-reported abstinence at 24 months was 68 of 244 (27.9%) and 56 of 238 (23.5%) participants in the high- and moderate-intensity disease management groups, respectively (OR, 1.33 [CI, 0.88 to 2.02]), and 56 of 244 (23.0%) participants in the pharmacotherapy-alone group (OR, 1.12 [CI, 0.78 to 1.61] for combined disease management vs. pharmacotherapy alone).

Limitation.—The effect of pharmacotherapy management cannot be separated from the provision of free pharmacotherapy, and cessation was validated in only 58% of self-reported quitters.

Conclusion.—Smokers are willing to make repeated pharmacotherapy-assisted quit attempts, leading to progressively greater smoking abstinence. Although point-prevalence abstinence did not differ at 24 months, analyses that incorporated assessments across the full 24 months of treatment suggest that higher-intensity disease management is associated with increased abstinence.

▶ People want to quit smoking, and they have to try multiple times even with reasonable help. The better the help and the more prolonged it is, the higher the success rate. So keep pushing all smokers in the preoperative clinic, and keep pushing all smokers in the postoperative visit to quit.

M. F. Roizen, MD

Caloric restriction delays disease onset and mortality in rhesus monkeys
Colman RJ, Anderson RM, Johnson SC, et al (Univ of Wisconsin, Madison)
Science 325:201-204, 2009

Caloric restriction (CR), without malnutrition, delays aging and extends life span in diverse species; however, its effect on resistance to illness and mortality in primates has not been clearly established. We report findings of a 20-year longitudinal adult-onset CR study in rhesus monkeys aimed at filling this critical gap in aging research. In a population of rhesus macaques maintained at the Wisconsin National Primate Research Center, moderate CR lowered the incidence of aging-related deaths. At the time point reported, 50% of control fed animals survived as compared with 80% of the CR animals. Furthermore, CR delayed the onset of age-associated pathologies. Specifically, CR reduced the incidence of diabetes, cancer, cardiovascular disease, and brain atrophy. These data demonstrate that CR slows aging in a primate species.

▶ Turning on the "sweet 16" gene complex—really the "DAF 16" gene complex—is what calorie restriction does. This involves, as the article implies, a series of different genes or steps, including SIRT 1, mTOR PGC-1 alpha, and potentially a myriad of others. Will activation of all of these by means other than calorie restriction also result in a 50% prolongation of lifespan, and decrease the diseases of aging such as Parkinsonism, heart failure, diabetes, cancer, and brain atrophy? We don't know, but the last conference I was at there were reported to be 14 drugs in phase 2 or 3 testing that activated parts of this "sweet 16" gene complex.

The implications for anesthesia education are spectacular, as they are for everything else in life. Three residencies, one at age 25 to 35 years, one at age 65 to 80 years, and the third at age 110 to 120 years as we would live on the life expectancy of retiring at 140 or so. And we will live with the quality of life that we now have at age 45 if this calorie restriction model is pertinent. In the meantime, what should we do? Calorie restriction is the item, but we have trouble even maintaining weights in America. So let's hope at least one of those 14 drug trials brings success.

M. F. Roizen, MD

Diet and Lifestyle Risk Factors Associated With Incident Hypertension in Women

Forman JP, Stampfer MJ, Curhan GC (Brigham and Women's Hosp and Harvard Med School, Boston, MA)

JAMA 302:401-411, 2009

Context.—Hypertension is an important preventable risk factor for death among women. While several modifiable risk factors have been identified, their combined risk and distribution in the population have not been assessed.

Objective.—To estimate the hypothetical fraction of hypertension incidence associated with dietary and lifestyle factors in women.

Design, Setting, and Participants.—Prospective cohort study of 83 882 adult women aged 27 to 44 years in the second Nurses' Health Study who did not have hypertension, cardiovascular disease, diabetes, or cancer in 1991, and who had normal reported blood pressure (defined as systolic blood pressure of ≤120 mm Hg and diastolic blood pressure of ≤80 mm Hg), with follow-up for incident hypertension for 14 years through 2005. Six modifiable lifestyle and dietary factors for hypertension were identified. The 6 low-risk factors for hypertension were a body mass index (BMI) of less than 25, a daily mean of 30 minutes of vigorous exercise, a high score on the Dietary Approaches to Stop Hypertension (DASH) diet based on responses to a food frequency questionnaire, modest alcohol intake up to 10 g/d, use of nonnarcotic analgesics less than once per week, and intake of 400 μg/d or more of supplemental folic acid. The association between combinations of 3 (normal BMI, daily vigorous exercise, and DASH-style diet), 4 (3 low-risk factors plus modest alcohol intake), 5 (4 low-risk factors plus avoidance of nonnarcotic analgesics), and 6 (folic acid supplementation ≥400 μg/d) low-risk factors and the risk of developing hypertension was analyzed.

Main Outcome Measures.—Adjusted hazard ratios for incident self-reported hypertension and population attributable risks (PARs).

Results.—A total of 12 319 incident cases of hypertension were reported. All 6 modifiable risk factors were independently associated with the risk of developing hypertension during follow-up after also adjusting for age, race, family history of hypertension, smoking status, and use of oral contraceptives. For women who had all 6 low-risk factors (0.3% of the population), the hazard ratio for incident hypertension was 0.22 (95% confidence interval [CI], 0.10-0.51); the hypothetical PAR was 78% (95% CI, 49%-90%) for women who lacked these low-risk factors. The corresponding hypothetical absolute incidence rate difference (ARD) was 8.37 cases per 1000 person-years. The PARs were 72% (95% CI, 57%-82%; ARD, 7.76 cases per 1000 person-years) for 5 low-risk factors (0.8% of the population), 58% (95% CI, 46%-67%; ARD, 6.28 cases per 1000 person-years) for 4 low-risk factors (1.6% of the population), and 53% (95% CI, 45%-60%; ARD, 6.02 cases per 1000 person-years) for 3 low-risk factors (3.1% of the population). Body mass index alone was the most powerful predictor of hypertension, with a BMI of 25 or greater having an adjusted PAR of 40% (95% CI, 38%-41%) compared with a BMI of less than 25.

Conclusions.—Adherence to low-risk dietary and lifestyle factors was associated with a significantly lower incidence of self-reported hypertension. Adopting low-risk dietary and lifestyle factors has the potential to prevent a large proportion of new-onset hypertension occurring among young women.

▶ This is a report from the second nurses' health study on what happened to the women who did not have hypertension, cardiovascular disease, diabetes, or cancer in 1991 and who had normal blood pressure. These healthy nurses were followed up for 14 years through 2005. Six modifiable lifestyle and dietary factors for hypertension were identified relating to weight gain, physical inactivity, lack of fruits and vegetables, non-use of a nonsteroidal analgesic, lack of modest alcohol use, and surprisingly, lack of intake of supplemental folic acid. It seems like these 6 factors are easy enough to do, with obviously the most difficult one being the presence of both fruit and vegetables and exercise in your daily activity, but for only 30 minutes a day, and only a modest amount of alcohol; all of those seem doable, and hypertension is such a huge risk factor for cardiovascular disease and mental dysfunction that we should all know our blood pressures, and we should all do or have these 6 easy activities to avoid hypertension and, by the way, heart failure as well.

M. F. Roizen, MD

Obesity, waist size and prevalence of current asthma in the California Teachers Study cohort

Von Behren J, Lipsett M, Horn-Ross PL, et al (Northern California Cancer Ctr; California Dept of Public Health, Richmond; et al)

Thorax 64:889-893, 2009

Background.—Obesity is a risk factor for asthma, particularly in women, but few cohort studies have evaluated abdominal obesity which reflects metabolic differences in visceral fat known to influence systemic inflammation. A study was undertaken to examine the relationship between the prevalence of asthma and measures of abdominal obesity and adult weight gain in addition to body mass index (BMI) in a large cohort of female teachers.

Methods.—Prevalence odds ratios (ORs) for current asthma were calculated using multivariable linear modelling, adjusting for age, smoking and race/ethnicity.

Results.—Of the 88 304 women in the analyses, 13% (n = 11 500) were obese (BMI $\geq$30 kg/m^2) at baseline; 1334 were extremely obese (BMI $\geq$40 kg/m^2). Compared with those of normal weight, the adjusted OR for adult-onset asthma increased from 1.40 (95% confidence interval

(CI) 1.31 to 1.49) for overweight women to 3.30 (95% CI 2.85 to 3.82) for extremely obese women. Large waist circumference (>88 cm) was associated with increased asthma prevalence, even among women with a normal BMI (OR 1.37, 95% CI 1.18 to 1.59). Among obese women the OR for asthma was greater in those who were also abdominally obese than in women whose waist was ≤88 cm (2.36 vs 1.57). Obese and overweight women were at greater risk of severe asthma episodes, measured by urgent medical visits and hospital admissions.

Conclusions.—This study confirms the association between excess weight and asthma severity and prevalence, and showed that a large waist was associated with increased asthma prevalence even among women considered to have normal body weight.

▶ This study clearly shows that when examining patients preoperatively, questions about asthma and wheezing should come up if the patient is obese.

M. F. Roizen, MD

Effects of Home-Based Diet and Exercise on Functional Outcomes Among Older, Overweight Long-Term Cancer Survivors: RENEW: A Randomized Controlled Trial

Morey MC, Snyder DC, Sloane R, et al (Duke Univ Older Americans Independence Ctr, Durham, NC; Duke Univ, Durham, NC; et al)

JAMA 301:1883-1891, 2009

Context.—Five-year survival rates for early stage colorectal, breast, and prostate cancer currently exceed 90% and are increasing. Cancer survivors are at greater risk for second malignancies, other comorbidities, and accelerated functional decline. Lifestyle interventions may provide benefit, but it is unknown whether long-term cancer survivors can modify their lifestyle behaviors sufficiently to improve functional status.

Objective.—To determine whether a telephone counseling and mailed print material–based diet and exercise intervention is effective in reorienting functional decline in older, overweight cancer survivors.

Design, Setting, and Participants.—Randomized controlled trial of 641 overweight (body mass index ≥25 and <40), long-term (≥5 years) survivors (aged 65-91 years) of colorectal, breast, and prostate cancer, who were randomly assigned to an intervention group (n = 319) or delayed intervention (control) group (n = 322) in Canada, the United Kingdom, and 21 US states. Individuals were recruited for the Reach out to Enhance Wellness (RENEW) trial from July 1, 2005, through May 17, 2007.

Intervention.—A 12-month, home-based tailored program of telephone counseling and mailed materials promoting exercise, improved diet quality, and modest weight loss. The control group was wait-listed for 12 months.

Main Outcome Measures.—Change in self-reported physical function on the Short-Form 36 physical function subscale (score range, 0-100; a high score indicates better functioning) from baseline to 12 months was the primary end point. Secondary outcomes included changes in function on the basic and advanced lower extremity function subscales of the Late Life Function and Disability Index (score range, 0-100), physical activity, body mass index, and overall health-related quality of life.

Results.—The mean baseline Short-Form 36 physical function score was 75.7. At the 12-month follow-up, the mean function scores declined less rapidly in the intervention group (−2.15; 95% confidence interval [CI], −0.36 to −3.93) compared with the control group (−4.84; 95% CI, −3.04 to −6.63) ($P = .03$). The mean baseline basic lower extremity function score was 78.2. The mean changes in basic lower extremity function were 0.34 (95% CI, −0.84 to 1.52) in the intervention group compared with −1.89 (95% CI, −0.70 to −3.09) in the control group ($P = .005$). Physical activity, dietary behaviors, and overall quality of life increased significantly in the intervention group compared with the control group, and weight loss also was greater (2.06 kg [95% CI, 1.69 to 2.43 kg] vs 0.92 kg [95% CI, 0.51 to 1.33 kg], respectively; $P < .001$).

Conclusion.—Among older, long-term survivors of colorectal, breast, and prostate cancer, a diet and exercise intervention reduced the rate of self-reported functional decline compared with no intervention.

Trial Registration.—clinicaltrials.gov Identifier: NCT00303875.

► Is the best it can be for a 5 year cancer survivor to survive five years? No, quite the contrary. While 5-year survival is great, cancer survivors, like all others, are coachable. Just small coaching, and by that I mean just a 12-month, home-based, based tailored program of telephone consulting increased cancer survivors' duration of strength training, daily servings of fruits and vegetables, significantly decreased saturated fat, weight, body mass index, and most importantly, improved measures of quality of life compared to the control group over 1 year. These were not small changes. I believe that such programs give a rationale for what anesthesiologists can do in preoperative clinic and in postoperative follow-up, although it might be said this is the responsibility of the operating surgeon or the oncologist or someone else. In fact, there is no one who is as responsible to the patient in the period as we are, and maybe we should be the one referring them to these services.

M. F. Roizen, MD

10-year follow-up of diabetes incidence and weight loss in the Diabetes Prevention Program Outcomes Study

Diabetes Prevention Program Research Group (George Washington Univ, Rockville, MD)

Lancet 374:1677-1686, 2009

Background.—In the 2·8 years of the Diabetes Prevention Program (DPP) randomised clinical trial, diabetes incidence in high-risk adults was reduced by 58% with intensive lifestyle intervention and by 31% with metformin, compared with placebo. We investigated the persistence of these effects in the long term.

Methods.—All active DPP participants were eligible for continued follow-up. 2766 of 3150 (88%) enrolled for a median additional follow-up of 5·7 years (IQR 5·5–5·8). 910 participants were from the lifestyle, 924 from the metformin, and 932 were from the original placebo groups. On the basis of the benefits from the intensive lifestyle intervention in the DPP, all three groups were offered group-implemented lifestyle intervention. Metformin treatment was continued in the original metformin group (850 mg twice daily as tolerated), with participants unmasked to assignment, and the original lifestyle intervention group was offered additional lifestyle support. The primary outcome was development of diabetes according to American Diabetes Association criteria. Analysis was by intention-to-treat. This study is registered with ClinicalTrials.gov, number NCT00038727.

Findings.—During the 10·0-year (IQR 9·0–10·5) follow-up since randomisation to DPP, the original lifestyle group lost, then partly regained weight. The modest weight loss with metformin was maintained. Diabetes incidence rates during the DPP were 4·8 cases per 100 person-years (95% CI 4·1–5·7) in the intensive lifestyle intervention group, 7·8 (6·8–8·8) in the metformin group, and 11·0 (9·8–12·3) in the placebo group. Diabetes incidence rates in this follow-up study were similar between treatment groups: 5·9 per 100 person-years (5·1–6·8) for lifestyle, 4·9 (4·2–5·7) for metformin, and 5·6 (4·8–6·5) for placebo. Diabetes incidence in the 10 years since DPP randomisation was reduced by 34% (24–42) in the lifestyle group and 18% (7–28) in the metformin group compared with placebo.

Interpretation.—During follow-up after DPP, incidences in the former placebo and metformin groups fell to equal those in the former lifestyle group, but the cumulative incidence of diabetes remained lowest in the lifestyle group. Prevention or delay of diabetes with lifestyle intervention or metformin can persist for at least 10 years.

▶ This, again, is one of the classic studies of our time. They looked at roughly 2700 people at risk who were followed for the average of 10 years in this study comparing lifestyle intervention, which really means diet and exercise, with metformin, and with placebo treatment. The amazing thing is that lifestyle treatment beat all of the others. Does the United States government, Medicare, or any insurance company now pay for lifestyle treatment of diabetes? No, but they pay through the nose for complications of diabetes and for metformin, when lifestyle treatment could reduce morbidity and reduce costs considerably. Is this a wonderful health care system or what? But before you condemn the United States health care system, it should be known that the United Kingdom, France, and Canada—ones I know about—don't pay for the most successful therapies as demonstrated by this study either. What are the implications for us? As individuals, if we get diabetes (or even if we don't) it means diet, exercise, and stress management should be our watchwords in everything we do personally. Maybe we should lean on others when we get a chance to do so, and to our insurance and government leaders to push such.

M. F. Roizen, MD

Combined effect of health behaviours and risk of first ever stroke in 20 040 men and women over 11 years' follow-up in Norfolk cohort of European Prospective Investigation of Cancer (EIPC Norfolk): prospective population study

Myint PK, Luben RN, Wareham NJ, et al (Univ of East Anglia, Norwich, UK; Univ of Cambridge, UK; MRC Epidemiology Unit, Cambridge, UK; et al)
BMJ 338:b349, 2009

Objective.—To quantify the potential combined impact of four health behaviours on incidence of stroke in men and women living in the general community.

Design.—Population based prospective study (EPIC-Norfolk).

Setting.—Norfolk, United Kingdom.

Participants.—20 040 men and women aged 40-79 with no known stroke or myocardial infarction at baseline survey in 1993-7, living in the general community, and followed up to 2007.

Main Outcome Measure.—Participants scored one point for each health behaviour: current non-smoking, physically not inactive, moderate alcohol intake (1-14 units a week), and plasma concentration of vitamin C $\geq$50 μmol/l, indicating fruit and vegetable intake of at least five servings a day, for a total score ranging from 0 to 4.

Results.—There were 599 incident strokes over 229 993 person years of follow-up; the average follow-up was 11. 5 years. After adjustment for age, sex, body mass index (BMI), systolic blood pressure, cholesterol concentration, history of diabetes and aspirin use, and social class, compared with people with the four health behaviours the relative risks for stroke for men and women were 1.15 (95% confidence interval 0.89 to 1.49) for three health behaviours, 1.58 (1.22 to 2.05) for two, 2.18 (1.63 to 2.92) for one, and 2.31 (1.33 to 4.02) for none ($P<0.001$ for trend). The relations were consistent in subgroups stratified by sex, age, body mass index, and social class, and after exclusion of deaths within two years.

Conclusion.—Four health behaviours combined predict more than a twofold difference in incidence of stroke in men and women.

▶ It seems pretty simple: if you are a non-smoker, physically active, have moderate alcohol intake, and eat a lot of fruits and vegetables, you decrease your risk of stroke by about 75%. I guess all of us should do this.

M. F. Roizen, MD

Cola-induced hypokalaemia: pathophysiological mechanisms and clinical implications

Tsimihodimos V, Kakaidi V, Elisaf M (Univ of Ioannina, Greece)

Int J Clin Pract 63:900-902, 2009

Background/Aims.—The consumption of soft drinks has increased considerably during the last decades. Among them, the cola-based preparations are possibly the refreshments with the largest sales worldwide. In addition to the possible detrimental effects of moderate, chronic cola consumption, it has been proposed that the consumption of large amounts of cola-based soft drinks may result in severe hypokalaemia.

Methods.—In this review, we discuss the clinical significance of these disturbances and summarise the pathophysiological mechanism that may underlie the development of this rare, but potentially severe, side effect.

Results/Conclusion.—Several lines of evidence suggest that the chronic consumption of large amounts of cola soft drinks may adversely affect potassium homeostasis and result in potentially severe conditions such as hypokalaemic myopathy.

▶ Wow. I did not realize my coffee habit, let alone my diet cola habit, could induce hypokalemia so severe that it could cause hypokalemic periodic paralysis. This hypokalemia occurred mainly with sugared soft drinks, promoted by the effect of sugar in causing hypokalemia, and with alkalosis, as alkalosis drives hypokalemia. The surprising effect to me: I didn't realize this really could occur. I guess it gives a reason to ask someone how much Coke or sugared soft drinks and caffeine they drink before operations.

M. F. Roizen, MD

Drug management for hypertension in type 2 diabetes in family practice

Putnam W, Buhariwalla F, Lacey K, et al (Dalhousie Univ, Halifax, Nova Scotia, Canada; Community health centre in Stanley, New Brunswick; et al)

Can Fam Physician 55:728-734, 2009

Objective.—To describe the number and classes of antihypertensive medications prescribed to patients with type 2 diabetes in community family practices, and to estimate the aggressiveness or "dosage intensity" of prescribing for hypertension in these situations.

Design.—Practice-based, cross-sectional observational study.

Setting.—Seventeen rural and urban family practices in the Maritime Family Practice Research Network in Nova Scotia, New Brunswick, and Prince Edward Island.

Participants.—A total of 670 patients with type 2 diabetes, ranging from 25 to 92 years of age.

Main Outcome Measures.—Number, classes, and combinations of classes of antihypertensive medications prescribed, as well as an index of each medication's dosage intensity.

Results.—Almost 80% of patients studied had hypertension. Participants with hypertension were taking an average of 2.5 medications, and 47.6% were taking 3 or more antihypertensive medications, but only 27.1% reached target blood pressure values of less than 130/80 mm Hg. Older patients took more antihypertensive medications, but there were no differences by sex. More than 90% were taking angiotensin-converting enzyme inhibitors or angiotensin receptor blockers, 66% were taking diuretics, 41% were taking β-blockers, and 38% were taking calcium channel blockers. We cannot describe the sequence in which antihypertensive medication classes were added, but analysis of patients taking multiple drug classes suggests that most patients were started on angiotensin-converting enzyme inhibitors or angiotensin receptor blockers, followed by diuretics, β-blockers, or calcium channel blockers. The most commonly used medications were prescribed at higher than two-thirds the maximum dose effective for hypertension.

Conclusion.—Hypertension is very common among family practice patients with type 2 diabetes; of those patients, few reach target blood pressures. Practice-based strategies to increase dosing and number of medications prescribed might be required.

▶ This study clearly implies that the weakening of the junction between endothelial cells which occurs in those being treated for diabetes, also occurs commonly in hypertension. Both make such potential tears between endothelial cells more common and lead to acceleration of atherosclerosis. This implies that the reason that this combination is so lethal—the combination of diabetes and hypertension—is not just because they both affect the same process, but it is because the essential mechanism, obesity, leads to both, and further that neither seems to get under control despite multiple drug attempts by their primary care physician. We should expect more of these to come into our practices, as the delayed effects of obesity take hold.

M. F. Roizen, MD

The Economic Burden of Insomnia: Direct and Indirect Costs for Individuals with Insomnia Syndrome, Insomnia Symptoms, and Good Sleepers

Daley M, Morin CM, LeBlanc M, et al (Université Laval, Québec, Canada; et al)

Sleep 32:55-64, 2009

Background and Purpose.—Insomnia is a highly prevalent problem that is associated with increased use of health care services and products, as well as functional impairments. This study estimated from a societal perspective the direct and indirect costs of insomnia.

Participants and Methods.—A randomly selected sample of 948 adults (mean age = 43.7 years old; 60% female) from the province of Québec, Canada completed questionnaires on sleep, health, use of health-care services and products, accidents, work absences, and reduced productivity. Data were also obtained from the Quebec government administered health insurance board regarding consultations and hospitalizations. Participants were categorized as having insomnia syndrome, insomnia symptoms or as being good sleepers using a standard algorithm. Frequencies of target cost variables were obtained and multiplied by unit costs to generate estimates of total costs for the adult population of the province of Quebec.

Results.—The total annual cost of insomnia in the province of Quebec was estimated at $6.6 billion (Cdn$). This includes direct costs associated with insomnia-motivated health-care consultations ($191.2 million) and transportation for these consultations ($36.6 million), prescription medications ($16.5 million), over the-counter products ($1.8 million) and alcohol used as a sleep aid ($339.8 million). Annual indirect costs associated with insomnia-related absenteeism were estimated at $970.6 million, with insomnia-related productivity losses estimated at $5.0 billion. The average annual per-person costs (direct and indirect combined) were $5,010 for individuals with insomnia syndrome, $1,431 for individuals presenting with symptoms, and $421 for good sleepers.

Conclusions.—This study suggests that the economic burden of insomnia is very high, with the largest proportion of all expenses (76%) attributable to insomnia-related work absences and reduced productivity. As the economic burden of untreated insomnia is much higher than that of treating insomnia, future clinical trials should evaluate the cost-benefits, cost-utility, and cost-effectiveness of insomnia therapies.

▶ Wow. And to think anesthesiologists administer good sleep and that we are relatively inexpensive compared with the overall cost, or as it was phrased on a famous t-shirt, "Wake up better." This study showed that it is roughly $5000 per person for insomnia syndrome, and $1400 extra for people presenting with symptoms in the Canadian system relating to insomnia—most of that from lost productivity. I guess this means that we really should take sleep history seriously in trying to evaluate people for sleep apnea (which is key and important, and now can be tested with home monitoring) and for overall insomnia from other causes. We probably should refer candidates at least postoperatively so that we can be regarded as boosters of productivity.

M. F. Roizen, MD

Comparative Effects of Three Popular Diets on Lipids, Endothelial Function, and C-Reactive Protein during Weight Maintenance

Miller M, Beach V, Sorkin JD, et al (Univ of Maryland School of Medicine, Baltimore; Univ of Maryland Med Ctr, Baltimore; et al)

J Am Diet Assoc 109:713-717, 2009

Although popular diets focus on weight loss and their favorable biochemical and physiological effects, fewer investigations have evaluated the biological impact of these diets during weight maintenance. To study this issue, three popular diets—Atkins, South Beach, and Ornish—were tested in a randomized and counterbalanced crossover study between January and December 2006. Participants completed each of the three 4-week isocaloric dietary intervention phases followed by a 4-week washout period. They were weighed weekly and caloric adjustments made if weight change exceeded 1 kg. At the completion of each dietary phase, 3-day food records were analyzed, fasting blood sampled, and brachial artery reactivity testing performed. Eighteen adults completed all three isocaloric dietary phases. During the South Beach and Ornish maintenance phase, there were significant reductions in low-density lipoprotein cholesterol (11.8%; $P=0.01$, 16.6%; $P=0.0006$, respectively) compared to prediet baseline. In addition, in contrast to the Atkins maintenance phase, significant reductions in low-density lipoprotein cholesterol and apolipoprotein B levels were observed after the South Beach ($P=0.003$, $P=0.05$; repeated measures analyses of variance) and Ornish maintenance phases ($P=0.0004$, $P=0.006$, repeated measures analyses of variance). Brachial artery testing revealed an inverse correlation between flow-mediated vasodilatation and intake of saturated fat ($r=-0.33$; $P=0.016$). These data suggest that during weight maintenance, less favorable biological effects are observed during a simulated, high-fat Atkins diet when compared to the South Beach and Ornish diet. The findings support additional study in subjects with visceral obesity and the metabolic syndrome, in whom an increased risk of coronary disease at baseline may be accentuated with chronic consumption of a diet that exhibits unfavorable effects on lipids and endothelial function.

▶ This article again speaks to the nonweight affects of food choices—saturated fat not only turns on genes that cause inflammation, but also inhibits vascular reactivity in a sustained enough fashion to cause things, such as impotence and misappropriation of blood flow. If all you care about is sex, wrinkles, and ability to move with energy, you should get saturated fat out of your diet, and we should urge it out of snack rooms and every other place in a hospital, including patient foods. Why is this important? This article isn't reviewed for your patients as much as it is for you and your own education. There are other effects of food choices than weight.

M. F. Roizen, MD

Comparison of Methods for Delivering a Lifestyle Modification Program for Obese Patients: A Randomized Trial

Digenio AG, Mancuso JP, Gerber RA, et al (South Lyme, CT; Pfizer, Inc., New London, CT; et al)

Ann Intern Med 150:255-262, 2009

Background.—Physicians frequently prescribe medications for weight loss but offer minimal lifestyle counseling despite the additional benefits of combining both interventions.

Objective.—To compare 5 methods of delivering a lifestyle modification program to obese patients receiving sibutramine.

Design.—Randomized, 6-month, open-label study. Participants were assigned to intervention groups by using a computer-generated schedule of randomly permuted blocks. Block length was 5.

Setting.—12 independent research clinics with experience running obesity trials.

Patients.—376 patients with obesity (body mass index ≥30 and <40 kg/m^2).

Intervention.—High-frequency face-to-face lifestyle modification counseling (HF-F2F) ($n = 74$), low-frequency face-to-face counseling (LF-F2F) ($n = 76$), high-frequency telephone counseling (HFTEL) ($n = 76$), high-frequency e-mail counseling (HF-EMAIL) ($n = 74$), or no dietitian contact (self-help [SELF]) ($n = 76$). All participants received sibutramine, 10 mg/d; a lifestyle manual; and access to a weight-loss Web site.

Measurements.—Percentage change in body weight at 6 months was the primary outcome. Secondary end points included changes in waist circumference; lipid, glucose, and insulin levels; blood pressure; weight-related symptoms; and quality of life at 6 months.

Results.—At 6 months, the mean weight loss, relative to baseline, in the HF-F2F and HF-TEL groups was similar (8.9% [95% CI, 8.0% to 9.8%] and 7.7% [CI, 6.8% to 8.7%]) and significantly greater than that in the other groups (LF-F2F, 6.4% [CI, 5.4% to 7.3%]; HF-EMAIL, 5.9% [CI, 5.0% to 6.8%]; and SELF, 5.2% [CI, 4.3% to 6.1%]). All groups showed significant improvements in waist circumference, high-density lipoprotein cholesterol and triglyceride levels, and measures of quality of life and weight-related symptoms. There were no serious adverse events and no differences in minor events among groups.

Limitation.—Most participants were women, and the attrition rate was 30%.

Conclusion.—High-frequency telephone contact with a dietitian was similar to HF-F2F contact for supporting lifestyle modification in obese patients trying to lose weight. The findings might be used by providers and health systems to promote healthy lifestyle changes for their patients.

▶ This article has many more implications than for just weight loss or weight maintenance; it speaks to what patients expect and what they respond to. Direct contact with you either through face to face or phone seemed to be the key in success here. But surprisingly, almost every maneuver seemed to have a benefit that was greater than I would have expected. Maybe that was because of the drug usage as well. If you seriously want to affect patient behavior, this article is worth your time.

M. F. Roizen, MD

2 Anesthesia-Related Pharmacology and Toxicology

Patient-controlled analgesia combined with either ondansetron or ondansetron plus prochlorperazine for control of pain and nausea and vomiting in patients undergoing abdominal surgery

Jellish WS, Owen K, Fluder E, et al (Loyola Univ Med Ctr, Maywood, IL)

J Clin Anesth 20:594-600, 2009

Study Objective.—To compare ondansetron with ondansetron plus prochlorperazine, added to a patient-controlled analgesia (PCA) solution for control of postoperative nausea and vomiting (PONV).

Design.—Prospective, randomized, double-blinded study.

Setting.—University hospital.

Patients.—150 ASA physical status I, II, and III patients undergoing abdominal surgery.

Interventions.—Patients were given a PCA morphine solution containing either 30 mg of ondansetron (Group O), 30 mg of ondansetron plus 20 mg of prochlorperazine (Group OP), or no antiemetic (Group C; control group).

Measurements.—Demographic data were recorded, along with anesthetic and surgical time, total fluid intake, frequency of Postanesthesia Care Unit (PACU) PONV, discharge time and length of stay, frequency of PONV while on the hospital floor, highest nausea scores, total PCA morphine use, and PCA utilization times.

Main Results.—Demographic and intraoperative variables were similar in all groups. In the first 24 hours after surgery, nausea was higher in Group C than Group OP. Emesis in Group C was twice that of either Group O or Group OP. No differences were noted between groups in PACU PONV. Patients receiving ondansetron plus prochlorperazine when on the hospital floor had a lower frequency of nausea, while patients receiving ondansetron alone had a lower frequency of vomiting than did the control group. The adjusted odds of vomiting doubled for every 12 hours for Group C patients when receiving PCA.

Conclusions.—Combination antiemetics added to PCA reduced emetic symptoms after abdominal surgery.

▶ This is an interesting study because of the import of postoperative nausea and vomiting in patient satisfaction surveys- as well as as well as their impact on the incidence of postoperative complications.[1,2,3] If not anticipated and treated in the postoperative period, efforts in the operating room to minimize postoperative nausea and vomiting, as well as pain, are negated with decreasing plasma concentrations of antiemetics and ongoing administration of opioids.

The results of this study, that the addition of ondansetron and prochlorperazine to a morphine patient-controlled analgesia (PCA) reduced vomiting in patients who had had abdominal surgery, while new, are not surprising. Whether or not the differences found in the combination of antiemetics are clinically significant remains to be determined. As noted by the authors, differences in morphine administration in the ondansetron and the ondansetron/prochlorperazine groups make that comparison in this study difficult. Clinical benefit would need to be demonstrated before widespread use of this combination of medications because of the potential costs associated with its implementation.

The potential benefits of this combination of antiemetic medications administered in conjunction with a morphine PCA include decreased nausea and vomiting, decreased costs for rescue medications, and decreased nursing time. These would have to outweigh the possible costs of this regimen—which include the costs associated with discarding unused PCA medications, the pharmacy costs of adding 2 additional medications to a morphine PCA, and the risks associated with giving all postoperative patients receiving a morphine PCA 2 antiemetic medications when not all of them would need them.

C. A. Lien, MD

References

1. Eberhart LH, Mauch M, Morin AM, Wulf H, Geldner G. Impact of multimodal anti-emetic prophylaxis on patient satisfaction in high-risk patients for postoperative nausea and vomiting. *Anaesthesia.* 2002;57:1022-1027.
2. Eryilmaz T, Sencan A, Camgoz N, Ak B, Yavuzer R. A challenging problem that concerns the aesthetic surgeon: postoperative nausea and vomiting. *Ann Plast Surg.* 2008;61:489-491.
3. Fortney JT, Gan TJ, Graczyk S, et al. A comparison of the efficacy, safety, and patient satisfaction of ondansetron versus droperidol as antiemetics for elective outpatient surgical procedures. *Anesth Analg.* 1998;86:731-738.

Pretreatment of rocuronium reduces the frequency and severity of etomidate-induced myoclonus

Choi JM, Choi IC, Jeong YB, et al (Univ of Ulsan, Seoul, Korea)
J Clin Anesth 20:601-604, 2009

Study Objective.—To investigate the effect of pretreatment with a low dose of rocuronium on the occurrence of etomidate-induced myoclonus.

Design.—Prospective, randomized, double-blinded study.

Setting.—Medical center in South Korea.

Patients.—110 ASA physical status I, II, and III patients scheduled for elective cardiac or pulmonary surgery with general anesthesia.

Interventions.—All patients were randomized to pretreatment with a low dose of rocuronium (0.06 mg/kg; Group R) or placebo (saline; Group S), followed three minutes later by etomidate (0.3 mg/kg).

Measurements.—Patients were monitored for myoclonic movements and pain on a scale of 0-3. Bispectral index (BIS) and electromyographic (EMG) activity were recorded continuously throughout the procedure.

Main Results.—Frequency of myoclonus was significantly lower in Group R (25%) than in Group S (63%). In the latter group, there was no difference in the frequency of male (59%) and female (68%) patients experiencing myoclonus. In Group S, EMG activity and BIS were significantly increased in patients who experienced severe myoclonus, and BIS was well correlated with EMG activity.

Conclusions.—Pretreatment with a small dose of rocuronium before induction of anesthesia with etomidate significantly reduced the frequency of myoclonus.

► Pretreatment with rocuronium decreases both the severity and frequency of myoclonus associated with etomidate administration. What is noteworthy in this study is that the authors used the technique of priming with a nondepolarizing neuromuscular blocking agent using one-tenth of 2 times the ED95 dose of rocuronium, and allowing it 3 minutes to have its effect before administering etomidate. Years ago, priming had been advocated to decrease the time to peak effect of an intubating dose of nondepolarizing neuromuscular blocker. This technique shortens the onset of block by approximately 30 seconds. Frequently with priming, especially with cisatracurium, too large a dose is administered. More frequently, insufficient time is allowed after administration of the priming dose of relaxant before induction medications are administered. The technique has largely fallen out of favor due to the risk of partial neuromuscular block with the priming dose of relaxant.

In this study, the authors did not monitor the depth of neuromuscular block with the priming dose. This information would have been very useful, as even priming doses of medications can cause significant neuromuscular block in patients. The authors reported that they did not see any evidence of neuromuscular block following the pretreatment dose of rocuronium (ptosis, regurgitation, or respiratory difficulty). While they did not observe any in their study population, signs and symptoms of partial neuromuscular block have been observed in patients and volunteers with train-of-four ratios of 90%.

Since medications as varied as opioids, benzodiazepines, and magnesium have been shown to decrease the frequency of myoclonus following etomidate administration, it would have been both interesting and useful to see how pretreatment with rocuronium compared with any of these medications in decreasing the severity and frequency of etomidate-induced myoclonus to determine which technique to consider applying to clinical practice.

C. A. Lien, MD

Admixture of ephedrine to offset side effects of propofol: a randomized, controlled trial

Austin JD, Parke TJ (Royal Berkshire Hosp, Reading, United Kingdom)
J Clin Anesth 21:44-49, 2009

Study Objective.—To determine whether adding ephedrine to propofol is as effective as adding lidocaine at reducing injection pain, and its effects on hemodynamics.

Design.—Randomized, double-blinded, controlled trial.

Setting.—District general hospital in the United Kingdom.

Patients.—156 adult, ASA physical status I, II, and III patients undergoing elective or emergency general anesthesia.

Interventions.—Patients were randomized to one of three groups to receive one mL of 1% lidocaine per 20 mL of 1% propofol (Group L), 15 mg of ephedrine per 20 mL of propofol (Group E15), or 30 mg of ephedrine per 20 mL of propofol (Group E30).

Measurements and Main Results.—Pain on injection, heart rate, and blood pressure at one-minute intervals for ten minutes were recorded. There was no significant difference in injection pain among groups. Group E30 had the least amount of hemodynamic change.

Conclusion.—Adding 30 mg of ephedrine to 20 mL of 1% propofol is as effective as adding lidocaine in preventing injection pain, and it results in a more stable hemodynamic profile.

▶ As stated in this study, propofol administration is associated with pain and hypotension—the latter being most problematic in geriatric patients. The incidence of pain on injection ranges from 10% to 100%, and is decreased by 40% to 80% with mixture of lidocaine to the propofol. Previous studies have looked at administration of ephedrine to decrease either the pain or hypotension associated with propofol administration. This study is the first to look at the effect of mixing 15 or 30 mg of ephedrine with 200 mg propofol on the pain with administration and the hypotension following administration. The idea is intriguing for the anesthesiologist who is concerned about the hypotension caused by propofol administration.

A problem with the study is that several pieces of information are missing. Some of the missing information includes the following:

- Neither the results nor the discussion section mentions that administration of a volatile anesthetic was allowed following induction if the anesthesiologist felt that it was necessary to maintain an adequate depth of anesthesia. Which agents were administered, and to which patients they were administered, is never described.
- Neither the dose of propofol nor the time course over which it was administered is recorded. How many times was each patient asked whether or not he or she was feeling pain and how severe it was? What was the dose of propofol each patient had received at the time the question was asked? Did it differ between the study groups?
- More complete report on the hemodynamic changes following administration of either the propofol-lidocaine or the propofol-ephedrine mixtures would have been helpful. Earlier studies have reported tachycardia following the administration of a combination of propofol and ephedrine. In this study, only the upper and lower 99.6% confidence intervals are reported. I wonder if any individual patient became tachycardic.

The results, as they are presented, are promising—less hypotension and similar incidence of discomfort with admixture of 30 mg ephedrine when compared with admixture of lidocaine. In light of missing data, however, the significance of the results is not known. A subsequent, more carefully controlled study seems warranted to determine whether or not this technique is something that should become part of routine clinical practice when administering propofol for induction of general anesthesia.

C. A. Lien, MD

Attenuation of a rocuronium-induced neuromuscular block in patients receiving prednisolone

Soltész S, Mencke T, Stunz M, et al (Hosp Leverkusen, Germany; Univ of Rostock, Germany; et al)

Acta Anaesthesiol Scand 53:443-448, 2009

Background.—This study tested the influence of continuous medication (more than 4 weeks) with prednisolone on a rocuronium-induced neuromuscular block.

Methods.—The time course of a rocuronium-induced neuromuscular blockade (0.3 mg/kg) was investigated in 40 patients with chronic inflammatory bowel disease undergoing elective abdominal surgery. The primary end point was the time from the start of injection of rocuronium until recovery of the TOF ratio to 0.9. Twenty patients received continuous medication with prednisolone (group A), and 20 were without glucocorticoid medication (group B). Additionally, another 20 patients without inflammatory bowel disease and without glucocorticoid medication served as control (group C).

Results.—The onset time was prolonged in group A [253 (51.2) s] compared with group B [187 (61.3) s]. Twitch height at the onset of the block was higher in group A [16.5 (0–61)%] than that in group B [5.0 (0–33)%]. The duration to 25% twitch height was shorter in group A [12.6 (0–20.7) min] compared with group B [16.7 (0–25.3) min] and group C [16.9 (0–29.3) min]. The recovery to a train-of-four ratio of 0.9 was reduced in group A [25.7 (23–34.3) min] compared with group B [34.7 (32.7–44.2) min] and group C [36.5 (31.7–42.3) min].

Conclusions.—Prednisolone treatment in patients with inflammatory bowel disease is associated with a delayed onset and a shorter duration of action of rocuronium. The presence of an inflammatory bowel disease did not influence the neuromuscular block.

▶ The reported effect of steroid administration on the dynamics of nondepolarizing neuromuscular blockade differs with some authors reporting potentiation of neuromuscular blockers by steroids and others reporting resistance to their effects.[1-3] This study is the second one by this group of authors reporting an attenuation of the effect on nondepolarizing neuromuscular blockers in patients receiving prednisolone.[4] The previous study described the impact of prednisolone on atracurium-induced neuromuscular block. This study, the effect of prednisolone on rocuronium-induced neuromuscular block, is identical in methodology and has similar results. In both studies the authors show that the effects of nondepolarizing neuromuscular blocking agents are attenuated by the administration of steroids. However, the results of the studies appear to be due to a decreased potency of the compounds in patients taking steroids rather than a change in onset of effect or duration of recovery.

In this study administration of rocuronium, 0.3 mg/kg caused 83.5% neuromuscular block in patients taking prednisolone and 95% block in patients not taking prednisolone. Of note, this dose is half or less than that recommended to facilitate endotracheal intubation. Not surprisingly, onset of block was shorter in the group of patients with the greater depth of block. Relatively larger doses of relaxants have shorter onsets of action, hence the relative overdose of nondepolarizing relaxants to allow for more rapid endotracheal intubation. Similarly not surprising, clinical duration of action and total duration of action (the times from administration of relaxant to 25% and 90% recovery of twitch response to stimulation) was more rapid in the group with a lesser degree of block—those patients taking prednisolone. The differences in results were small (4 minutes and 9 minutes, respectively) but statistically significant. Interestingly, the recovery interval of 25% to 75% recovery was not impacted by steroid therapy. While this may have been due to under powering of the study, had these patients truly been resistant to neuromuscular block, one might have expected that their 25% to 75% recovery interval would have been shorter.

What would have been more useful in terms of clinically relevant results would have been either of 2 different studies: 1) a dose-response study to determine the impact of long-term steroid therapy on the potency of rocouronium, or 2) the pharmacodynamics of a rocuronium dose typically administered for endotracheal intubation. This would have at least guided clinicians in their use of the drug in patients taking steroids.

C. A. Lien, MD

References

1. Kindler CH, Verotta D, Gray AT, Gropper MA, Yost CS. Additive inhibition of nicotinic acetylcholine receptors by corticosteroids and the neuromuscular blocking drug vecuronium. *Anesthesiology.* 2000;92:821-832.
2. Paradiso K, Sabey K, Evers AS, Zorumski CF, Covey DF, Steinbach JH. Steroid inhibition of rat neuronal nicotinic alpha4beta2 receptors expressed in HEK 293 cells. *Mol Pharmacol.* 2000;58:341-351.
3. Leeuwin RS, Veldsema-Currie RD, van Wilgenburg H, Ottenhof M. Effects of corticosteroids on neuromuscular blocking actions of d-tubocurarine. *Eur J Pharmacol.* 1981;69:165-173.
4. Soltesz S, Menke T, Mey C, Röhrig S, Diefenbach C, Molter GP. Influence of a continuous prednisolone medication on the time course of neuromuscular block of atracurium in patients with chronic inflammatory bowel disease. *Br J Anaesth.* 2008;100:798-802.

Reversal of Profound Rocuronium-induced Blockade with Sugammadex: A Randomized Comparison with Neostigmine

Jones RK, Caldwell JE, Brull SJ, et al (Saddleback Memorial Med Ctr, Laguna Hills, CA; Univ of California, San Francisco; College of Medicine, Jacksonville, FL)
Anesthesiology 109:816-824, 2008

Background.—Traditionally, reversal of nondepolarizing neuromuscular blocking agents was achieved using acetylcholinesterase inhibitors, but these are unable to adequately reverse profound blockade. Sugammadex is a novel reversal agent, reversing the effects of rocuronium by encapsulation. This study assessed the efficacy and safety of sugammadex *versus* neostigmine for reversal of profound rocuronium-induced neuromuscular blockade.

Methods.—This phase III, randomized study enrolled surgical patients, aged 18 yr or older with American Society of Anesthesiologists physical status I–IV. Patients were randomized to receive sugammadex (4.0 mg/kg) or neostigmine (70 μg/kg) plus glycopyrrolate (14 μg/kg). Anesthetized patients received an intubating dose of rocuronium (0.6 mg/kg), with maintenance doses (0.15 mg/kg) as required. Neuromuscular monitoring was performed by acceleromyography. Sugammadex or neostigmine was administered at reappearance of 1–2 posttetanic counts (profound neuromuscular blockade). The primary efficacy parameter was the time from sugammadex or neostigmine–glycopyrrolate administration to return of the train-of-four ratio to 0.9.

Results.—In the intent-to-treat population ($n = 37$ in each group), geometric mean time to recovery to a train-of-four ratio of 0.9 with sugammadex was 2.9 min *versus* 50.4 min with neostigmine–glycopyrrolate

($P < 0.0001$) (median, 2.7 min *vs.* 49.0 min). Most sugammadex patients (97%) recovered to a train-of-four ratio of 0.9 within 5 min after administration. In contrast, most neostigmine patients (73%) recovered between 30 and 60 min after administration, with 23% requiring more than 60 min to recover to a train-of-four ratio of 0.9.

Conclusions.—Recovery from profound rocuronium-induced neuromuscular blockade was significantly faster with sugammadex *versus* with neostigmine, suggesting that sugammadex has a unique ability to rapidly reverse profound rocuronium neuromuscular blockade.

▶ What is presented in this study confirms information that has been previously published. Regardless of the depth of block, sugammadex antagonizes block more rapidly than does neostigmine. Additionally, sugammadex administration, even in appropriate doses, does not guarantee rapid and complete recovery in all patients.

It's difficult to interpret how the results of this study can be applied to the clinical setting. Depth of neuromuscular block was maintained at deeper levels than recommended with a volatile anesthetic. Patients received up to 1.5 times the MAC concentration of sevoflurane and had depth of block maintained at a profound enough level that the reversal agent, either neostigmine or sugammadex, could be administered at a post-tetanic count of 2. Typically when volatile agents are used for maintenance of anesthesia, depth of block is maintained at a train-of-four count of 2 or 3. These more profound levels of neuromuscular block, where even the diaphragm—that is resistant to neuromuscular block—is paralyzed, if used at all, are found in areas such as the intensive care unit before tracheal suctioning in a patient with increased intracranial pressure.

That neostigmine did not effectively antagonize this profound level of block is hardly surprising. There is a ceiling with regard to what anticholinesterases can do in reversing neuromuscular block, and a significant degree of spontaneous recovery has to have occurred for them to be effective antagonists.[1] Additionally, earlier studies of reversal of rocuronium-induced block have found sugammadex to work more quickly and effectively than either neostigmine or edrophonium.[2]

As demonstrated by White in an earlier study,[3] administration of sugammadex does not guarantee that all patients recover neuromuscular strength completely within a few minutes. In this study by Jones, 1 patient who received sugammadex required more than 16 minutes to recover to a train-of-four ratio of 0.9. Interestingly, the times to recovery to train-of-four ratios of 0.7, 0.8, and 0.9 following administration of sugammadex were not that different from one another (1.8, 2.3, and 2.7 minutes, respectively). The range of responses, however, increased as a greater degree of recovery was sought.

What this study very clearly delineates is that even when sugammadex is widely available for clinical use, classic teaching in terms of appropriate dosing of neuromuscular blocking agents and the import of use of monitors of neuromuscular blockade should not be discarded.

C. A. Lien, MD

References

1. Beemer GH, Bjorksten AR. Pharmacodynamics of atracurium in clinical practice: effect of plasma potassium, patient demographics, and concurrent medication. *Anesth Analg*. 1993;76:1288-1295.
2. Sacan O, White PF, Tufanogullari B, Klein K. Sugammadex reversal of rocuronium-induced neuromuscular blockade: a comparison with neostigmine-glycopyrrolate and edrophonium-atropine. *Anesth Analg*. 2007;104:569-574.
3. White PF, Tufanogullari B, Sacan O, et al. The effect of residual neuromuscular blockade on the speed of reversal with sugammadex. *Anesth Analg*. 2009;108: 846-851.

Reversal of Rocuronium-induced Neuromuscular Blockade with Sugammadex in Pediatric and Adult Surgical Patients

Plaud B, Meretoja O, Hofmockel R, et al (Centre Hospitalier Universitaire de Côte-de-Nacre, Caen, France; Univ of Helsinki, Finland; Klinik und Poliklinik főr Anästhesiologie und Intensivtherapie, Rostock, Germany; et al)

Anesthesiology 110:284-294, 2009

Background.—Sugammadex reverses neuromuscular blockade by chemical encapsulation of rocuronium. This phase IIIA study explored efficacy and safety of sugammadex in infants (28 days to 23 months), children (2–11 yr), adolescents (12–17 yr), and adults (18–65 yr).

Methods.—Anesthetized patients (American Society of Anesthesiologists class 1–2) received 0.6 mg/kg rocuronium and were randomized to receive sugammadex (0.5, 1.0, 2.0, or 4.0 mg/kg) or placebo at reappearance of T2. Neuromuscular monitoring was performed using acceleromyography. Primary endpoint was time from sugammadex/placebo administration to recovery of the train-of-four ratio to 0.9. Adverse events and electrocardiograms were recorded, and blood samples were collected for safety and determination of sugammadex and rocuronium plasma concentrations.

Results.—A dose-response relation was demonstrated in children (n = 22), adolescents (n = 28), and adults (n = 26), but not infants because of the small sample size (n = 8). After placebo, median recovery time of train-of-four to 0.9 was 21.0, 19.0, 23.4, and 28.5 min in infants, children, adolescents, and adults, respectively. After 2.0 mg/kg sugammadex train-of-four 0.9 was attained in 0.6, 1.2, 1.1, and 1.2 min, respectively. The sugammadex plasma concentrations were similar for the children, adolescent, and adult age groups across the dose range. Sugammadex was well tolerated: No reoccurrence of blockade, inadequate reversal, significant QT prolongation, or other abnormalities were observed.

Conclusions.—Sugammadex is a new reversal agent that rapidly, effectively, safely, and with similar recovery times reverses rocuronium-induced

neuromuscular blockade in children, adolescents, adults, and the small number of infants studied.

▶ Not surprisingly, sugammadex appears to effectively antagonize residual neuromuscular block after the reappearance of the second twitch in the train-of-four count in infants and children. In the 2 infants in this study receiving sugammadex, either 2 mg/kg or 4 mg/kg, the time required for recovery to a train-of-four ratio of 0.9 was approximately half that required in adolescents and adults. Doubling the dose that the first infant received did not shorten recovery time in the second infant. In children, as the dose of sugammadex is increased from 0.5 mg/kg to 4 mg/kg the time required for recovery of the train-of-four ratio becomes progressively shorter. Interestingly, in adolescents and adults, recovery to a train-of-four ratio of 0.9 is not shortened any further by increasing the dose from 2 mg/kg to 4 mg/kg—indicating that when administering sugammadex at this degree of recovery (two twitches in response to train-of-four stimulation) the smaller dose of 2 mg/kg is likely to be adequate. Any conclusions about dosing in infants would be speculative at best as the total number of infants studied was only 8. It is clear, though, even in this age group, that administration of a dose of sugammadex as small as 0.5 mg/kg shortens recovery when compared with the administration of placebo.

With only 30 infants and children studied, it is impossible to comment on the safety of sugammadex in young patients. Two things stand out in the authors' reporting of complications. First, the incidence of adverse events seems higher in infants and children than it is in older patients. This may be due to the nature of events reported—such as pyrexia, viral gastroenteritis, pharyngitis, and rhinitis—that were not observed in adolescents and adults. While hypoglycemia and anemia were reported only in the 2 youngest age groups studied, these events did not appear to be related to sugammadex. Although there were no serious adverse events in the adults and adolescent study groups, there were 2 serious adverse events reported in the "infant" and "children" study groups (3 days of postoperative vomiting in one and diarrhea and hematuria in another). Whether these differences in severity and incidence of adverse events can be attributed to the differences in age of the 4 study populations is not known. Certainly, additional studies in infants and children are warranted to document not only the pharmacodynamics of sugammadex, but its safety.

C. A. Lien, MD

Reversal of Neuromuscular Blockade by Sugammadex after Continuous Infusion of Rocuronium in Patients Randomized to Sevoflurane or Propofol Maintenance Anesthesia

Rex C, Wagner S, Spies C, et al (Klinik für Anästhesiologie und Operative Intensivmedizin, Klinikum am Steinenberg, Reutlingen, Germany; Universitätsklinikum, Marburg, Germany; Charité – Universitätsmedizin, Berlin, Germany; et al)

Anesthesiology 111:30-35, 2009

Background.—Sugammadex rapidly reverses neuromuscular blockade induced by bolus rocuronium doses, but it has not been investigated after continuous rocuronium infusion in surgical patients. We therefore examined the clinical effect of sugammadex for neuromuscular blockade induced by continuous rocuronium infusion in adults undergoing surgery under maintenance anesthesia with sevoflurane or propofol.

Methods.—This four-center, comparative, parallel-group study, randomly assigned 52 adult patients (American Society of Anesthesiologists Class I-III) to maintenance anesthesia with sevoflurane or propofol. Neuromuscular blockade was induced by bolus injection of 0.6 mg/kg rocuronium followed by continuous infusion of 7 $\mu g \cdot kg^{-1} \cdot min^{-1}$ rocuronium adjusted to maintain a neuromuscular blockade depth of zero response to train-of-four and a posttetanic count of no more than 10 responses. A single dose of 4 mg/kg sugammadex was administered at first twitch (T_1) 3–10%. The primary clinical effect variable was recovery time to a train-of-four ratio of 0.9.

Results.—Median recovery time from start of sugammadex administration to a train-of-four ratio of 0.9 in the sevoflurane and propofol groups was 1.3 and 1.2 min, respectively. The estimated difference in recovery time between groups was 9 s (95% confidence interval −6 to 20 s), entirely within the predefined equivalence interval. Median plasma rocuronium concentration just before sugammadex administration was 33% lower during maintenance anesthesia with sevoflurane than with propofol. Sugammadex was well tolerated. One adverse event (procedural hypotension) was considered to be probably related to sugammadex.

Conclusions.—Single-dose sugammadex (4 mg/kg) after continuous rocuronium infusion is equally effective and well tolerated during maintenance anesthesia with sevoflurane or propofol.

▶ By the time sugammadex becomes available for clinical use in the United States, its pharmacodynamic properties will likely have been more completely characterized than any other neuromuscular blocking agent or reversal compound at the time of its Food and Drug Administration (FDA) approval. This is the first study in patients, of all of those published to date, to examine the efficacy of sugammadex in restoring neuromuscular function following discontinuation of a rocuronium infusion during a sevoflurane or propofol anesthetic. The dose of sugammadex used in this trial was moderate (4 mg/kg) and this dose quickly restored neuromuscular function even though it was administered at reappearance of the first twitch in the train-of-four. In contrast to recovery after anticholinesterase administration, speed of recovery was not affected by the anesthetic administered. Neuromuscular function in patients in both the sevoflurane and the propofol groups were completely recovered (train-of-four ratio = 0.9) within 2.4 minutes. With this rocuronium: sugammadex dosing paradigm allowing for maintenance of profound block intraoperatively and rapid recovery of neuromuscular strength, it will be the time required for emergence from anesthesia rather than the time to recover from neuromuscular block that defines the time to extubation after completion of surgery. Whether or not recovery is even shorter when depth of block during the rocuronium infusion is maintained at a level more frequently used in the operating rooms (train-of-four count = 1 or 2) remains to be determined.

Of note, one patient in this series of 52 developed hypotension following the administration of sugammadex. Whether or not this decrease in blood pressure was accompanied by an increase in heart rate was not reported. Based on this occurrence, though, additional studies of the safety of sugammadex seem warranted.

C. A. Lien, MD

Rapid injection of rocuronium reduces withdrawal movement on injection

Lee YC, Jang YH, Kim JM, et al (Keimyung Univ, School of Medicine, Korea)

J Clin Anesth 21:427-430, 2009

Study Objective.—To test whether rapid injection of rocuronium reduces withdrawal movement on injection.

Design.—Randomized, prospective trial.

Setting.—Operating room in a university hospital.

Patients.—150 ASA physical status I and II patients aged 18 to 60 years, undergoing general anesthesia.

Interventions.—Patients were randomized to three groups. After undergoing anesthesia induction with thiopental sodium, then 5 seconds later receiving a rubber tourniquet applied to the mid-forearm to stop intravenous (IV) flow by gravity, the pretreatment drug was injected. The tourniquet was held for 15 seconds then released, and 1.0 mg/kg of 1% rocuronium was injected IV. Group C patients (n = 50) were pretreated with 0.1 mL/kg of 0.9% NaCl and then injected with rocuronium slowly within 10 seconds. Group L patients (n = 50) were pretreated with 0.1 mL/kg of preservative-free 1% lidocaine and then injected with rocuronium slowly within 10 seconds. Group R patients (n = 50) were pretreated with 0.1 mL/kg of 0.9% NaCl and then rapidly injected with rocuronium within approximately one second (as quickly as possible).

Measurements.—After injection of the patient with the study drug, a single anesthesiologist with no knowledge of the study protocol graded each patient's response as follows: 0 = no response; 1 = mild movement limited to the wrist only; 2 = moderate movement involving the elbow and shoulder; and 3 = severe movement involving more than one extremity.

Main Results.—Group C had the most intense and frequent withdrawal response. The frequency and intensity of withdrawal movement was significantly less in Groups L and R than Group C. No significant difference in withdrawal response between Groups L and R was noted.

Conclusions.—Withdrawal response can be significantly reduced for rocuronium injection without lidocaine pretreatment, simply through rapid injection.

▶ Like propofol, intravenous administration of rocuronium causes pain. Since rocuronium, though, is not a sedative hypnotic, it is not the first medication administered to patients. Maneuvers such as deepening the level of anesthesia before administration of rocuronium will eliminate the withdrawal response to its administration. There are, however, situations in which the neuromuscular blocking agent has to be administered under a relatively light plane of anesthesia or before the administration of other anesthetic adjuncts. In these situations, application of a tourniquet to the extremity, intravenous administration of lidocaine, and then release of the tourniquet 15 seconds later has been demonstrated to reduce the withdrawal response.[1] Dilution of rocuronium to 0.5 mg/kg has also been found to completely eliminate the pain associated with administration.[2]

These authors have identified yet another means of reducing the withdrawal response associated with administration of rocuronium. Application of a tourniquet to an arm shortly after the administration of a sedative hypnotic would seem impractical to many clinicians. Rapid administration of rocuronium is more consistent with the commonplace, day to day administration of medications in the operating room—and, as found in this study, as effective as pretreatment with lidocaine in reducing the withdrawal response.

While the effect of rapid administration is not as pronounced as that of dilution with sodium chloride, which completely eliminates the withdrawal response, it is more practical than other maneuvers described to date and as effective as pretreatment with lidocaine. Consider the volume of medication required with the dilution method to give a 20 kg child a 1 mg/kg dose of rocuronium if it has been diluted to 0.5 mg/kg (40 mL). Rapid administration of the equivalent dose of rocuronium without dilution reduces the pain associated with administration and is both as effective as and less cumbersome than placing a tourniquet on the arm with the intravenous line, administering lidocaine, releasing the tourniquet, and then administering the rocuronium. It is also more likely to be used as part of routine anesthetic practice than other maneuvers that have been previously studied.

C. A. Lien, MD

References

1. Shevchenko Y, Jocson JC, McRae VA, et al. The use of lidocaine for preventing the withdrawal associated with the injection of rocuronium in children and adolescents. *Anesth Analg.* 1999;88:746-748.
2. Tuncali B, Karci A, Tuncali BE, et al. Dilution of rocuronium to 0.5 mg/kg with 0.9% NaCl eliminates the pain during intravenous injection in awake patients. *Anesth Analg.* 2004;99:740-743.

3 Anesthesia Techniques and Monitors

Effects of tracheal tube orientation on the success of intubation through an intubating laryngeal mask airway: study in Mallampati class 3 or 4 patients

Ye L, Liu J, Wong DT, et al (Sichuan Univ, People's Republic of China; Univ of Toronto, Ontario, Canada)

Br J Anaesth 102:269-272, 2009

Background.—We evaluated the effects of conventional tracheal tube orientation on success of intubation through an intubating laryngeal mask airway (ILMA) in Mallampati class 3 or 4 patients.

Methods.—Two hundred adults, ASA I–II, Mallampati class 3 or 4, undergoing elective surgery under general anaesthesia were enrolled. All the patients were randomly allocated to either normal or reverse group based on the orientation of the tracheal tube as it was initially inserted into the ILMA. Tracheal intubation was considered successful, if proper tracheal positioning was attained within three insertion attempts. χ^2 analysis was used to compare categorical variables.

Results.—Tracheal intubation through the ILMA was successful in 183 of 200 patients (91.5%): 157 (78.5%) on the first attempt. Seventeen (8.5%) were intubated using direct laryngoscopy. The first-attempt success rate was higher in the reverse than in the normal group (85.0% *vs* 72.0%, $P=0.025$), although the overall success rate was similar between the reverse and the normal groups (93.0% *vs* 90.0%). The incidence of sore throat was comparable in the normal group and the reverse group (22.0% *vs* 12.0%, NS).

Conclusions.—Overall, tracheal intubation was successful in 91.5% of patients through an ILMA with a conventional tracheal tube in Mallampati class 3 or 4 patients. The first-attempt success rate was higher in the reverse group compared with the normal group, but the overall success rate was similar between the reverse and the normal groups.

► Study of optimal management of the unanticipated difficult airway is difficult. However, few situations are more anxiety provoking than an unanticipated difficult intubation. Knowing what has proven useful in patients with potentially difficult airways may be helpful in this situation. In this large trial, the authors studied 200 patients with Mallampati 3 or 4 airways to determine the success with reversing the orientation of an endotracheal tube as it is passed through an intubating laryngeal mask airway (ILMA) to intubate a patient's trachea. Their finding confirmed those of other investigators in patients with Mallampati 1 or 2 airways. Reversing the orientation of the endotracheal tube, when using an ILMA, increases the success of endotracheal intubation on the first attempt. Interestingly, this maneuver, rotating the endotracheal tube 180°, also allows an endotracheal tube to pass easily over a fiber optic bronchoscope through the vocal cords when it doesn't with conventional orientation.

The study was carefully designed to eliminate some of the other factors associated with difficult intubation, such as morbid obesity, that will increase a patient's risk of regurgitation and aspiration, and limited mouth opening, which may make it difficult to insert the ILMA into the patient's mouth. Other indicators of a potentially difficult intubation, such as a long, narrow mouth with a high arched palate, a large tongue, impaired mandibular protrusion, limited neck mobility, and a short, thick neck are predictive of a difficult intubation and were not considered in this study. Additional evaluation of endotracheal tube orientation through the ILMA in patients with any of these additional factors may further define the potential impact of this maneuver in facilitating intubation in the difficult airway.

The results of this trial do not guarantee success when using the ILMA and reverse orientation of the endotracheal tube in a patient with a difficult airway, and it is not an endorsement of a cavalier approach to the difficult airway. While 75% of patients were intubated on the first attempt, 7% could not be intubated within 3 attempts. This study defines, though, another maneuver that may prove useful in intubating the trachea of the patient with an unanticipated difficult airway.

C. A. Lien, MD

Factors associated with delayed postsurgical voiding interval in ambulatory spinal anesthesia patients: a prospective cohort study in 3 types of surgery

Gil MJL, Gómez AE, Vargas DB, et al (Viladecans Hosp, Barcelona, Spain; Hospital Universitari Germans Trias i Pujol, Barcelona, Spain; et al)

Am J Surg 197:182-188, 2009

Background.—Spinal anesthesia has been considered inappropriate for ambulatory surgery patients because of concern about voiding dysfunction. The purpose of this study was to analyze the relationship between voiding interval and type of surgery under spinal anesthesia with lidocaine and to identify other nonanesthetic risk factors for delayed voiding.

Patients and Methods.—A prospective study of 406 patients undergoing ambulatory surgery under spinal anesthesia with lidocaine was performed. Voiding interval was defined as the time in minutes from the injection of local anesthetic to the patient's first spontaneous voiding. Univariate and multivariate linear regression models were constructed to identify risk factors associated with length of voiding interval.

Results.—A total of 187 patients underwent herniorrhaphy; 187 patients underwent lower limb surgery; and 32 patients went benign anorectal surgery. The mean ± sd voiding interval was 230 ± 50.5 minutes. Factors associated with length of voiding interval in the univariate analysis were sex, body mass index (BMI), type and duration of surgery, lidocaine dose, and volume of fluid administered. Factors that remained significant in the multivariate model were sex, BMI, lidocaine dose and type of surgery: spontaneous voiding came later after inguinal herniorrhaphy surgery than after lower-limb surgery (regression coefficient 20 minutes; 95% confidence interval 11.5–29.8). Multivariate models performed for each type of surgery separately identified sex and lidocaine dose as factors related to length of voiding interval in all types of surgery.

Conclusions.—A longer voiding interval was associated with inguinal herniorrhaphy, spinal lidocaine dose, and male sex.

▶ Increasingly, surgery is being done on an ambulatory basis. Additionally, the patients undergoing ambulatory surgery can have significant comorbidities. While discharging patients home promptly after surgery is a goal of ambulatory surgery, there are other factors that should be taken into account when caring for patients.

In this study, the authors demonstrated that surgery type, lidocaine dose, and male gender were independent risk factors for a longer time to voiding after surgery. Lidocaine was dosed on a mg/kg basis, and patient positioning was used to achieve the desired anesthetic level—T8 for inguinal herniorrhaphy, T10 for lower extremity surgery, and L3 for anorectal surgery. The results, a 15-minute delay in voiding with a 10 mg increase in lidocaine dose, are, from a clinical point-of-view, neither pronounced nor surprising. The effects of larger doses of local anesthetics and higher levels of spinal anesthesia will dissipate more slowly than will those resulting from smaller doses.

Interestingly, the authors did not comment on the use of opioids or any medications other than midazolam in the perioperative period. Certainly, administration of supplementary medications may have contributed to prolonged voiding times.

Not all hospitals or surgical centers require that patients void before discharge. In this case, time to discharge will be dependent on other factors, including the patient's ability to understand postoperative instructions, the availability of an escort, the return of sensation and strength to the lower extremities, as well as the presence of nausea and vomiting or pain. This study did not look at these factors; If it had, the study results would have been applicable to more ambulatory surgical settings.

C. A. Lien, MD

Comparison of blood pressure measured at the arm, ankle and calf

Moore C, Dobson A, Kinagi M, et al (South Manchester Univ Hosps NHS Trust, Wythenshawe, UK)

Anaesthesia 63:1327-1331, 2008

The suitability of alternative sites for non-invasive blood pressure (NIBP) measurement was investigated in 100 awake healthy volunteers. The calf and the ankle were chosen for comparison with the arm, and the results analysed subjected to Bland–Altman analysis. Discomfort was graded using a Visual Analogue Scale. There was a poor agreement between the different sites with respect to systolic blood pressure: the agreement was closer for diastolic and mean measurements. The mean blood pressure calf measurement was on average 4 mmHg (95% limits of agreement−12 to 20), higher than the arm. The ankle was 8 mmHg higher (−8 to 24) than the arm. ANOVA demonstrated a statistically significant difference in the discomfort scores between the sites ($p < 0.001$). The calf demonstrated the highest discomfort score and the ankle the lowest. We suggest that the ankle should be considered in preference to the calf as an alternative site for NIBP measurement if use of an arm is undesirable or impossible.

▶ Not infrequently, clinicians monitor blood pressure by placing a blood pressure cuff somewhere other than the upper arm. Sites that can and have been used include any portion of an upper or lower extremity. This study examined the differences in systolic, diastolic, and mean arterial pressure measured at the upper arm, the calf, and the ankle in volunteers not receiving an anesthetic.

A lack of specifics regarding methodology make interpretation of the authors results difficult. They found that having blood pressure taken at the calf is more painful than having it taken at either the arm or the ankle; yet the blood pressure measured at either the calf or ankle was elevated relative to that measured at the arm. The authors do not describe the order in which blood pressures were measured at the different sites and whether or not this may have impacted blood pressure measurements in the study. Additionally, the authors did not report the number of times that the cuff had to be inflated more than once in each subject at each site and, without knowing the actual measured blood pressures, it is impossible to ascertain how many times this may have happened or if it happened. Findings regarding relative blood pressures at each of the sites are not consistent with what has been reported, where one would have expected that systolic pressures measure at the ankle should have been higher than at the calf and diastolic blood pressure lower. Rather, there was substantial variability in blood pressure measured at any of the sites. The body mass index of patients, and whether or not blood pressure at each site was measured with the same size cuff, would have also been useful pieces of information in interpreting the significance of the results.

While knowing a patient's real blood pressure is important in deciding to treat either hyper- or hypotension, relative changes in blood pressure with induction of anesthesia and changing surgical stimuli and blood loss are also important.

Patient management decisions are made based on these relative changes. This article does not contribute to our understanding of whether one site or another is preferable for detecting changes in blood pressure over the course of an anesthetic or operation. Based on these results, clinicians may continue to monitor blood pressure on any accessible extremity when access to the arms is limited.

C. A. Lien, MD

Use of a leucocyte filter to remove tumour cells from intra-operative cell salvage blood

Catling S, Williams S, Freites O, et al (Singleton Hosp, Swansea, UK)
Anaesthesia 63:1332-1338, 2008

The intra-operative blood loss of 50 consecutive gynae-oncology patients undergoing surgery for endometrial, cervical or ovarian cancer was cell salvaged and filtered. In each case blood samples were taken from the effluent tumour vein, a central venous line, the cell saver reservoir, the cell salvage re-transfusion bag after processing but before filtration and from the cell salvage re-transfusion bag after processing and filtration. Samples were examined using immunohisto-chemical monoclonal antibody markers for epithelial cell lines. Viable, nucleated malignant cells were detected in 2/50 central venous samples, 34/50 reservoir samples and 31/50 unfiltered cell salvaged samples. After passage through a Pall RS leucocyte depletion filter no remaining viable, nucleated malignant cells were detected in any sample. The clinical risks of cell salvage in these circumstances should be reviewed in the light of the risks of allogeneic blood transfusion.

▶ The authors provided a nice overview of the history of intraoperative cell salvage, including an acknowledgement of initial assumptions that cell salvage is "contra-indicated in any situation in which there [is] a risk of contamination of the re-infused blood — particularly with amniotic fluid, infectious agents, and malignant cells." The authors then stated that the contra-indications, while sensible and intuitive at a time when cell salvage was new, were not supported by any evidence, and are now being revised with the benefit of the results of studies on the ability of cell salvage systems to remove such contaminants. The authors concluded that "the theoretical risk of reinfusion of salvaged blood containing tumor cells that are not detectable by current methods must be balanced against the recent encouraging clinical studies of disease recurrence rates and mortality in patients receiving salvaged blood, and against the well documented risks of allergenic transfusion."

D. H. Chestnut, MD

Prevalence of difficult intubation in a bariatric population, using the beach chair position

Fox WTA, Harris S, Kennedy NJ (Musgrove Park Hosp, Taunton, Somerset, UK)

Anaesthesia 63:1339-1342, 2008

We retrospectively reviewed the anaesthetic charts of patients who had undergone bariatric surgery in our regional centre since the start of the service. We identified Cormack and Lehane grade of laryngoscopy, any difficulties associated with tracheal intubation, and the impact of age, gender and body mass index on laryngoscopy grade. The patients were anaesthetised in the 'beach chair' position prior to laryngoscopy. One hundred and ninety-two patients' notes were available for review out of a total of 198. Mean age was 43.3 years (SD 10.3) and mean BMI 50.8 (SD 8.0). Grade of laryngoscopy was unrecorded in 20 patients. Of the 192 patients, 162 (84%) had a Cormack and Lehane grade of 1 or 2. Nine (4.7%) patients were graded as 3 and only one patient had a grade 4 laryngoscopy. There were two cases (1%) of difficulty in intubation. A bougie was used 16 times (8%). Logistic regression showed that age was a significant factor for increasing laryngoscopy grade ($p = 0.0102$) but that BMI was not ($p = 0.6271$).

▶ This retrospective analysis of practice was limited by the information available through chart review. Interestingly, while the authors commented on the Cormack and Lehane grade of the view available with laryngoscopy, they did not comment on which of these patients were, in fact, difficult to intubate. While 1 patient had a Cormack and Lehane grade of 4, 2 were described as being a difficult intubation, and an additional 17 patients were intubated using an airway adjuvant. Neither the Cormack and Lehane grade of these patients nor the indication for the use of alternative airway techniques was noted.

The authors' finding that advanced age, rather than body mass index (BMI), is associated with more difficult intubation is surprising in light of other data suggesting that neck circumference is the best predictor of a difficult intubation in the morbidly obese patient.[1] The explanation for this finding may reside in data that was not available, such as neck circumference, thyromental distance, mouth opening, and neck extension.

Most surprisingly, the authors described using the same induction regimen for all patients, regardless of the findings on airway exam. I wonder if the authors had considered any of these patients as difficult airways before induction of anesthesia. If they had, would their approach to induction and airway management have changed? Certainly, while many obese patients can be intubated, they can be difficult to ventilate with a mask. This difficulty ventilating patients after loss of consciousness, coupled with rapid arterial desaturation due to oxygen consumption and decreased functional residual capacity, can make induction of anesthesia in obese patients very challenging.

C. A. Lien, MD

Reference

1. Brodsky JB, Lemmons HJM, Brock-Utne JG, Vierra M, Saidman LJ. Morbid obesity and tracheal intubation. *Anesth Analg.* 2002;94:732.

Cervical spine motion during flexible bronchoscopy compared with the Lo-Pro GlideScope®

Wong DM, Prabhu A, Chakraborty S, et al (Toronto Western Hosp, Canada; et al)

Br J Anaesth 102:424-430, 2009

Background.—The most appropriate device for tracheal intubation in patients with potential cervical spine injury remains controversial. We hypothesized that the Lo-Pro GlideScope® (LP-G) videolaryngoscope would not cause significantly greater cervical spine movement than fibreoptic bronchoscopy even in the non-immobilized spine.

Methods.—Twenty-eight healthy adults requiring intubation for radiographic procedures were randomized to either the LP-G or the flexible bronchoscope (FB) devices. Continuous fluoroscopy was used to assess cervical spine movement during tracheal intubation. The point of maximum movement was compared with baseline for change in angulation between Occiput (Occ)-C1, Occ-C2, Occ-C4, Occ-C5, C1–2, C2–4, and C4–5. Measurements were made by two independent observers. The change in angulation was also measured for tongue pull and jaw thrust, manoeuvres for enlarging the pharyngeal space, before FB intubation.

Results.—LP-G resulted in greater cervical extension compared with FB for every angle calculated, statistically significant between Occ-C1 ($P<0.05$), Occ-C2 ($P<0.05$), and Occ-C4 ($P<0.01$). Tongue pull resulted in significantly less cervical spine motion than FB intubation at Occ-C1, Occ-C2, Occ-C4, and Occ-C5 ($P<0.05$). When jaw thrust was added to tongue pull, there was a tendency for greater movement than FB intubation at Occ-C1, Occ-C2, and Occ-C3. This was statistically significant at Occ-C1 and Occ-C3 ($P<0.05$) for one of the two observers.

Conclusions.—During intubation under general anaesthesia, LP-G resulted in greater cervical movement than FB when no cervical immobilization was used in adults without cervical disease. Airway manoeuvres performed before FB, especially jaw thrust, also resulted in cervical spine movement.

▶ Maintaining an aligned cervical spine during intubation in patients with cervical spine injury is of obvious import. Previous studies have looked at the degree of movement in the cervical cord in cadavers or patients using different techniques of airway manipulation for intubation. The results of this study confirm previous studies, in that fiberoptic intubation causes the least movement of the cervical cord. The lower profile of the Lo-Pro GlideScope videolaryngoscope does not render it a preferable means of accomplishing endotracheal intubation in patients with compromise of the cervical cord.

Interestingly, in this study the investigators did not rely on 1 physician to determine the degree of movement at each portion of the cervical cord with each form of airway manipulation. Both a radiologist and a neurosurgeon interpreted the images obtained through fluoroscopy. While there were differences in their determination of the maximal degree of movement, similar trends, in terms of whether greater movement occurred during fiberoptic bronchoscopy for intubation or use of the Lo-Pro GlideScope, were noted by both physicians.

Of note, the investigators responsible for intubation were both experienced in the use of the fiberoptic bronchoscope and the Lo-Pro GlideScope for intubation. Even with their experience in using these techniques, cervical neck movement could not be minimized with the latter. The authors did not look at the degree of movement when in-line stabilization is used—as it might commonly be in the patient with an unstable cervical spine—leaving questions unanswered. How much less would the degree of movement during laryngoscopy and intubation have been with the Lo-Pro GlideScope? Would it have been equivalent to that observed during intubation with a fiberoptic bronchoscope? As noted by the authors of this article and others, in patients with compromise of the cervical cord, clinicians should use the intubation techniques with which they are most comfortable. As found in this study, for the clinician requiring a jaw thrust to facilitate fiberoptic intubation, a significant degree of movement of the cervical cord can occur—potentially negating the beneficial effects of fiberoptic bronchoscopy.

C. A. Lien, MD

The use of desflurane or propofol in combination with remifentanil in myasthenic patients undergoing a video-assisted thoracoscopic-extended thymectomy

Gritti P, Carrara B, Khotcholava M, et al (Ospedali Riuniti di Bergamo, Italy)
Acta Anaesthesiol Scand 53:380-389, 2009

Background.—Although several studies of the use of desflurane in anesthesia have revealed many desirable qualities, there are no data on the use and effects especially on the neuromuscular function of desflurane on myasthenia gravis (MG) patients. The purpose of this study was to evaluate the use of either desflurane or propofol, both combined with remifentanil, in patients with MG undergoing a video-assisted thoracoscopic-extended thymectomy (VATET).

Methods.—Thirty-six MG patients who underwent VATET were enrolled. Nineteen patients were anesthetized with remifentanil and propofol infused with a target-controlled infusion plasma model, and 17 patients with desflurane and remifentanil. No muscle relaxant was used. The intubating conditions, hemodynamic and respiratory changes, neuromuscular transmission and post-operative complications were evaluated.

Results.—Neuromuscular transmission was significantly decreased in the desflurane group (6.7%, from 3% to 9% during anesthesia $P = <0.05$). The intubating conditions were good in all 36 patients and 35 patients were successfully extubated in the operating room. The time-to-awakening, post-operatory pH and base excess were significantly different in the two groups, with a decreasing mean arterial pressure in the group administered with desflurane. No patients required reintubation due to myasthenic or cholinergic crisis, or respiratory failure. No other significant differences between the two groups studied were observed.

Conclusion.—Our experience indicates that anesthesia with desflurane plus remifentanil in patients with MG could determine a reversible muscle relaxation effect, but with no clinical implication, allowing a faster recovery with no difference in extubation time and post-operative complications in the two groups.

► In this study, 36 patients with myasthenia gravis received 1 of 2 different anesthetics for their video-assisted thoracoscopic-extended thymectomy (VATET) procedure. This study is noteworthy because there are relatively few studies in these patients with compromised muscle strength who undergo such relatively invasive surgical procedures. As their muscle strength is influenced by so many different factors including their underlying disease process, their medication regimen and changes in that regimen, and many anesthetic medications including nondepolarizing neuromuscular blocking agents and volatile anesthetics, definition of better ways of providing care for myasthenic patients during surgical procedures would be useful. These authors have demonstrated that in this small group of patients, the 2 anesthetics were comparable in terms of postoperative respiratory failure.

The study results, however, should be interpreted with caution. As the authors of the study note, volatile anesthetics, even in patients with no neuromuscular disease, interfere with neuromuscular transmission. Their effects are more pronounced in patients with myasthenia gravis. While healthy patients will have minimal decrement in the train-of-four (TOF) response to stimulation, those with myasthenia gravis will have a substantially more pronounced effect.[1] The influence of desflurane on neuromuscular transmission has been documented in the presence and absence of nondepolarizing neuromuscular blockers.[2,3] It appears to potentiate neuromuscular block more than isoflurane and, in contrast to other volatile agents, has been shown to cause significant fade in the TOF response of a patient with no neuromuscular disease when administered at MAC concentrations as used in this study.[3] Therefore, one has to be cautious when concluding that patients receiving desflurane will not be at greater risk of respiratory failure than those receiving propofol. The author's results support the use of caution.

The muscle strength of patients was appropriately measured in a quantitative fashion using the TOF-Watch,®[4] which describes a period of 5 to 20 minutes as being required to establish a stable baseline. Patients with myasthenia will likely develop fade in the TOF with repetitive stimulation.

As noted by the authors, all volatile anesthetics interfere with neuromuscular transmission—potentiating nondepolarizing neuromuscular blockers. As noted previously, desflurane may have a greater impact than other anesthetics. In agreement with this, the authors' results indicate that fade in the TOF response is greater in patients receiving desflurane than it is in those receiving propofol. At 60 minutes, and at the conclusion of the procedure, there is significantly more fade in the TOF response in those patients that had received desflurane—although the mean TOF responses appear similar. In order to provide a more complete description of the effect of desflurane in patients with myasthenia, the authors should have provided the range of TOF responses at the different time points defined in their study. This would have contributed significantly to the body of literature on the effects of desflurane in patients with myasthenia gravis. Finally, studies have shown that large numbers of patients are required to define differences in outcome with varying degrees of neuromuscular blockade.[5] This study was too small to define the impact of different anesthetic regimens on clinical outcomes in patients with myasthenia gravis.

C. A. Lien, MD

References

1. Mann R, Blobner M, Jelen-Esselborn S, Busley R, Werner C. Preanesthetic train-of-four fade predicts the atracurium requirement of myasthenia gravis patients. *Anesthesiology.* 2000;93:346-350.
2. Wright PM, Hart P, Lau M, et al. The magnitude and time course of vecuronium potentiation by desflurane versus isoflurane. *Anesthesiology.* 1995;82:404-411.
3. Kelly R, Lien CA, Savarese JJ, et al. Depression of neuromuscular function in a patient during desflurane anesthesia. *Anesth Analgesia.* 1993;76:868-871.
4. Fuchs-Buder T, Skovgaard LT, Eriksson LI, Mirakhur RK, Viby-Mogensen J. Good clinical research practice in pharmacodynamics studies of neuromuscular blocking agents II: the Stockholm revision. *Acta Anaesthsiol Scand.* 2007;51:789-808.
5. Murphy GS, Szokol JW, Marymount JH, Greenberg SB, Avram MJ, Vender JS. Residual neuromuscular blockade and critical respiratory events in the postanesthesia care unit. *Anesthesiology.* 2008;107:130-137.

Efficacy of oropharyngeal lidocaine instillation on hemodynamic responses to orotracheal intubation

Sun H-L, Wu T-J, Ng C-C, et al (Cathay General Hosp, Taipei, Taiwan; et al)
J Clin Anesth 21:103-107, 2009

Study Objective.—To determine whether oropharyngeal instillation of lidocaine after anesthetic induction modifies the hemodynamic response to intubation.

Design.—Prospective, randomized, double-blind, placebo-controlled study.

Setting.—Operating room of a university hospital.

Patients.—56 ASA physical status I and II adult patients scheduled for elective surgery requiring orotracheal intubation and general anesthesia.

Interventions.—Patients were randomized to receive oropharyngeal instillation with either 5 mL 2% lidocaine (n = 28, lidocaine group) or 5 mL normal saline (n = 28, control group) 45 seconds after anesthetic induction bolus. Orotracheal intubation was attempted three minutes later.

Measurements.—Systolic (SBP), diastolic (DBP), mean arterial pressure (MAP), and heart rate (HR) were recorded at baseline, just before intubation, and for three minutes postintubation at one-minute intervals. Occurrence of adverse events such as arrhythmias, ischemic changes in electrocardiography, and bronchospasm after intubation were also documented.

Main Results.—All postintubation values of SBP, DBP, MAP, and HR were significantly lower in the lidocaine group than the control group ($P < 0.01$). In both groups, postintubation HRs were significantly higher than baseline values ($P < 0.05$). More patients ($P < 0.001$) became hypertensive postintubation in the control group (14/28, 50%) than the lidocaine group (2/28, 7%).

Conclusion.—Oropharyngeal instillation of lidocaine for three minutes before intubation attenuates the cardiovascular responses to intubation.

▶ This article offers yet another means of minimizing increases in blood pressure and heart rate occurring as a result of endotracheal intubation. Avoiding hypertension and tachycardia resulting from intubation—especially in those patients at risk for myocardial ischemia—provides the rationale for many induction regimens. Oropharyngeal instillation of 5 mL of 2% lidocaine 3 minutes before laryngoscopy blunted the increases in heart rate and blood pressure observed in patients intubated almost 4 minutes following induction of anesthesia with propofol, fentanyl, and rocuronium.

How well this technique works relative to other means of avoiding hemodynamic changes with laryngoscopy such as: instillation of lidocaine directly into the trachea, administering intravenous lidocaine, providing a deeper level of anesthesia, or administering β-blockers before intubation is not clear. However, when faced with a patient who can be ventilated for 3 minutes following induction of anesthesia, this technique may provide an option. Of note, it does not eliminate entirely the hypertension and tachycardia observed following intubation. Additionally, whether or not it will improve tolerance of the endotracheal tube during emergence from anesthesia is not known and will depend, among other things, on the duration of surgery.

C. A. Lien, MD

Acceleromyography and mechanomyography for establishing potency of neuromuscular blocking agents: a randomized-controlled trial

Claudius C, Skovgaard LT, Viby-Mogensen J (Copenhagen Univ Hosp, Rigshospitalet, Denmark; Copenhagen Univ, Denmark)

Acta Anaesthesiol Scand 53:449-454, 2009

Background.—Acceleromyography (AMG) is increasingly being used in neuromuscular research, including in studies establishing the potency of neuromuscular blocking and reversal agents. However, AMG is insufficiently validated for use interchangeably with the gold standard, mechanomyography (MMG) for this purpose. The aim of this study was to compare AMG and MMG for establishing dose–response relationship and potency, using rocuronium as an example.

Methods.—We included 40 adult patients in this randomized-controlled single-dose response study. Anaesthesia was induced and maintained with propofol and opioid. Neuromuscular blockade was induced with rocuronium 100, 150, 200 or 250 μg/kg. Neuromuscular monitoring was performed with AMG (TOF-Watch® SX) with pre-load (Hand Adapter) at one arm and MMG (modified TOF-Watch® SX) on the other, using 0.1 Hz single twitch stimulation. Dose–response relationships were determined for both recording methods using log (dose) against probit (maximum block). The obtained slopes of the regression lines, ED_{50}, ED_{95} and the maximum block were compared.

Results.—The ED_{50} and ED_{95} [95% confidence interval (CI)] for AMG were 185 μg/kg (167–205 μg/kg) and 368 μg/kg (288–470 μg/kg), compared with 174 μg/kg (159–191 μg/kg) and 338 μg/kg (273–418 μg/kg) for MMG. There were no statistically significant biases in maximum block, ED_{50}, ED_{95} or slopes obtained with the two methods.

Conclusion.—Our results indicate that any possible difference between AMG and MMG is so small that it justifies AMG to be used for establishing the potency of neuromuscular blocking agents. However, the wide CIs show that we cannot rule out a 13% higher ED_{50} and a 26% higher ED_{95} for AMG.

▶ The question of whether or not to use acceleromyography or mechanomyography to monitor muscle strength while determining the potency of neuromuscular blocking agents has, at last, been put to rest. Acceleromyography provides data comparable with that of mechanomyography when determining ED_{50} (the dose that will, on average, provide 50% depression of twitch response) and the ED_{95} (the dose that will provide 95% depression of twitch response) for rocuronium—the steroidal neuromuscular blocking agent for which the ED_{95} has, in multiple studies, been found to be between 0.3 and 0.4 mg/kg. Historically, dose response data was derived through mechanomyography that measured the strength of abduction of the thumb in response to ulnar nerve stimulation. The equipment required to do this type of monitoring was bulky and required a significant amount of time and expertise for calibration. More recently, acceleromyography has been used in studies of neuromuscular function in the presence of neuromuscular blocking agents. The acceleromyograph measures the acceleration of the thumb as it abducts in response to ulnar nerve stimulation. In contrast to the mechanomyograph, the acceleromyograph is easily portable, small, and simple to calibrate. Since its introduction into the clinical practice, questions have been raised regarding its validity as a monitor of muscle strength.

The confidence intervals found for the ED_{95} are large. However, as noted by the authors, the doses chosen for administration were closer to the ED_{50} than the ED_{95} of the compound, and the ED_{50} is a more robust measure. ED_{95} more likely to be influenced by the doses administered. Three patients in this study developed either 0% or 100% neuromuscular block in response to administered doses; others developed >85% or less than 5% block. Patients developing no or complete block are not discarded in calculating the potency. Rather, they are assigned values of 0.5% and 99.5%, respectively. Choice of doses, therefore, can very much influence calculation of the potency of a compound. Dose-response data is not linear and there is not agreement on a single way to work with the data. A number of ways can be used to linearize data, including log values of doses, probit, logit, or arcsine values of percentage responses are among accepted techniques to report and analyze data.[1] Claudius used a probit transformation of the data for his analysis. While their confidence intervals were wide, reported ED_{50} and ED_{95} values are not dissimilar to what has been reported previously.

What is perhaps most striking about this dose-response study is that it was preceded by a power analysis. This has not previously been done in any study of determination of neuromuscular blocking agent potency, and many earlier studies have been done with far fewer than 40 subjects. This study has set a new standard for studies of this type, and has raised the question of how best to determine the appropriate "n" for a muscle relaxant trial.

While at the outset this study will catch the attention of clinicians interested in neuromuscular pharmacology and monitoring, its results (that the acceleromyograph is a valid monitor of muscle strength) should interest all clinicians who use nondepolarizing neuromuscular blocking agents.

C. A. Lien, MD

Reference

1. Fuchs-Buder T, Claudius C, Skovgaard LT, Eriksson LI, Mirakhur RK, Viby-Mogensen J. Good clinical research practices in pharmacodynamic studies of neuromuscular blocking agents II: the Stockholm revision. *Acta Anaesthesiol Scand.* 2007;51:789-808.

Randomized clinical trial of Entonox® *versus* midazolam–fentanyl sedation for colonoscopy

Maslekar S, Gardiner A, Hughes M, et al (Univ of Hull Hosp, Cottingham, UK)
Br J Surg 96:361-368, 2009

Background.—Intravenous sedation for colonoscopy is associated with cardiorespiratory complications and delayed recovery. The aim of this randomized clinical trial was to compare the efficacy of Entonox® (50 per cent nitrous oxide and 50 per cent oxygen) and intravenous sedation using midazolam–fentanyl for colonoscopy.

Methods.—Some 131 patients undergoing elective colonoscopy were included. Patients completed a Hospital Anxiety and Depression questionnaire, letter cancellation tests and pain scores on a 100-mm visual analogue scale before, immediately after the procedure and at discharge. They also completed a satisfaction survey at discharge and 24 h after the procedure.

Results.—Sixty-five patients were randomized to receive Entonox® and 66 to midazolam–fentanyl. Completion rates were similar (94 *versus* 92 per cent respectively; $P = 0{\cdot}513$). Patients receiving Entonox® had a shorter time to discharge. They reported significantly less pain (mean score 16·7 *versus* 40·1; $P < 0{\cdot}001$), and showed better recovery of psychomotor function immediately after the procedure and at discharge. Patient satisfaction was higher among patients who received Entonox® (median score 96 *versus* 89; $P = 0{\cdot}001$).

Conclusion.—Entonox® provides better pain relief and faster recovery than midazolam–fentanyl and so is more effective for colonoscopy. Registration number: ISRCTN81142957 (http://www.controlledtrials.com).

▶ This is an interesting study comparing patient, physician, and nurse satisfaction with different sedation regimens for colonoscopy. Patients received a 50% oxygen/nitrous oxide combination or midazolam and fentanyl. There are many factors that contribute to satisfaction for a particular medication regimen, some of which were assessed in this study. Certainly, reasons for satisfaction or dissatisfaction differ between patients, surgeons, and nurses. In this study, all study groups were quite satisfied with both medication regimens—with median satisfaction scores ranging from 89 to 96. While physicians were equally satisfied with both sedation regimens, the patients and nurses were more satisfied with the oxygen/nitrous oxide than the combination of intravenous medications. The different results between practitioners may have been due to the greater level of sedation in the nitrous oxide treatment group and the more rapid recovery from nitrous oxide sedation than the intravenous agents—facilitating their nursing care. Decreased patient ability to cooperate with requests for them to move when receiving the intravenous medications may have also contributed to the nurse's greater satisfaction with the nitrous oxide regimen. In contrast, the endoscopists were able to complete the colonoscopies within the same time frame regardless of the sedation regimen, and the difficulty in completing the colonoscopy was similar in both treatment groups.

While the depth of sedation that can be achieved through administration of opioids and benzodiazepines is potentially greater than that achieved through inhalation of 50% nitrous oxide, patients receiving nitrous oxide were able to control their intake of the medication and, thereby, control their depth of sedation—perhaps accounting, at least in part, for their satisfaction with this regimen. Interestingly, in spite of the greater satisfaction scores with nitrous oxide—with scores ranging from 90 to 100—7 of 65 patients would choose a different sedation regimen for their next colonoscopy.

Because many patients currently receive propofol for their colonoscopies rather than intravenous sedation or nitrous oxide, the results of this study may not be relevant to a large number of practices. How this regimen would compare in terms of recovery, sedation, and satisfaction surveys would be a very interesting study.

C. A. Lien, MD

Dexmedetomidine suppresses the decrease in blood pressure during anesthetic induction and blunts the cardiovascular response to tracheal intubation

Kunisawa T, Nagata O, Nagashima M, et al (Asahikawa Med College, Hokkaido, Japan; Tokyo Metropolitan Police Hosp, Japan; Massachusetts General Hosp and Harvard Med School, Boston)
J Clin Anesth 21:194-199, 2009

Study Objective.—To evaluate the effect of dexmedetomidine combined with fentanyl on hemodynamics.

Design.—Prospective, double-blinded, randomized study.

Setting.—Operating room of a university hospital.

Patients.—30 ASA physical status II and III patients with mild-to-moderate cardiovascular disease.

Interventions.—Patients were assigned to one of three groups: Group D-F2 [dexmedetomidine, effect-site concentration (ESC) of fentanyl = two ng/mL]; Group F2 (placebo, ESC of fentanyl = two ng/mL), or Group F4 (placebo, ESC of fentanyl = 4 ng/mL).

Measurements.—Dexmedetomidine (an initial dose of 1.0 μg/kg for 10 min, followed by a continuous infusion of 0.7 $\mu g \cdot kg^{-1} \cdot hr^{-1}$) or placebo saline was administered 15 minutes before anesthetic induction. Anesthesia was induced with propofol and fentanyl using a target-controlled infusion system. Hemodynamic parameters: systolic (SBP) and diastolic blood pressures (DBP), and heart rate (HR) during anesthetic induction were measured and the percent changes were calculated for both induction and intubation.

Main Results.—After inducing anesthesia, SBP was significantly higher in Group D-F2 (127 ± 24 mmHg) than Group F2 (90 ± 20 mmHg) or Group F4 (77 ± 21 mmHg). The SBP in Groups F2 and F4 reached 160 ± 31 mmHg and 123 ± 36 mmHg, respectively, after intubation, but no significant change in SBP was noted in Group D-F2. The percent increase in SBP due to tracheal intubation in Group D-F2 was 3% ± 4% and was significantly lower than that of Group F2 (70% ± 34%) or Group F4 (45% ± 36%).

Conclusion.—Dexmedetomidine combined with fentanyl during anesthetic induction suppresses the decrease in blood pressure due to anesthetic induction and also blunts the cardiovascular response to tracheal intubation.

▶ How to induce anesthesia so as not to decrease blood pressure in patients at risk for the adverse effects of hypotension and yet have an adequate depth of anesthesia to avoid hypertension and tachycardia during laryngoscopy and intubation is an ongoing challenge for the anesthesiologist. All sedative hypnotics are to varying degrees myocardial depressants and vasodilators. Some of these effects can be mitigated by administering vasopressors shortly after induction or by administering smaller doses of the sedative hypnotic, risking an inadequate depth of anesthesia for laryngoscopy and intubation. While etomidate may not cause the decreases in blood pressure that accompany administration of other sedative hypnotics, it does not eliminate the increases in blood pressure and heart rate that accompany laryngoscopy and endotracheal intubation.

Dexmedetomidine, an alpha agonist, has been described as an anesthetic adjuvant that decreases MAC and allows for maintenance of hemodynamic stability.

This small study in American Society of Anesthesiologists (ASA) physical status II and III patients demonstrated that when dexmedetomidine, 0.7 μg/kg/hr following a loading dose of 1 mg/kg, was used as part of an induction with propofol and fentanyl, decreases in blood pressure after induction and increases in blood pressure after intubation were significantly less than those occurring after induction of anesthesia with propofol and fentanyl. Of note, patients in this study did not receive any premedication. If these results are applicable to patients with more severe comorbidities and to patients in whom dosing of induction agents is not so rigidly controlled, they present an intriguing option for induction of anesthesia in the patient in whom hypo- and hypertension must be avoided.

C. A. Lien, MD

Comparison of the adductor pollicis, orbicularis oculi, and corrugator supercilii as indicators of adequacy of muscle relaxation for tracheal intubation

Lee HJ, Kim KS, Jeong JS, et al (Hanyang Univ Hosp, Seoul, Republic of Korea)

Br J Anaesth 102:869-874, 2009

Background.—The purpose of this study was to verify which muscle among the adductor pollicis (AP), orbicularis oculi (OO), and corrugator supercilii (CS) is a better predictor of optimal intubating conditions after administration of rocuronium.

Methods.—In this prospective trial, 201 patients were randomized into six groups to receive rocuronium at a dose of 0.6 or 1.0 mg kg^{-1} during propofol–remifentanil–nitrous oxide anaesthesia. The tracheal intubation was performed after maximal neuromuscular block by acceleromyography at the thumb (AP), the eyelid (OO), and the superciliary arch (CS). The onset time, intubating conditions, peak vital signs, and bispectral index were assessed.

Results.—The onset time of rocuronium in the OO and CS muscle was significantly shorter than in the AP muscle ($P<0.001$), but excellent intubating conditions were significantly increased in the AP (87) and the CS (77) compared with the OO (32) after a dose of 0.6 mg kg^{-1} of rocuronium ($P<0.05$).

Conclusions.—After administration of rocuronium, twitch monitoring at the OO allows a faster intubation but is associated with an unacceptable incidence of inadequate intubating conditions. Excellent intubating conditions are observed most frequently with AP monitoring but with the longest delay before intubation is attempted. Monitoring of the CS allows intubation earlier than that of AP with fewer patients having excellent but no patients having inadequate intubating conditions.

▶ The quest for ways to intubate the trachea more quickly is a fascinating one. It has fueled the development of compounds that have faster onsets of effect, and it has caused us to increase the doses of neuromuscular blocking agents used for endotracheal intubation to 3 or 4 times the ED95 value. While allowing for a faster onset of neuromuscular blockade, this increase in dose is also associated with a longer duration of effect, and may be associated with greater side effects. In addition to depth of neuromuscular blockade, ease of endotracheal intubation depends on several other factors, including patient airway anatomy, experience of the person doing the laryngoscopy, patient position, and depth of anesthesia. To further complicate the issue, depth of neuromuscular block is not the same in all muscle groups.[1]

As clinicians, we do not routinely monitor depth of neuromuscular block at the orbicularis oculi. While onset of block in this muscle group has been reported to allow good or excellent intubating conditions,[2,3] as noted in this study, reports are conflicting. Many different muscle groups need to be relaxed to allow for excellent intubating conditions (relaxed jaw, abducted vocal cords, lack of cough response, and patient movement to intubation). These include, at a minimum, relaxation of the following: masseter muscle, laryngeal adductors, and diaphragm. Onset in each neuromuscular block in each of these muscle groups is different and precedes that in the adductor pollicis.[1]

As found in this study, while onset of block is most rapid in the orbicularis oculi—which is similar to onset of block in the larynx, intubating conditions are better when the clinician waits for complete block at the corrugator supercilii and even better with waiting a bit longer for complete relaxation at the adductor pollicis. Interestingly, waiting the additional minute to 1.5 minutes significantly increases the frequency of excellent intubating conditions. Given these data, one has to wonder, why is there such a rush to intubate the trachea? The only time when rapid intubation is essential is when a patient is at risk of regurgitation. In that case, the patient will likely receive either succinylcholine or rocuronium, 1 to 1.2 mg/kg, and be intubated at 1 minute regardless of the results of monitoring depth of neuromuscular blockade. If a patient is anticipated to be difficult to intubate or ventilate, he will likely not receive a neuromuscular blocking agent.

Finally, waiting 1 or 2 additional minutes may lessen the complications of endotracheal intubation, which range from abrasion of the tracheal mucosa to granuloma formation to tracheal perforation. Minimizing the trauma associated with laryngoscopy and intubation by waiting an extra minute or 2 after administration of the neuromuscular blocking agent for intubation may decrease the risk of a patient developing an airway-related anesthetic complication.

C. A. Lien, MD

References

1. Donati F, Meistelman C, Plaud B. Vecuronium neuromuscular blockade at the adductor muscles of the larynx and adductor pollicis. *Anesthesiology.* 1991;74:833.
2. Debaene B, Beaussier M, Meistelman C, Donati F, Lienhart A. Monitoring the onset of neuromuscular block at the orbicularis oculi can predict good intubating conditions during atracurium-induced neuromuscular block. *Anesth Analg.* 1995;80:360.
3. Le Corre F, Plaud B, Benhamou E, Debaene B. Visual estimation of onset time at the orbicularis oculi after five muscle relaxants: Application to clinical monitoring of tracheal intubation. *Anesth Analg.* 1999;89:1305.

Relaxing music as pre-medication before surgery: a randomised controlled trial

Bringman H, Giesecke K, Thörne A, et al (Södertälje Hosp, Sweden; et al)
Acta Anaesthesiol Scand 53:759-764, 2009

Introduction.—Patients who await surgery often suffer from fear and anxiety, which can be prevented by anxiolytic drugs. Relaxing music may be an alternative treatment with fewer adverse effects. This randomised clinical trial compared pre-operative midazolam with relaxing music.

Method.—Three hundred and seventy-two patients scheduled for elective surgery were randomised to receive pre-operative prevention of anxiety by 0.05–0.1 mg/kg of midazolam orally or by relaxing music. The main outcome measure was the State Trait Anxiety Inventory (STAI X-1), which was completed by the patients just before and after the intervention.

Results.—Of the 177 patients who completed the music protocol, the mean and (standard deviation) STAI-state anxiety scores were 34 (8) before and 30 (7) after the intervention. The corresponding scores for the 150 patients in the midazolam group were 36 (8) before and 34 (7) after the intervention. The decline in the STAI-state anxiety score was significantly greater in the music group compared with the midazolam group ($P < 0.001$, 95% confidence interval range −3.8 to −1.8).

Conclusion.—Relaxing music decreases the level of anxiety in a pre-operative setting to a greater extent than orally administrated midazolam. Higher effectiveness and absence of apparent adverse effects makes pre-operative relaxing music a useful alternative to midazolam for pre-medication.

▶ Most patients are somewhat apprehensive about pending surgery. Relief of perioperative anxiety may improve patient satisfaction with a surgical experience. As we learned years ago, the preoperative visit is an important anxiolytic; this trial reinforces the concept that not all patients benefit from perioperative administration of benzodiazepines. While easy to administer, their use is not without adverse effects such as agitation, excessive sedation, and postoperative amnesia.

As shown in this study, anxiolysis can be provided through nonpharmacologic means. Patients listening to the music of their choice for the hour before their surgery had significant decreases in their anxiety scores relative to patients receiving midazolam. While decreases in heart rate, systolic, and mean arterial pressures were statistically significant compared with decreases in the midazolam group, they were clinically similar and one would not use this intervention for its hemodynamic effects.

Unfortunately, the benefits of preoperative exposure to music—decreased sedation and postoperative amnesia—are difficult to quantitate. The cost of being able to offer and maintain this therapeutic modality, however, is substantial. Whether or not its benefits warrant the cost of being able to offer and maintain this option for those desiring it remains to be determined. Additionally, just as midazolam should not be given to all patients, this holistic approach to anxiolysis may not be appropriate for all. A preoperative assessment of the patient's anxiety level and his or her expectations for the perioperative experience will remain important factors in deciding how to provide the best perioperative care for patients.

C. A. Lien, MD

Avoidance of neuromuscular blocking agents may increase the risk of difficult tracheal intubation: a cohort study of 103 812 consecutive adult patients recorded in the Danish Anaesthesia Database

Lundstrøm LH, the Danish Anaesthesia Database (Copenhagen Univ Hosp, Herlev, Denmark; et al)

Br J Anaesth 103:283-290, 2009

Background.—Previous studies indicate that avoiding neuromuscular blocking agents (NMBAs) may be a risk factor for difficult tracheal intubation (DTI). We investigated whether avoiding NMBA was associated with DTI.

Methods.—A cohort of 103 812 consecutive patients planned for tracheal intubation by direct laryngoscopy was retrieved from the Danish Anaesthesia Database. We used an intubation score based upon the number of attempts, change from direct laryngoscopy to a more advanced technique, or intubation by a different operator. We retrieved data on age, sex, ASA physical status classification, priority of surgery, time of surgery, previous DTI, modified Mallampati score, BMI, and the use of NMBA. Using logistic regression, we assessed whether avoiding NMBA was associated with DTI.

Results.—The frequency of DTI was 5.1 [95% confidence interval (CI): 5.0–5.3]%. In a univariate analysis, avoiding NMBA was associated with DTI, odds ratio (OR) 1.52 (95% CI: 1.43–1.61)%, *P*<0.0001. Using multivariate analysis, avoiding NMBA was associated with DTI, OR 1.48 (95% CI: 1.39–1.58), *P*<0.0001. Among patients intubated using NMBA, a multivariate analysis identified patients anaesthetized with only non-depolarizing NMBA to be more at risk for DTI than those anaesthetized with depolarizing NMBA alone.

Conclusions.—Avoiding NMBA may increase the risk of DTI. However, confounding by indication may be a problem in this observational study and systematic reviews with meta-analysis or more randomized clinical trials are needed.

▶ Access to a national database, such as that available in Denmark, provides unparalleled access to practice information across a country. However, analysis of retrospective data is limited by the data that were collected.

The findings of this study are not really surprising. The administration of neuromuscular blockers to facilitate intubation is relatively routine. They relax the jaw, which allows the mouth to be opened for laryngoscopy and paralyzes the vocal cords so that an endotracheal tube can easily be passed into the trachea. Many different investigative groups have found that adequate intubating conditions, comparable with those associated with neuromuscular blockade, can be obtained through the administration of a combination of sedative hypnotics, opioids, and volatile anesthetics.[1-6] This, though, is not routine practice, and the required doses of agents to achieve comparable intubating conditions are, depending on an individual's practice, somewhat larger than those that would typically be used in the induction of anesthesia when a neuromuscular blocking agent was to be included.

While it is tempting to take the findings of this study (ie, that the avoidance of neuromuscular blocking agents is associated with difficult tracheal intubation) at face value, there are situations in clinical practice where neuromuscular blocking agents are not used as part of the induction regimen. One of these occurs when providing care for a patient with a known difficult airway. In this case, clinicians may not administer a neuromuscular blocking agent until the patient's airway has been secured. In this scenario an awake or sedated intubation with topical anesthesia and either direct laryngoscopy, fiberoptic bronchoscopy, or visualization of the vocal cords through the use of another airway device would likely be used to facilitate endotracheal intubation. General anesthesia would be induced after correct positioning of the endotracheal has been confirmed. This practice, induction after intubation, may have contributed to the findings, in that patients known to have difficult airways did not receive a neuromuscular blocking agent to facilitate endotracheal intubation.

What is interesting in this article is that while the use of neuromuscular blocking agents decreased over the 3 years of the study, the frequency of difficult intubations remained constant at just over 5%, suggesting the use of neuromuscular blocking agents and the incidence of difficult intubations are not related. These findings would confirm those of Bouvet et al[7]—that neither laryngeal injuries nor intubation conditions are associated with neuromuscular blocking agent administration.

C. A. Lien, MD

References

1. Klemola UM, Mennander S, Saarnivaara L. Tracheal intubation without the use of muscle relaxants: remifentanil or alfentanil in combination with propofol. *Acta Anaesthesiol Scand.* 2000;44:465-469.
2. Durmus M, Ender G, Kadir BA, Nurcin G, Erdogan O, Ersoy MO. Remifentanil with thiopental for tracheal intubation without muscle relaxants. *Anesth Analg.* 2003;96:1336-1339.
3. Grant S, Noble S, Woods A, Murdoch J, Davidson A. Assessment of intubating conditions in adults after induction with propofol and varying doses of remifentanil. *Br J Anaesth.* 1998;81:540-543.
4. Alexander R, Olufolabi AJ, Booth J, El-Moalem HE, Glass PS. Dosing study of remifentanil and propofol for tracheal intubation without the use of muscle relaxants. *Anaesthesia.* 1999;54:1037-1040.
5. Jabbour-Khoury SI, Dabbous AS, Rizk LB, et al. A combination of alfentanil-lidocaine-propofol provides better intubating conditions than fentanyl-lidocaine-propofol in the absence of muscle relaxants. *Can J Anaesth.* 2003;50:116-120.
6. Scheller MS, Zornow MH, Saidman LJ. Tracheal intubation without the use of muscle relaxants: a technique using propofol and varying doses of alfentanil. *Anesth Analg.* 1992;75:788-793.
7. Bouvet L, Stoian A, Jacquot-Laperrière S, Allaouchiche B, Chassard D, Boselli E. Laryngeal injuries and intubating conditions with or without muscular relaxation: an equivalence study. *Can J Anaesth.* 2008;55:674-684.

A comparison of Postoperative Throat and Neck Complaints After the Use of the i-gel® and the La Premiere® Disposable Laryngeal Mask: A Double-Blinded, Randomized, Controlled Trial

Keijzer C, Buitelaar DR, Efthymiou KM, et al (The Netherlands Cancer Inst–Antoni Van Leeuwenhoek Hosp, Amsterdam; et al)
Anesth Analg 109:1092-1094, 2009

Background.—Many supralaryngeal airway devices are available. Because of the absence of an inflatable cuff, we hypothesized that use of the i-gel® should produce fewer postoperative throat and neck complaints compared with a standard disposable laryngeal mask (LM).

Methods.—Two hundred eighteen patients were randomized to have either an i-gel or La Premiere® LM airway placed for airway management. Patients were interviewed postoperatively for throat and neck complaints at 1, 24, and 48 h. Interviewers and patients were blinded to the device used.

Results.—One hundred nine patients had an i-gel and 103 had a La Premiere supraglottic device inserted. The incidence of sore throat was significantly lower with the i-gel than with LM at 1 (6 vs 32), 24 (7 vs 48), and 48 h (5 vs 25). Similar results were seen for dysphagia. The incidence of neck pain was also lower for the i-gel at 24 (1 vs 7) and 48 h (1 vs 7).

Conclusion.—In this randomized study, the i-gel supraglottic device resulted in a lower incidence of throat and neck complaints than the La Premiere LM airway.

▶ Potential implications of this study are large. Laryngeal masks are commonly used to maintain an airway in any variety of surgical procedures. The I-gel is a relatively new potential alternative to the laryngeal mask. As demonstrated in this study, it is easier to place in that it takes less time to insert the I-gel than the La Premiere laryngeal mask, and its use results in fewer patient complaints up to 48 hours postoperatively.

Differences in ease of use, while not apparently different, may have existed. The authors do not report on the range or average number of insertion attempts to seat each device successfully. Additionally, while it is likely that there were no differences in patient head position for surgery or average duration of surgery in each patient group—head position is not explicitly described in the article. It may have been a factor in differences in postoperative patient discomfort.

The purpose of this study was to identify differences in patient comfort following an anesthetic with either the I-gel or the laryngeal mask for maintenance of the airway. Ultimately, though, it is important to know whether patient difference in discomfort resulted in functional differences in the 2 study groups. Did patients return to work more slowly, have difficulty eating, or require more analgesics after having a laryngeal mask airway rather than an I-gel used during their anesthetic? Were they less satisfied with their anesthetic because of postoperative discomfort? Did they require more analgesics after they were discharged to home because of airway discomfort? These factors are important as patient satisfaction plays a significant role in the anesthetic management chosen for each patient.

The authors did not do a cost comparison on the use of the I-gel versus the laryngeal mask. Cost analyses are complex in that they optimally involve the cost of all of the confounding factors and complications as well as the acquisition costs for any anesthetic technique. Should the I-gel be no more expensive to purchase than the laryngeal mask, the results presented in this study would indicate that the use of the I-gel would be preferred over that of the La Premiere disposable laryngeal mask. Given the lower complication rate associated with its use, though, clinicians may choose to use it even if it is more expensive to acquire.

C. A. Lien, MD

Obstructive Sleep Apnea Is Not a Risk Factor for Difficult Intubation in Morbidly Obese Patients

Neligan PJ, Porter S, Max B, et al (Hosp of Univ of Pennsylvania; Univ of Pennsylvania School of Medicine, Philadelphia)

Anesth Analg 109:1182-1186, 2009

Background.—Morbid obesity (MO), obstructive sleep apnea (OSA), and neck circumference (NC) are widely believed to be independent risk factors for difficult tracheal intubation. In this study, we sought to determine whether these factors were associated with increased risk of difficult intubation in patients undergoing bariatric surgery. The predictive factors tested were OSA and its severity, as determined by apnea-hypopnea index (AHI), gender, NC, and body mass index (BMI).

Methods.—All sequentially enrolled MO patients underwent preoperative polysomnography. Severity of OSA was quantified using AHI and the American Society of Anesthesiologists' OSA severity scale. All patients had a standardized anesthetic that included positioning in the "ramped position" for direct laryngoscopy.

Results.—One hundred eighty consecutive patients were recruited, 140 women and 40 men. The incidence of OSA was 68%. The mean BMI was 49.4 kg/m^2. The mean AHI was 31.3 (range, 0–135). All the patients' tracheas were intubated successfully without the aid of rescue airways by anesthesiology residents. Six patients required three or more intubation attempts, a difficult intubation rate of 3.3%. There was an 8.3% incidence of difficult laryngoscopy, defined as a Cormack and Lehane Grade 3 or 4 view. There was no relationship between NC and difficult intubation (odds ratio 1.02, 95% confidence interval 0.93–1.1), between the diagnosis of OSA and difficult intubation ($P = 0.09$), or between BMI and difficult intubation (odds ratio 0.99, 95% confidence interval 0.92–1.06, $P = 0.8$). There was no relationship between number of intubation attempts and BMI ($P = 0.8$), AHI ($P = 0.82$), or NC ($P = 0.3$). Mallampati Grade III or more predicted difficult intubation ($P = 0.02$), as did male gender ($P = 0.02$). Finally, there was no relationship between Cormack and Lehane grade and BMI ($P = 0.88$), AHI ($P = 0.93$), or OSA ($P = 0.6$). Increasing NC was associated with difficult laryngoscopy but not difficult intubation ($P = 0.02$).

Conclusions.—In MO patients undergoing bariatric surgery in the "ramped position," there was no relationship between the presence and severity of OSA, BMI, or NC and difficulty of intubation or laryngoscopy grade. Only a Mallampati score of 3 or 4 or male gender predicted difficult intubation.

▶ In this prospective trial the authors attempted to define the impact of factors associated with obstructive sleep apnea that have been shown in other trials to be associated with a difficult intubation on the ease of intubation and laryngoscopy. Patients were carefully positioned in a ramped up position. Interestingly, all of the patients in this study were intubated; the vast majority of them received their first laryngoscopy from junior residents, and only 6 of 180 patients required 3 to 4 laryngoscopies. Although not reported, it would have been useful for the authors to more completely outline the demographics of the patients who were difficult to intubate compared with the 174 patients intubated during their first laryngoscopy to compare these groups. Knowing whether or not there were any similarities in terms of predisposing identifiable patient characteristics contributing to a difficult intubation would have been very useful. That being said, the authors found that a history of obstructive sleep apnea did not predict a difficult intubation.

As noted by the authors, this study is more a comment on the import of careful positioning in facilitating a potentially difficult intubation. Intubations in settings other than the operating room can be difficult because of inadequate lighting, unfamiliar equipment, and inadequate patient positioning. Use of a ramped position has previously been described as rendering bariatric patients easier to intubate.[1,2] A more recent trial[3] described a variation of this using the operating room table to recreate a ramped up position. An advantage of the beach chair position[3] is that pillows do not have to be removed from beneath a patient to position the patient for surgery. In the anesthetized obese patient, movement of the patient for repositioning may be especially difficult. With the positioning described in these studies, adjustment of the table after intubation is all that is required for positioning before the beginning of surgery.

Anesthesiologists are, in large part, responsible for patient positioning in the operating room. Proper positioning is important, and when not done correctly it may lead to neuropathies and difficulty in line placement. As suggested by this study, careful attention to detail in positioning for endotracheal intubation is also important. It may result in the frequency of difficult intubations, even in a patient population historically noted to be difficult, falling to less than 4%.

C. A. Lien, MD

References

1. Collins JS, Lemmens HJ, Brodsky JB, Brock-Utne JG, Levitan RM. Laryngoscopy and morbid obesity: a comparison of the "sniff" and "ramped" positions. *Obes Surg.* 2004;14:1171-1175.
2. Greenland KB, Eley V, Edwards MJ, Allen P, Irwin MG. The origins of the sniffing position and the three axes alignment theory for direct laryngoscopy. *Anaesth Intensive Care.* 2008;36:23-27.
3. Fox WTA, Harris S, Kennedy NJ. Prevalence of difficult intubation in a bariatric population, using the beach chair position. *Anaesthesia.* 2008;63:1339-1342.

Infusion requirements and reversibility of rocuronium at the corrugator supercilii and adductor pollicis muscles

Suzuki T, Mizutani H, Miyake E, et al (Surugadai Nihon Univ Hosp, Chiyoda-Ku, Tokyo, Japan)

Acta Anaesthesiol Scand 53:1336-1340, 2009

Background.—The aim of this study is to compare the infusion rates required to maintain a constant neuromuscular block and the reversibility of rocuronium at the corrugator supercilii muscle (CSM) and the adductor pollicis muscle (APM).

Methods.—We randomly allocated 30 female patients into two groups of 15 patients each to monitor neuromuscular block at either the CSM or the APM. After induction of anaesthesia and laryngeal mask insertion, contraction of the CSM to the facial nerve stimulation or that of the APM to the ulnar nerve stimulation was quantified using an acceleromyograph during 1.0–1.5% end-tidal sevoflurane anaesthesia. All the patients received a bolus of 1 mg/kg rocuronium. When the first twitch (T1) of train-of-four (TOF) recovered to 10% of the control, rocuronium infusion was commenced and maintained at T1 of 10% of the control at the CSM or APM for 120 min. Immediately after rocuronium infusion was discontinued, the time required for 0.04 mg/kg neostigmine- facilitated recovery to a TOF ratio of 0.9 was recorded.

Results.—Rocuronium infusion dose after a lapse of 120 min was significantly larger in the CSM than in the APM [7.1 (2.3) vs. 4.7 (2.6) μg/kg/min; $P = 0.001$]. The time for facilitated recovery was shorter in the CSM than in the APM [11.4 (3.8) vs. 16.2 (6.0) min; $P = 0.016$].

Conclusion.—A larger rocuronium infusion dose was required to maintain a constant neuromuscular block at the CSM. Neostigmine-mediated reversal was faster at the CSM.

► This study confirms that centrally located neuromuscular units, such as those on the face and those involved with respiration, have a faster onset of block and are relatively resistant to nondepolarizing neuromuscular blockade than those located more peripherally, such as the adductor pollicis. As is observed during spontaneous recovery of neuromuscular function following nondepolarizing neuromuscular blockade, neostigmine-facilitated recovery occurs more quickly in the centrally located neuromuscular units than in the more peripheral ones.

Although the authors did not find any cumulation of rocuronium when monitoring the depth of block at the corrugator supercilii, with no decrease in infusion rate required to maintain a stable depth of block, they did decrease the rocuronium infusion rate, when dosed based on monitoring at the adductor pollicis. The decrease in the infusion rate was, on average, 0.6 μg/kg/min over the course of a 2-hour infusion. Whether or not this change in the infusion rate was statistically significant was not determined. Based on modeling work comparing recovery from benzylisoquinolinium neuromuscular blocking agents from steroidal neuromuscular blocking agents,[1] a significant decrease in the infusion requirement to maintain a stable depth of neuromuscular block at the adductor pollicis would not have been surprising.

Quantitative monitoring of depth of block at the corrugated supercilii, such as described in this article, is not commonly practiced. Because clinicians frequently have access only to the face for monitoring, perhaps it should be. Even techniques for quantitative monitoring at the adductor pollicis, which are more widely available, are not commonly employed.[2] If monitoring at the corrugator supercilii were to be used more commonly, the depth of block that would have to be maintained to allow rapid and complete anticholinesterase-facilitated recovery at the adductor pollicis would have to be defined because strength in the adductor pollicis recovers more slowly than that in the corrugator supercilii. As noted by Dr Suzuki, a train-of-four ratio of 0.9 at the corrugator supercilii was associated with a significantly deeper level of block at the adductor pollicis.

Clinical monitoring of muscle strength with a qualitative monitor (one that does not interpret response to train-of-four stimulation) is more widely available than quantitative monitoring. Incorporation of qualitative monitoring of twitch response at the face is fraught with many potential shortcomings. Some of these include direct muscle stimulation, relative overdosing of neuromuscular blocking agents, and inability to quantify fade in response to train-of-four stimulation. Use of quantitative monitoring—as long as the depth of block can be correlated with that at the adductor pollicis—may eliminate some of these issues.

C. A. Lien, MD

References

1. Wright PM, Hart P, Lau M, Sharma ML, Gruenke L, Fisher DM. Cumulative characteristics of atracurium and vecuronium. a simultaneous clinical and pharmacokinetic study. *Anesthesiology.* 1994;81:59-68.
2. Naguib M, Kopman AF, Lien CA, Hunter JM, Lopez A, Brull SJ. A survey of current management of neuromuscular block in the United States and Europe [published online ahead of print Nov 12 2009]. *Anesth Analg.* 2009.

A Randomized, Clinical Trial of Frozen Versus Standard Nasogastric Tube Placement

Chun D-H, Kim NY, Shin Y-S, et al (CHA Univ, Sungnam, Korea; Yonsei Univ College of Medicine, Seoul, Korea)
World J Surg 33:1789-1792, 2009

Background.—Insertion of a nasogastric tube (NGT) in an anesthetized, paralyzed, and intubated patient is difficult, and many methods have been proposed to aid in the procedure. We present a simple insertion technique.

Methods.—A silicone NGT was made rigid by filling it with distilled water and freezing it. Patients were randomized into either the control or the frozen group, and an NGT was inserted after intubation.

Results.—A total of 100 patients (50 in each group) were included in this study. The success rate increased significantly by making the tube more rigid (control:frozen = 58%:88%; $p = 0.001$). There was no difference between groups in the incidence of nasal bleeding.

Conclusions.—A simple method of freezing an NGT with distilled water increased the success rate of insertion for intubated patients.

▶ The placement of nasogastric tubes (NGTs) is associated with a number of complications, including ulceration of the nose, epistaxis, sinusitis, fistula formation, vomiting and aspiration, bronchial placement and resultant pneumonia, bronchial perforation and pneumothorax or pulmonary hemorrhage, intravascular penetration, enteric perforation, NGT breakage or obstruction and rupture,[1] and knotting over the epiglottis.[2] The incidence of complications following NGT placement ranges from 0.3% to 8%.[1] This being said, the perioperative placement of NGTs is a fairly common practice. The indications, absolute and relative, for the procedure are numerous. They range from providing a means of administering medications or enteral feeding to aspiration of stomach contents—whether secretions, poisons, or air.

An incidence of 17% failure in placement of NGTs has been reported in awake patients using a swallowing technique.[3] In having placed many NGTs and observed the placement of many more in anesthetized patients, the incidence of failure seems to be considerably less. It may be easier to place a NGT in an anesthetized patient because these patients do not respond with coughing or gagging to attempted placement. Furthermore, passage of a NGT can be facilitated with any of several different maneuvers, including a jaw lift, tongue thrust, closing off the peritonsillar space and piriform fossa, or laryngoscopy.

This article describes another technique to facilitate passing a NGT that is otherwise difficult or impossible to insert. Although interesting, flushing NGTs with saline and freezing them to provide an alternative for a rare event does not seem practical. Both time and space would be required to prepare and store the NGTs. Even if this solution is manageable as an option for the difficulty to place NGT, the complications associated with use of frozen NGTs have to be defined. This study focused on the success, rather than the complications, associated with their use.

C. A. Lien, MD

References

1. Pillai JB, Vegas A, Brister S. Thoracic complications of nasogastric tube: review of safe practice. *Interact Cardiovasc Thorac Surg*. 2005;4:429-433.
2. Agarwal A, Gaur A, Sahu D, Singh PK, Pandey CK. Nasogastric knotting over the epiglottis: a cause of respiratory distress. *Anesth Analg*. 2002;94:1659-1660.
3. Inoue K, Horohisa T, Yamada T, Yoshikawa T. Nasogastric tubes in patients with dysphagia. *The Lancet*. 2002;359:81.

Local Anesthetic Hernia Repair in Overweight and Obese Patients

Reid TD, Sanjay P, Woodward A (Princess of Wales Hosp, Bridgend, UK; Ninewells Hosp, Dundee, UK; Royal Glamorgan Hosp, Llantrisant, UK)

World J Surg 33:138-141, 2009

Background.—Inguinal hernia repair under local anesthesia (LA) has many advantages and is associated with high patient satisfaction. However, there are concerns of exceeding the maximum safe dose of LA agents in overweight and obese patients. The aim of the present study was to establish whether inguinal hernia repair could be safely performed under LA in overweight and obese patients.

Methods.—Patients who underwent elective LA hernia repair under a single consultant surgeon were studied retrospectively. Each patient received the same LA mixture developed at our hospital specifically for hernia repair. The mixture includes lignocaine and bupivocaine, both with adrenaline, made up to a volume of 100 ml with saline. Data were collected by case note review, and by postal and telephone surveys.

Results.—A total of 125 patients who underwent LA hernia repair, in whom body mass index (BMI) was measured, were studied. Based on the World Health Organization (WHO) classification, there were 35 (28%) normal weight patients and 63 (72%) overweight (BMI $\geq 25 < 30$) or obese (BMI ≥ 30) patients. The median BMI was 27 (range 19–38). The mean volumes of LA mixture used for each group were 58 ml and 62 ml, respectively. High day case rates of 91% and 84% were obtained for the two groups, respectively. Complications included three wound hematomas and three simple wound infections, with no significant differences between groups. One patient developed a recurrent hernia (<1%).

Conclusion.—Local anesthetic inguinal hernia repair in the obese is safe and well tolerated. Use of a large volume local anesthetic mixture is recommended in overweight and obese patients.

▶ This study is potentially very interesting for 2 reasons. Increasingly, surgery is being done on an ambulatory basis and the population is becoming increasingly obese. Bariatric patients provide multiple challenges for the anesthesiologist because of changes in airway anatomy, the presence of comorbidities, difficulties in placing a regional anesthetic, or invasive monitors because of body habitus and altered medication pharmacology. This study, which addressed none of these issues, was a descriptive report of the result of a survey of obese and overweight patients, as well as those with a normal body habitus. All patients had undergone hernia repair with local anesthesia. They were queried regarding their satisfaction with the procedure. Patient records were also reviewed for complications such as infection and hematoma formation. The authors' conclusions were that 125 patients had undergone hernia repair by a single surgeon, and the complication rate was the same in the obese and overweight patients and nonobese patients. No patient developed urinary retention in either study group; 1 or 2 in each group developed a wound hematoma and 1 or 2 in each group developed a wound infection or required admission to the hospital. Most interesting when considering these results is that all patients, regardless of weight, received similar doses of local anesthetic.

In reporting and comparing results, the authors put both overweight and obese patients in the same group. As a result, there may have been differences in the results of the overweight group (25 < body mass index [BMI] < 30) and in the obese group (BMI ≥ 30) that were lost in considering the patients the same. Certainly, complications and risks of anesthesia vary for the 2 groups—with risk increasing with increasing weight. Additionally, many details are lacking in this report. What postoperative analgesics were administered is not reported. No details of the anesthetic management are provided. This information could have provided some understanding regarding the source of patient satisfaction or not. Also missing is information regarding surgeon satisfaction, times to discharge following surgery, and details regarding administration of the local anesthetic. Had this information been provided, readers would have had a better understanding of the implications of providing local anesthesia for hernia repair in obese patients.

C. A. Lien, MD

4 Cardiothoracic and Vascular Anesthesia

Variation in perioperative vasoactive therapy in cardiovascular surgical care: Data from the Society of Thoracic Surgeons

Hernandez AF, Li S, Dokholyan RS, et al (Duke Univ School of Medicine, Durham, NC; et al)

Am Heart J 158:47-52, 2009

Background.—The appropriate use of vasoactive cardiovascular drugs in high-risk coronary artery bypass grafting (CABG) patients has not been well characterized.

Methods.—We performed a detailed chart analysis on 2,390 randomly selected patients undergoing CABG between January 2004 and June 2005 at 55 hospitals participating in the Society of Thoracic Surgeons' National Adult Cardiac Surgery Database. Patients were eligible if they had elective/urgent CABG with an ejection fraction (EF) <40%, or if they had an elective or urgent CABG at ≥65 years with diabetes, or a glomerular filtration rate <60 mL/min per 1.73 m^2. Logistic regression modeling was used to determine predictors of and provide risk-adjusted frequencies of postoperative vasoactive therapies.

Results.—Vasoactive therapy was used in 90% of patients. Inotropes/vasopressors were used in 28% (668), vasodilators in 18% (430), and the combination in 43% (1,037). Predictors of any inotrope use were preoperative atrial fibrillation (odds ratio [OR] 1.48), other arrhythmia (OR 2.09), EF (OR 1.09 per 5-unit decrease), severe mitral regurgitation (OR 2.56), 3-vessel coronary artery disease (OR 1.35), New York Heart Association class IV (1.38), on-pump (OR 1.86), other procedure (OR 2.51), and peripheral vascular disease (OR 1.28) (all OR $P < .05$). Hospital-level risk-adjusted rates of any inotrope use varied significantly from 100% to 35% ($P < .01$) and vasodilator rates varied from 100% to 10% ($P < .01$).

Conclusions.—There is marked hospital variation in the use of vasoactive therapies in high-risk CABG patients in clinical practice, indicating an important area for further research to better clarify best practice.

▶ This study involving 48 cardiac surgical centers in essence measures the popularity of the various vasoactive drugs used during coronary artery bypass grafting (CABG) in patients who have low left ventricular ejection fractions.

Unsurprisingly, the presence of substantial variation in vasoactive drug use across institutions despite a fairly homogeneous patient population indicates that physician biases contribute importantly to decisions about vasoactive drug use. Fig 1, as seen in the original article, the relative frequency of use of these drugs, except that the bar representing nitroprusside is too high by a factor of 10. The apparent inclusion of the preoperative and precardiopulmonary bypass (CPB) periods also clouds interpretation because nitroglycerin and phenylephrine are probably used most frequently at those times. The presence of severe mitral regurgitation and simultaneous performance of a cardiac operation in addition to CABG were the 2 strongest predictors of vasoactive drug use. As the authors suggest, prospective comparisons of different vasoactive drug choices are needed, but this is unlikely to transpire in the absence of a new competing drug for which a pharmaceutical company seeks FDA approval. In the absence of such prospective comparisons, evidence-based improvement in clinical decision-making about the use of these drugs will partly depend on recording more information about the decisions being made, eg, blood pressure, cardiac output, and left ventricular contractility. Such analyses would be further aided by stratification of vasoactive drug selection decisions into preCPB, postCPB, and postoperative epochs.

G. P. Gravlee, MD

Estimated Radiation Dose Associated With Cardiac CT Angiography

Hausleiter J, Meyer T, Hermann F, et al (Klinik an der Technischen Universität München, Germany; et al)

JAMA 301:500-507, 2009

Context.—Cardiac computed tomography (CT) angiography (CCTA) has emerged as a useful diagnostic imaging modality in the assessment of coronary artery disease. However, the potential risks due to exposure to ionizing radiation associated with CCTA have raised concerns.

Objectives.—To estimate the radiation dose of CCTA in routine clinical practice as well as the association of currently available strategies with dose reduction and to identify the independent factors contributing to radiation dose.

Design, Setting, and Patients.—A cross-sectional, international, multicenter, observational study (50 study sites: 21 university hospitals and 29 community hospitals) of estimated radiation dose in 1965 patients undergoing CCTA between February and December 2007. Linear regression analysis was used to identify independent predictors associated with dose.

Main Outcome Measure.—Dose-length product (DLP) of CCTA.

Results.—The median DLP of 1965 CCTA examinations performed at 50 study sites was 885 mGy × cm (interquartile range, 568-1259 mGy × cm), which corresponds to an estimated radiation dose of 12 mSv (or 1.2 × the dose of an abdominal CT study or 600 chest x-rays). A high variability in DLP was observed between study sites (range of median DLPs per site,

331-2146 mGy × cm). Independent factors associated with radiation dose were patient weight (relative effect on DLP, 5%; 95% confidence interval [CI], 4%-6%), absence of stable sinus rhythm (10%; 95% CI, 2%-19%), scan length (5%; 95% CI, 4%-6%), electrocardiographically controlled tube current modulation (−25%; 95% CI, −23% to −28%; applied in 73% of patients), 100-kV tube voltage (−46%; 95% CI, −42% to −51%; applied in 5% of patients), sequential scanning (−78%; 95% CI, −77% to −79%; applied in 6% of patients), experience in cardiac CT (−1%; 95% CI, −1% to 0%), number of CCTAs per month (0%; 95% CI, 0%-1%), and type of 64-slice CT system (for highest vs lowest dose system, 97%; 95% CI, 88%-106%). Algorithms for dose reduction were not associated with deteriorated diagnostic image quality in this observational study.

Conclusions.—Median doses of CCTA differ significantly between study sites and CT systems. Effective strategies to reduce radiation dose are available but some strategies are not frequently used. The comparable diagnostic image quality may support an increased use of dose-saving strategies in adequately selected patients.

▶ Interestingly, when one flies in the air one gets about 1/30th of a dose of a chest X-ray. So if you fly 100 hours a year, you are getting 3 chest X-rays, not an inconsequential amount of radiation for your risk of cancer. But here is the amazing thing: the average dose of cardiac CT is 600 chest X-rays, and even in the ones that had the most careful shielding and used the most techniques including β- blockers to minimize exposure time, it is over 350 chest X-ray equivalents. Don't get a cardiac CT if you are not serious about the reason for getting it.

M. F. Roizen, MD

Ionizing Radiation in Cardiac Imaging: A Science Advisory From the American Heart Association Committee on Cardiac Imaging of the Council on Clinical Cardiology and Committee on Cardiovascular Imaging and Intervention of the Council on Cardiovascular Radiology and Intervention

Gerber TC, Carr JJ, Arai AE, et al

Circulation 119:1056-1065, 2009

Background.—The medical uses of radiation have increased, producing a more than 700% increase in the collective dose received since 1980. Computed tomography (CT) studies accounted for about 50% of the collective dose in 2006, with 1.5% from cardiac CT. Nuclear medicine studies accounted for about 25% of the 2006 collective dose, with about 85% coming from cardiac imaging. Risks to the patient from these exposures to ionizing radiation must be weighed against the risks of missing important diagnoses or treatment decisions by not performing these tests. A Science Advisory from the American Heart Association Committee on Cardiac Imaging offered recommendations to guide the use of ionizing radiation for patients.

Definitions.—Exposure refers to the amount of ionization produced in air by photon irradiation and is readily measured for CT and fluoroscopy. *Absorbed radiation dose* is the energy absorbed per unit of mass by some part of the patient's body after exposure to ionizing radiation. The absorbing material and the energy of the photons contribute. Absorbed dose is not readily quantified for internal organs. *Effective dose* (E) reflects the risk of biological effects from ionizing radiation. E is widely used in studies of medical imaging but is designed only for use in a radiation protection context. It is not measured directly but rather estimated based on *organ dose*, or the dose received by an individual organ; *radiation weighting factor*, which represents the relative biological effectiveness of ionizing radiation, a value that differs with type and energy of radiation; and *tissue-specific weighting factors*, which express the radiation sensitivity of each organ or tissue. Weighting factor changes between 1991 and 2007 have raised E estimates for coronary CT angiograms by 30% to 50%. The *activity* of radionuclides reflects the number of nuclear disintegrations per second. An older dosimetry concept, *whole-body dose*, is often used in package inserts prepared before the concept of E was widely used. This represents the total energy absorbed by the body divided by the mass of the standard reference human body; values are typically 50% or less of the E value.

Key Findings.—Radiation dose to internal organs cannot be measured directly but are estimated using generic modeling techniques. These broadly indicate risk and are not patient specific. E values differ because of recent changes in calculation methods and cannot be easily compared to previous reported values. The potential for and degree of carcinogenesis linked to radiation from medical imaging are not yet determined. The recommended course is to assume a conservative linear no-threshold relationship exists between radiation dose and risk of malignancies, although this relationship is neither scientifically confirmed nor observed.

Recommendations.—Physicians should be educated to order cardiac imaging studies that expose patients to ionizing radiation only after carefully considering the potential benefit to the patient and the degree of compliance with established criteria for appropriate use. The risk of missing important diagnoses if the tests are not performed is an important factor in this decision. To ensure that they do not subject patients to repeated exposure to ionizing radiation, healthcare providers should diligently evaluate each patient's records, including those from other medical institutions, to see what tests have been performed. Physicians and patients should discuss the risks and benefits of planned imaging procedures whenever it is practical and appropriate. Asymptomatic patients at low risk for ischemic heart disease do not need routine surveillance radionuclide stress tests or cardiac CTs. Should a cardiac imaging study be deemed necessary, practitioners should make every effort to minimize the dose of ionizing radiation while balancing image noise and quality sufficient to permit accurate interpretation of the study. No system currently tracks an individual's cumulative lifetime dose. Imaging experts and manufacturers need to continue efforts to improve the ability to produce consistent radiation output metrics for all diagnostic modalities and record the information automatically as part of the imaging experience. Diagnostic reference levels for radiation doses from cardiac radiographic imaging procedures must be determined to establish benchmark radiation doses that can be compared nationally.

▶ This seems to be an awful self-serving guideline from the Imaging and Intervention Council where they compare the risk of imaging with the risk from other things. So the lifetime risk from a cancer of the breast is in fact 12.45% that goes up to something on the order of 13.15% after 1 CT angiogram. This is more than the risk of taking estrogens or progestins; it is dismissed by this group. Let's just be clear from other studies we have reviewed, one CT cardiac angiogram is the equivalent of 600 chest X-rays, and substantially increases cancer risk—10 over a lifetime doubles your risk of breast cancer.

M. F. Roizen, MD

Impact of Smoking Cessation Before Resection of Lung Cancer: A Society of Thoracic Surgeons General Thoracic Surgery Database Study

Mason DP, Subramanian S, Nowicki ER, et al (Cleveland Clinic, OH; Duke Univ, Durham, NC)

Ann Thorac Surg 88:362-371, 2009

Background.—Smoking cessation is presumed to be beneficial before resection of lung cancer. The effect of smoking cessation on outcome was investigated.

Methods.—From January 1999 to July 2007, in-hospital outcomes for 7990 primary resections for lung cancer in adults were reported to the Society of Thoracic Surgeons General Thoracic Surgery Database. Risk of hospital death and respiratory complications was assessed according to timing of smoking cessation, adjusted for clinical confounders.

Results.—Hospital mortality was 1.4% (n = 109), but 1.5% in patients who had smoked (105 of 6965) vs 0.39% in those who had not (4 of 1025). Compared with the latter, risk-adjusted odds ratios were 3.5 ($p = 0.03$), 4.6 ($p = 0.03$), 2.6 ($p = 0.7$), and 2.5 ($p = 0.11$) for those whose timing of smoking cessation was categorized as current smoker, quit from 14 days to 1 month, 1 to 12 months, or more than 12 months preoperatively, respectively. Prevalence of major pulmonary complications was 5.7% (456 of 7965) overall, but 6.2% in patients who had smoked (429 of 6941) vs 2.5%% in those who had not (27 of 1024). Compared with the latter, risk-adjusted odds ratios were 1.80 ($p = 0.03$), 1.62

($p = 0.14$), 1.51 ($p = 0.20$), and 1.29 ($p = 0.3$) for those whose timing of smoking cessation was categorized as above.

Conclusions.—Risks of hospital death and pulmonary complications after lung cancer resection were increased by smoking and mitigated slowly by preoperative cessation. No optimal interval of smoking cessation was identifiable. Patients should be counseled to stop smoking irrespective of surgical timing.

▶ The Society of Thoracic Surgeons database continues to yield interesting, clinically useful information. In this instance, the impact of smoking and smoking cessation on resections for lung cancer was retrospectively assessed. The authors chose to interpret their findings conservatively, although the data suggest an inflection point for improved mortality at a preoperative smoking cessation duration of 1 month or longer. The findings also suggest the possibility that smoking cessation for 14 days to 1 month might be worse than continued smoking. Because the accuracy of patient reporting of smoking cessation intervals is dubious, I agree with the authors that these findings should be interpreted with caution. Nevertheless, if one can use the need for surgery as a springboard for smoking cessation, patients will benefit. Anesthesiologists are encouraged to participate actively in smoking cessation counseling and in referrals to smoking cessation programs.

G. P. Gravlee, MD

A comparison of volatile and non volatile agents for cardioprotection during on-pump coronary surgery

De Hert S, Vlasselaers D, Barbé R, et al (Univ of Amsterdam, Netherlands; VACMAN (Volatile Anaesthetics and Cardioprotection Multicentre ANalysis) study group; et al)

Anaesthesia 64:953-960, 2009

A randomised study of 414 patients undergoing coronary artery surgery with cardiopulmonary bypass was conducted to compare the effects of a volatile anaesthetic regimen with either deesflurane or sevoflurane, and a total intravenous anaesthesia (TIVA) regimen on postoperative troponin T release. The primary outcome variable was postoperative troponin T release, secondary outcome variables were hospital length of stay and 1-year mortality. Maximal postoperative troponin T values did not differ between groups (TIVA: 0.30 [0.00–4.79] $ng.ml^{-1}$ (median [range]), sevoflurane: 0.33 [0.02–3.68] $ng.ml^{-1}$, and desflurane: 0.39 [0.08–3.74] $ng.ml^{-1}$). The independent predictors of hospital length of stay were the EuroSCORE ($p < 0.001$), female gender ($p = 0.042$) and the group assignment ($p < 0.001$). The one-year mortality was 12.3% in the TIVA group, 3.3% in the sevoflurane group, and 6.7% in the desflurane

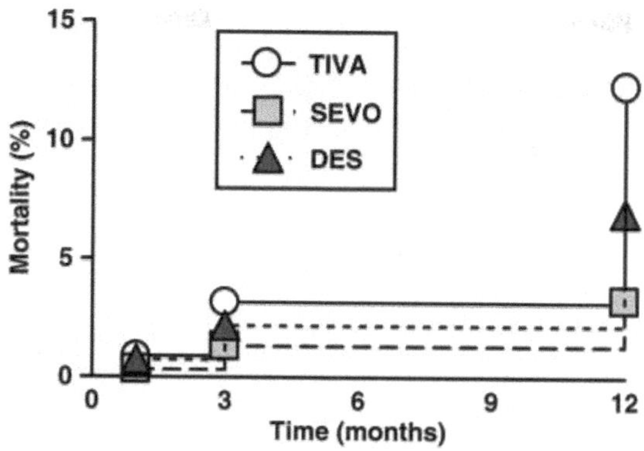

FIGURE 2.—Mortality curves of the patients in the three different study groups. (Reprinted from De Hert S, Vlasselaers D, Barbé R, et al. A comparison of volatile and non volatile agents for cardioprotection during on-pump coronary surgery. *Anaesthesia*. 2009;64:953-960, with permission from John Wiley & Sons.)

group. The EuroSCORE ($p = 0.003$) was the only significant independent predictor of 1-year mortality (Fig 2).

▶ The authors admit that this study is a bit "dirty" design-wise, because neither the anesthetic nor surgical techniques were standardized outside of one component. The single standardized component was the use of a 0.5 MAC or higher concentration of sevoflurane or desflurane from 30 minutes before application of the aortic cross-clamp to 10 minutes after its release. This seemed to be enough to reduce the length of hospital stay and probably to reduce 1-year mortality, even though there was no difference in troponin T release between groups. Troponin T is a highly sensitive marker for myocardial injury, but not for injury to other organs or for the generalized inflammatory response to surgery or cardiopulmonary bypass, hence the differences observed may be attributable to noncardiac factors. When variables were analyzed individually, the use of a volatile agent reduced 1-year mortality (Relative risk 0.95, 95% CI 0.90-0.99, $P = .018$), as suggested by Fig 2. When a stepwise multivariate model was applied, however, only EuroSCORE emerged as an independent predictor of 1-year mortality. Evidence continues to emerge that volatile anesthetic agents in clinically relevant doses provide protection to the heart and to other organs, for example, brain, kidney, and liver. This evidence has become sufficiently compelling that I believe anesthesiologists should preferentially use 0.5 MAC or higher dosing of a volatile agent (isoflurane, sevoflurane, or desflurane) for anesthesia in procedures where there is a relatively high risk of mortality or postoperative clinically important organ dysfunction. Obvious exceptions exist, such as a patient in shock whose blood pressure is too low to tolerate a volatile agent.

G. P. Gravlee, MD

Incidence and Patterns of Adverse Event Onset During the First 60 Days After Ventricular Assist Device Implantation

Genovese EA, Dew MA, Teuteberg JJ, et al (Univ of Pittsburgh Med Ctr, PA; Univ of Pittsburgh School of Medicine, PA; Univ of Pittsburgh, PA)

Ann Thorac Surg 88:1162-1170, 2009

Background.—Although ventricular assist devices (VADs) provide effective treatment for end-stage heart failure, VAD support remains associated with significant risk for adverse events (AEs). To date there has been no detailed assessment of the incidence of a full range of AEs using standardized event definitions. We sought to characterize the frequency and timing of AE onset during the first 60 days of VAD support, a period during which clinical observation suggests the risk of incident AEs is high.

Methods.—A retrospective analysis was performed utilizing prospectively collected data from a single-site clinical database including 195 patients aged 18 or greater receiving VADs between 1996 and 2006. Adverse events were coded using standardized criteria. Cumulative incidence rates were determined, controlling for competing risks (death, transplantation, recovery-wean).

Results.—During the first 60 days after implantation, the most common AEs were bleeding, infection, and arrhythmias (cumulative incidence rates, 36% to 48%), followed by tamponade, respiratory events, reoperations, and neurologic events (24% to 31%). Other events (eg, hemolysis, renal, hepatic events) were less common (rates <15%). Some events (eg, bleeding, arrhythmias) showed steep onset rates early after implantation. Others (eg, infections, neurologic events) had gradual onsets during the 60-day period. Incidence of most events did not vary by implant era (1996 to 2000 vs 2001 to 2006) or by left ventricular versus biventricular support.

Conclusions.—Understanding differential temporal patterns of AE onset will allow preventive strategies to be targeted to the time periods when specific AE risks are greatest. The AE incidence rates provide benchmarks against which future studies of VAD-related risks may be compared.

▶ This single-center report includes primarily left ventricular assist device (LVAD) patients in whom this device was being used as a "bridge" to cardiac transplantation. This is a very high-risk group in which one would expect high morbidity and mortality even without placement of an LVAD or biventricular assist device. The center reporting these outcomes has a very strong reputation for excellence in circulatory assist devices. Nevertheless, the morbidities reported are staggering, and this probably explains reluctance on the part of many patients to submit themselves to this intervention or of cardiologists to suggest it. As the authors point out, previous work supports the concept that things tend to go better when LVADs are implanted earlier in the progression of advanced left ventricular failure, but with these kinds of numbers one might suggest that this is analogous to Sophie's choice. The good news is that these data do not reflect the ever-increasing use of smaller, nonpulsatile pumps, which are easier to place, induce less blood trauma, and require less anticoagulation.

G. P. Gravlee, MD

Blood transfusion for acute decompensated heart failure—friend or foe?

Garty M, Cohen E, Zuchenko A, et al (Rabin Med Ctr, Petah Tiqwa, Israel; et al)
Am Heart J 158:653-658, 2009

Background.—In acute coronary syndromes (ACSs), blood transfusion (BT) has been associated with worse outcomes. The impact of BT among patients with acute decompensated heart failure (ADHF) remains unknown.

Methods.—Propensity score analysis of patients with ADHF with and without BT in a national heart failure (HF) survey was used in this study.

Results.—Of the 4,102 enrolled patients, 2,335 had ADHF, of whom 166 (7.1%) received BT. These patients were older (75.6% vs 73.6%, $P = .04$), more likely to be females (54.8% vs 43.9%, $P = .007$), more likely to have diabetes (59.0% vs 51.1%, $P = .04$) and renal dysfunction (59.0% vs 40.2%, $P < .001$), and more likely to receive inotropes (16.9% vs 8.0%, $P < .001$), but they had similar rates of ACS (41.0% vs 39.4%, $P = .69$) and prior HF (64.5% vs 70.0%, $P = .23$). Nadir hemoglobin levels were commonly <10 g/dL in BT patients (92.7% vs 8.0%); 15 BT patients had bleeding complications, of which 10 are major bleeding. Major predictors for BT were ACS (OR 1.85, 95% CI 1.15-2.96), inotropes use (OR 2.36, 95% CI 1.22-4.55), and nadir hemoglobin (OR 0.18 per 1 g/dL increase, 95% CI 0.14-0.22). In-hospital, 30-day, 1-year, and 4-year unadjusted mortality rates were higher for BT patients (10.8% vs 5.2%, $P = .02$; 11.0% vs 8.5%, $P = .27$; 39.6% vs 28.5%, $P = .03$; 69.5% vs 59.5%, $P = .01$, respectively). However, in 103 propensity-matched pairs (c-statistic 0.97), short-term mortality tended to be lower with BT (8.7% vs 14.6%, $P = .20$; 9.7% vs 18.4%, $P = .08$; 38.8% vs 42.7%, $P = .59$; and 72.8% vs 76.7%, $P = .52$, respectively).

Conclusions.—Acute decompensated HF patients receiving BT had worse clinical features and unadjusted outcomes, but BT per se seemed to be safe and perhaps even beneficial.

► Our heads are spinning with accumulating studies about the pros and cons of anemia versus blood transfusion. Several retrospective studies correlate anemia with worse outcomes in decompensated heart failure at the time of acute myocardial infarction. Many prospective and retrospective studies associate transfusion with adverse outcomes, such as an increased incidence of infections or cancer recurrences. Investigating patients with decompensated congestive heart failure, this study retrospectively compares outcomes in transfused and untransfused patients. When comparing case-matched transfused patients to untransfused ones, outcomes were not different (Fig 1 in the original article). Of course, case-matching techniques are fraught with difficulties, eg, potentially important variables may be unintentionally excluded from the matching process. Nevertheless, it is encouraging to see the pendulum swing slightly back toward a concept that critically ill patients who are anemic may benefit from blood transfusion.

G. P. Gravlee, MD

Early On-Cardiopulmonary Bypass Hypotension and Other Factors Associated With Vasoplegic Syndrome

Levin MA, Lin H-M, Castillo JG, et al (Mount Sinai School of Medicine, NY)
Circulation 120:1664-1671, 2009

Background.—Vasoplegic syndrome is a form of vasodilatory shock that can occur after cardiopulmonary bypass (CPB). We hypothesized that the severity and duration of the decline in mean arterial pressure immediately after CPB is begun can be used as a predictor of patients will develop vasoplegia in the immediate post-CPB period and of poor clinical outcome. We quantified the decline in mean arterial pressure by calculating an area above the mean arterial blood pressure curve.

Methods and Results.—We retrospectively analyzed 2823 adult cardiac surgery cases performed between July 2002 and December 2006. Of these 2823, 577 (20.4%) were vasoplegic after separation from CPB. We found that 1645 patients (58.3%) had a clinically significant decline in mean arterial pressure after starting CPB (area above the mean arterial blood pressure curve >0) and were significantly more likely to become vasoplegic (23.0% versus 16.9%; odds ratio, 1.26; 95% confidence interval, 1.12 to 1.43; $P < 0.001$). These patients were also far more likely either to die in hospital or to have a length of stay >10 days (odds ratio, 3.30; 95% confidence interval, 1.44 to 7.57; $P = 0.005$). Additional risk factors for developing vasoplegia that were identified included the additive euroSCORE, procedure type, prebypass mean arterial pressure, length of bypass, administration of pre-CPB vasopressors, core temperature on CPB, pre-and post-CPB hematocrit, the preoperative use of β-blockers or angiotensin-converting enzyme inhibitors, and the intraoperative use of aprotinin.

Conclusions.—The results of this investigation suggest that it is possible to predict vasoplegia intraoperatively before separation from CPB and that the presence of a clinically significant area above the mean arterial blood pressure curve serves as a predictor of poor clinical outcome.

▶ This interesting retrospective analysis associates hypotension at the onset of cardiopulmonary bypass (CPB) with vasoplegia after CPB. Vasoplegia after CPB was defined as a requirement for high doses of vasopressors (including norepinephrine, epinephrine, dopamine, and/or vasopressin) on separation from CPB. This definition suffers somewhat from the absence of data on systemic vascular resistance because clinicians may initiate high doses of epinephrine or dopamine because of a low cardiac output states without necessarily invoking the presence of a vasoplegic state. Similarly, the presence of a low mean arterial pressure at the onset of CPB does not insure a diagnosis of vasoplegia because there may be mechanical problems, such as hypovolemia, restricted venous return, or arterial outflow. Despite these limitations, it seems reasonable to conclude that sustained low mean arterial pressures in the presence of adequate CPB total perfusion flows serves as a predictor of profound vasodilation on separation from CPB. Given that situation, clinicians should probably prepare for that possibility.

G. P. Gravlee, MD

Morphine-Based Cardiac Anesthesia Provides Superior Early Recovery Compared with Fentanyl in Elective Cardiac Surgery Patients

Murphy GS, Szokol JW, Marymont JH, et al (NorthShore Univ HealthSystem, Evanston, IL)

Anesth Analg 109:311-319, 2009

Background.—Experimental and clinical data suggest that morphine possesses unique cardioprotective and antiinflammatory properties. In this clinical investigation, we sought to determine whether the choice of intraoperative opioid (morphine or fentanyl) influences early recovery after cardiac surgery.

Methods.—Ninety patients undergoing cardiac surgery with cardiopulmonary bypass were randomized to receive either morphine (40 mg) or fentanyl (600 μg) as part of a standardized opioid-isoflurane anesthetic. Quality of recovery was assessed using the QoR-40 questionnaire administered preoperatively and daily on postoperative days 1–3. During the first three postoperative days, pain was measured using a 100-mm visual analog scale, and the use of IV and oral pain medications (morphine or acetaminophen/hydrocodone) was quantified. Hemodynamic variables, duration of tracheal intubation, postoperative febrile reactions, organ morbidities, and intensive care unit (ICU) and hospital length of stay were evaluated.

Results.—Compared with patients given fentanyl, those receiving morphine had higher global QoR-40 scores on postoperative days 1 (173 vs 160, $P < 0.0001$), 2 (174 vs 164, $P < 0.0001$), and 3 (177 vs 167, $P < 0.001$). Differences between the groups were observed in the QoR-40 dimensions of emotional state, physical comfort, and pain (all $P < 0.01$–0.0001). Postoperative visual analog scale pain scores, use of pain medication in the ICU and surgical ward, and postoperative febrile reactions were reduced significantly in the morphine group (all $P < 0.01$). No differences between the groups were noted in duration of tracheal intubation, ICU and hospital length of stay, or postoperative complications.

Conclusions.—In patients undergoing elective cardiac surgery with cardiopulmonary bypass, postoperative quality-of-life measures and pain control during recovery were enhanced when morphine (40 mg) was administered intraoperatively as part of a balanced anesthetic technique compared with fentanyl.

▶ Having trained in the high-dose morphine era, I found this article especially interesting. These authors used what I would call medium doses of morphine. Intraoperative differences were minor and clinically insignificant. The most striking finding was the impressively lower incidence of postoperative fever in the morphine group. Although this finding may seem minor, fever is quite unfriendly to a post-cardiopulmonary bypass (CPB) brain that has experienced a shower of microemboli and probably a stunned myocardium as well. Why might intraoperative morphine reduce postoperative fever? The answer could be that morphine is more promiscuous than fentanyl in that it binds to a wider array of opioid receptor subtypes.[1]

G. P. Gravlee, MD

Reference

1. Bilfinger TV, Fimiani C, Stefano GB. Morphine's immunoregulatory actions are not shared by fentanyl. *Int J Cardiol.* 1998;64:S61-S66.

Minimally Invasive Coronary Artery Bypass Grafting: Dual-Center Experience in 450 Consecutive Patients

McGinn JT Jr, Usman S, Lapierre H, et al (Staten Island Univ Hosp, NY; Univ of Ottawa Heart Inst, Canada)
Circulation 120:S78-S84, 2009

Background.—Minimally invasive coronary artery bypass grafting (MICS CABG) is a novel coronary operation that does not require infrastructure and is potentially available to all cardiac surgeons. It aims at decreasing the invasiveness of conventional CABG while preserving the applicability and durability of surgical revascularization, We examined the feasibility and safety of MICS CABG in the first large series of this operation to date.

Methods and Results.—All myocardial territories are accessed via a 4- to 6-cm left fifth intercostal thoracotomy. An apical positioner and epicardial stabilizer are introduced into the chest through the subxyphoid and left seventh intercostal spaces, respectively. The left internal thoracic artery is used to graft the left anterior descending artery, and radial artery or saphenous vein segments are used to graft the lateral and inferior myocardial territories. Proximal anastomoses are performed directly onto the aorta or from the left internal thoracic artery as a T-graft. In the first 450 consecutive MICS CABG procedures at our 2 centers, mean ± SD age was 62.3 ± 10.7 years and 123 patients were female (27%). The average number of grafts was 2.1 ± 0.7, with complete revascularization in 95% of patients. There were 34 patients in whom cardiopulmonary bypass was used (7.6%), 17 conversions to sternotomy (3.8%), and 10 reinterventions for bleeding (2.2%). Perioperative mortality occurred in 6 patients (1.3%).

Conclusions.—MICS CABG is feasible and has excellent procedural and short-term outcomes. This operation could potentially make multivessel minimally invasive coronary surgery safe, effective, and more widely available.

▶ This report features a creative adaptation of the minimally invasive direct coronary artery bypass (MIDCAB) approach, which has typically been used for single-vessel left anterior descending revascularization using the left internal mammary artery. By adding 2 small supplemental incisions for placement of a tissue stabilizer and an apical positioner, the authors gained access to the circumflex marginal and right coronary arteries as well (Fig 1 in the original article). By manipulation of the pulmonary artery and the use of selective right-lung ventilation with positive end-expiratory pressure (PEEP), access is obtained to the ascending aorta for the performance of proximal anastomoses using saphenous vein or radial artery segments. The authors also report selective use of paravertebral nerve blocks for postoperative pain control. Early graft patency appears equivalent to that of off-pump coronary artery bypass grafts (OPCABGs) conducted via a median sternotomy. The authors admit that they tended to select patients who needed 1 or 2 distal grafts, and that 50% of their total CABG procedures were performed using median sternotomy. It seems likely that patients' return to normal life activities would be faster after this approach as opposed to a median sternotomy with or without cardiopulmonary bypass (CPB). That type of follow-up information was not provided. It would be interesting to obtain the anesthesiologists' perspectives on this creative approach to CABG.

G. P. Gravlee, MD

Microcirculatory Alterations in Cardiac Surgery: Effects of Cardiopulmonary Bypass and Anesthesia

De Backer D, Dubois M-J, Schmartz D, et al (Free Univ of Brussels, Belgium)
Ann Thorac Surg 88:1396-1403, 2009

Background.—Heterogeneity in microvascular perfusion is associated with impaired tissue oxygenation. We hypothesized that cardiac surgery with or without cardiopulmonary bypass (CPB) could induce microvascular alterations.

Methods.—We used an orthogonal polarization spectral imaging technique to evaluate the sublingual microcirculation in patients undergoing cardiac surgery with ($n = 9$) or without ($n = 6$) CPB. We also included, as a control group, 7 patients undergoing thyroidectomy with the same anesthetic procedure. Hemodynamic and microcirculatory variables were obtained the day before surgery, after induction of anesthesia, during CPB, on admission to the intensive care unit or the recovery room, and 6

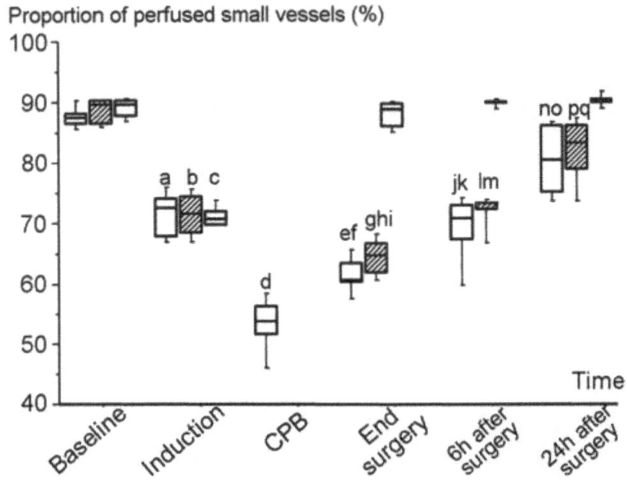

FIGURE 1.—Evolution of the proportion of perfused small vessels in patients undergoing cardiac surgery with (white boxes, n = 9) and without (hatched boxes, n = 6) cardiopulmonary bypass (CPB), and in patients undergoing thyroid surgery (dotted boxes, n = 7). Analysis of variance: group × time interaction $p < 0.0001$, group comparisons $p < 0.0001$, and time effect $p < 0.0001$. Post-hoc comparisons: $^{a}p = 0.008$; $^{b}p = 0.03$; $^{c}p = 0.04$; $^{d}p = 0.002$; $^{e}p = 0.008$; $^{g}p = 0.03$; $^{i}p = 0.012$; $^{l}p = 0.03$; $^{n}p = 0.008$; $^{p}p = 0.04$, compared with baseline; $^{h}p = 0.03$, without versus with CPB; and $^{f}p = 0.0015$; $^{j}p = 0.004$; $^{k}p = 0.0019$; $^{m}p = 0.004$; $^{o}p = 0.0015$; $^{q}p = 0.004$, versus thyroid surgery. (Reprinted from De Backer D, Dubois M-J, Schmartz D, et al. Microcirculatory alterations in cardiac surgery: effects of cardiopulmonary bypass and anesthesia. *Ann Thorac Surg*. 2009;88:1396-1403, with permission from The Society of Thoracic Surgeons.)

and 24 hours after the end of the surgical procedure. Data are presented as median (25th to 75th percentile).

Results.—No differences in hemodynamic variables were observed between the two cardiac surgery groups. The proportion of perfused vessels was similar in all three groups at baseline (89% [87% to 90%]), and decreased similarly after induction of anesthesia to 71% (69% to 74%). It decreased further during CPB to 53% (50% to 56%). On admission to the intensive care unit or recovery room, alterations were more severe in CPB than in off-pump patients (60% [59% to 62%] versus 64% [61% to 65%]; $p = 0.03$), whereas they had already normalized in thyroidectomy patients (89% [86% to 90%]; $p = 0.0005$ versus cardiac surgery). In both cardiac surgery groups these microcirculatory alterations decreased with time, but persisted at 24 hours. The severity of microvascular alterations correlated with peak lactate levels after cardiac surgery ($y = 11.5 - 0.15x$; $r^2 = 0.65$; $p < 0.05$).

Conclusions.—Microcirculatory alterations are observed in cardiac surgery patients whether or not CPB is used. Anesthesia contributes to these alterations, but its effects are transient (Fig 1).

▶ This elegantly simple clinical study has some very interesting findings. The most surprising one was that, despite identical anesthetic management, off-pump and on-pump coronary artery bypass graft patients had comparable reductions in microcirculation at the end of surgery, and that patients undergoing thyroidectomy lacked these changes. As shown in Fig 1, induction of anesthesia alone modestly reduced microcirculation in all 3 groups. The authors chose a total intravenous anesthetic technique, including propofol and remifentanil for all 3 groups, and it seems reasonable to speculate that replacing propofol with a potent inhalational anesthetic would improve microcirculation.

G. P. Gravlee, MD

A prospective, randomized, crossover pilot study of inhaled nitric oxide versus inhaled prostacyclin in heart transplant and lung transplant recipients

Khan TA, Schnickel G, Ross D, et al (UCLA School of Medicine, Los Angeles, CA)

J Thorac Cardiovasc Surg 138:1417-1424, 2009

Objective.—Inhaled nitric oxide has been shown to reduce pulmonary vascular resistance in patients undergoing cardiothoracic surgery, but it is limited by toxicity, the need for special monitoring, and cost. Inhaled prostacyclin also decreases pulmonary artery pressure, is relatively free of toxicity, requires no specific monitoring, and is less expensive. The objective of this study was to compare nitric oxide and prostacyclin in the treatment of pulmonary hypertension, refractory hypoxemia, and right ventricular dysfunction in thoracic transplant recipients in a prospective, randomized, crossover pilot trial.

Methods.—Heart transplant and lung transplant recipients were randomized to nitric oxide or prostacyclin as initial treatment, followed by a crossover to the other agent after 6 hours. Pulmonary vasodilators were initiated in the operating room for pulmonary hypertension, refractory hypoxemia, or right ventricular dysfunction. Nitric oxide was administered at 20 ppm, and prostacyclin was administered at 20,000 ng/mL. Hemodynamic and oxygenation parameters were recorded before and after initiation of pulmonary vasodilator therapy. At 6 hours, the hemodynamic and oxygenation parameters were recorded again, just before discontinuing the initial agent. Crossover baseline parameters were measured 30 minutes after the initial agent had been stopped. The crossover agent was then started, and the hemodynamic and oxygenation parameters were measured again 30 minutes later.

Results.—Heart transplant and lung transplant recipients ($n = 25$) were randomized by initial treatment (nitric oxide, $n = 14$; prostacyclin, $n = 11$). Nitric oxide and prostacyclin both reduced pulmonary artery pressure and central venous pressure, and improved cardiac index and mixed venous oxygen saturation on initiation of therapy. More importantly, at the 6-hour crossover trial, there were no significant differences between nitric oxide and prostacyclin in the reduction of pulmonary artery pressures or central venous pressure, or in improvement in cardiac index or mixed venous oxygen saturation. Nitric oxide and prostacyclin did not affect the oxygenation index or systemic blood pressure. There were no complications associated with nitric oxide or prostacyclin.

Conclusion.—In heart transplant and lung transplant recipients, nitric oxide and prostacyclin similarly reduce pulmonary artery pressures and central venous pressure, and improve cardiac index and mixed venous oxygen saturation. Inhaled prostacyclin may offer an alternative to nitric oxide in the treatment of pulmonary hypertension in thoracic transplantation.

▶ Nitric oxide (NO) serves as an important component of our therapeutic arsenal for the management of heart, lung, or heart-lung transplant patients. However, it is expensive and difficult to administer. Nonrandomized studies have suggested similar benefits with other inhaled vasodilators, such as prostacyclin, nitroglycerin, and nitroprusside, but this appears to be the first prospective comparison. Prostacyclin was as effective as NO and did not induce systemic hypotension, which often occurs when prostacyclin is administered intravenously. It is possible that inhaled prostacyclin may yet be shown to increase bleeding via its platelet inhibition activity, but that did not appear to be a problem in this small preliminary study. Nebulization of prostacyclin has its own technical difficulties, but this very promising approach deserves continued study.

G. P. Gravlee, MD

Does an Obese Body Mass Index Affect Hospital Outcomes After Coronary Artery Bypass Graft Surgery?

Engel AM, McDonough S, Smith JM (Inst for Res and Education, Cincinnati, OH; Good Samaritan Hosp, Cincinnati, OH)

Ann Thorac Surg 88:1793-1800, 2009

Background.—More than one third of adults in the United States are obese. Coronary artery bypass graft surgery (CABG) has become necessary for many obese persons. We evaluated the effect of this procedure on in-hospital mortality and morbidity of patients based on their body mass index (BMI).

Methods.—Data in a cardiac surgery database were examined retrospectively. Data selected from the database included CABG surgery from January 2003 to December 2007. The resulting cohort included a total of 10,590 patients. The BMI was grouped into four categories: underweight (BMI $\leq$ 19), normal weight (BMI 20 to 29), obese (BMI 30 to 39), and morbidly obese (BMI $\geq$ 40). Regression analysis was conducted to determine whether BMI was an independent predictor of morbidity and mortality after CABG.

Results.—Our results indicate that patients with an obese BMI are not at greater risk for morbidity or mortality after CABG. Logistic regression analysis found that CABG patients in the underweight body mass index group had the greatest risk of mortality, prolonged ventilation, reoperation for bleeding, and renal failure. Linear regression indicated length of hospital stay and intensive care unit stay after surgery were the longest for patients with an underweight BMI.

Conclusions.—Despite the comorbidities that are often present with obesity, an obese BMI was not found to be an independent predictor of morbidity or mortality after CABG. On the contrary, the underweight patients are at greater risk for mortality and complications after CABG surgery.

▶ This database review of over 10 000 coronary artery bypass graft surgery (CABG) patients showed very little effect of obesity or morbid obesity on most outcomes, although there was a small effect on total length of hospital stay and on duration of postoperative ventilation. The most interesting findings involved underweight patients, defined as those with a body mass index below 20 kg/m^2. Underweight patients had a higher incidence of several adverse outcomes, but patients in this group were also slightly older than patients in the other weight groups and were more likely to be female and to have chronic obstructive pulmonary disease (COPD). In a multivariate model, all of these risk factors independently predicted higher mortality, but the strongest predictor was underweight status, with an adjusted odds ratio of 2.21 (95% confidence interval 1.08-4.52). This study suggests that we should worry as much or more about very thin patients as we do about the morbidly obese.

G. P. Gravlee, MD

Narrowing the gap: Early and intermediate outcomes after percutaneous coronary intervention and coronary artery bypass graft procedures in California, 1997 to 2006

Carey JS, Danielsen B, Milliken J, et al (California Society of Thoracic Surgeons, Sacramento; Health Information Solutions, Sacramento; et al)
J Thorac Cardiovasc Surg 138:1100-1107, 2009

Objective.—Percutaneous coronary intervention is increasingly used to treat multivessel coronary artery disease. Coronary artery bypass graft procedures have decreased, and as a result, percutaneous coronary intervention has increased. The overall impact of this treatment shift is uncertain. We examined the in-hospital mortality and complication rates for these procedures in California using a combined risk model.

Methods.—The confidential dataset of the Office of Statewide Health Planning and Development patient discharge database was queried for 1997 to 2006. A risk model was developed using International Classification of Diseases, Ninth Revision, Clinical Modification procedures and diagnostic codes from the combined pool of isolated coronary artery bypass graft and percutaneous coronary intervention procedures performed during 2005 and 2006. In-hospital mortality was corrected for "same-day" transfers to another health care institution. Early failure rate was defined as in-hospital mortality rate plus reintervention for another percutaneous coronary intervention or cardiac surgery procedure within 90 days.

Results.—Coronary artery bypass graft volume decreased from 28,495 (1997) to 15,520 (2006), whereas percutaneous coronary intervention volume increased from 38,098 to 53,703. Risk-adjusted mortality rate decreased from 4.7% to 2.1% for coronary artery bypass graft procedures and from 3.4% to 1.9% for percutaneous coronary intervention. Expected mortality rate increased for both procedures. Early failure rate decreased from 13.1% to 8.0% for percutaneous coronary intervention and from 6.5% to 5.4% for coronary artery bypass graft. For the years 2004 and 2005, the risk of recurrent myocardial infarction or need for coronary artery bypass graft during the first postoperative year was 12% for percutaneous coronary intervention and 6% for coronary artery bypass grafts.

Conclusion.—This study shows that as volume shifted from coronary artery bypass grafts to percutaneous coronary intervention, expected mortality increased for both procedures. Risk-adjusted mortality rate decreased for both procedures, more so for coronary artery bypass grafts, so that corrected in-hospital mortality rates essentially equalized at approximately 2.0% in 2006. The post-procedural risk of reintervention, death, or myocardial infarction within the first year was twice as high for percutaneous coronary intervention as for coronary artery bypass grafts.

▶ Since the dawn of the current millennium, cardiothoracic surgery has been losing ground to stent placement in the treatment of atherosclerotic coronary artery disease. This has occurred despite evidence that outcomes are better with coronary artery bypass grafting (CABG) than with stent placement(s) in 2-vessel and 3-vessel disease. In England, the National Health Service has placed some restrictions on the use of stents and has taken an active role in directing patients toward the most appropriate therapy for their severity of coronary artery disease. Such direction has not taken place in the United States, but it appears to be needed, as supported by this report. The data presented derive from an enormous administrative database for the state of California. Like most administrative databases, this one lacks detailed analysis of comorbidities. As expected, early mortality remains higher for CABG than for percutaneous interventions, but the gap has narrowed over time to the point of virtual equivalence. Long-term freedom from reintervention among survivors has always been better for CABG than for stent placement.

G. P. Gravlee, MD

The effect of biventricular pacing on cardiac function after weaning from cardiopulmonary bypass in patients with reduced left ventricular function: A pressure–volume loop analysis

Hanke T, Misfeld M, Heringlake M, et al (Univ of Lübeck, Germany; San Raffaele Hosp, Milan, Italy)

J Thorac Cardiovasc Surg 138:148-156, 2009

Objective.—Patients with severely reduced left ventricular function undergoing coronary artery bypass grafting have increased complication rates. We hypothesized that temporary postoperative atrial synchronous biventricular pacing would improve left ventricular function after cardiopulmonary bypass.

Methods.—A left ventricular pressure–volume catheter was placed in 21 patients undergoing coronary artery bypass grafting (ejection fraction 29% ± 5%). Pressure–volume loops were obtained after weaning from cardiopulmonary bypass with atrial synchronous biventricular, left ventricular, and right ventricular outflow tract pacing and atrial-only stimulation at 90 beats/min.

Results.—Steady-state systolic and preload-independent parameters were superior for atrial synchronous biventricular and left ventricular pacing and atrial-only pacing relative to atrial synchronous right ventricular outflow tract pacing ($P < .05$). Diastolic parameters, excepting maximum negative rate of left ventricular pressure change, were unaffected. No significant differences were observed between atrial synchronous biventricular and left ventricular pacing and atrial-only pacing. Systolic dyssynchrony was significantly lower for atrial synchronous biventricular pacing (21% ± 5%), atrial synchronous left ventricular pacing (20% ± 6%), and atrial-only pacing (20% ± 6%) versus atrial synchronous right ventricular outflow tract pacing (25% ± 7%, $P < .05$). Atrioventricular interval during atrial-only stimulation was positively correlated with difference in stroke work between atrial synchronous biventricular pacing and atrial-only pacing ($r^2 = 0.78$, $P > .001$).

Conclusion.—Postoperative atrial synchronous biventricular and left ventricular pacing and atrial-only stimulation significantly improve systolic function relative to atrial synchronous right ventricular outflow tract pacing. If atrioventricular conduction is prolonged, atrial synchronous biventricular pacing is preferable to atrial-only pacing.

► In patients who have poor left ventricular function and require a permanent pacemaker, increasing evidence points to improved functional status when synchronized biventricular pacing is used rather than univentricular (right-sided) pacing. Often, patients who undergo cardiac surgery benefit from temporary DDD or DOO pacing, for which epicardial right ventricular pacing is predominantly used. Astute clinicians have long recognized that right ventricular pacing induces dyssynchronous left ventricular systolic wall motion observed by transesophageal echocardiography. Hanke et al have conducted a very interesting study showing that this pattern is physiologically suboptimal, although they did not assess clinical outcomes. The most appealing aspect of the study was its demonstration that, even with univentricular pacing, left ventricular physiology is enhanced by pacing the left rather than the right ventricle. This means that one need not apply technologically sophisticated biventricular atrioventricular temporary pacing during cardiac surgery to achieve improved left ventricular physiologic function. Simply placing the temporary epicardial ventricular pacing wire(s) along the lateral left ventricular wall achieves the same benefit. This simple step proved physiologically superior to placing the ventricular wire on the right ventricle, so it seems appropriate to apply this finding to most cardiac surgical patients who require ventricular pacing.

G. P. Gravlee, MD

Renal and Hepatic Function Improve in Advanced Heart Failure Patients During Continuous-Flow Support With the Heartmate II Left Ventricular Assist Device

Russell SD, Rogers JG, Milano CA, et al (Johns Hopkins Hosp, Baltimore, MD; Duke Univ Medl Ctr, Durham, NC; et al)
Circulation 120:2352-2357, 2009

Background.—The effects of continuous blood flow and reduced pulsatility on major organ function have not been studied in detail.

Methods and Results.—We evaluated renal (creatinine and blood urea nitrogen) and hepatic (aspartate transaminase, alanine transaminase, and total bilirubin) function in 309 (235 male, 74 female) advanced heart failure patients who had been supported with the HeartMate II continuous-flow left ventricular assist device for bridge to transplantation. To determine whether patients with impaired renal and hepatic function improve over time with continuous-flow left ventricular assist device support or whether there are any detrimental effects in patients with normal organ function, we divided patients into those with above-normal and normal laboratory values before implantation and measured blood chemistry over time during left ventricular assist device support. There were significant improvements over 6 months in all parameters in the above-normal groups, with values in the normal groups remaining in the normal range over time. Mean blood urea nitrogen and serum creatinine in the above-normal groups decreased significantly from 37 ± 14 to 23 ± 10 mg/dL ($P < 0.0001$) and from 1.8 ± 0.4 to 1.4 ± 0.8 mg/dL ($P < 0.01$), respectively. There were decreases in aspartate transaminase and alanine transaminase in the above-normal groups from 121 ± 206 and 171 ± 348 to 36 ± 19 and 31 ± 22 IU ($P < 0.001$), respectively. Total bilirubin for the above-normal group was 2.1 ± 0.9 mg/dL at baseline; after an acute increase at week 1, it decreased to 0.9 ± 0.5 mg/dL by 6 months ($P < 0.0001$). Both renal and liver values from patients in the normal groups remained normal during support with the left ventricular assist device.

Conclusions.—The HeartMate II continuous-flow left ventricular assist device improves renal and hepatic function in advanced heart failure patients who are being bridged to transplantation, without evidence of detrimental effects from reduced pulsatility over a 6-month time period.

► In bridge-to-transplantation patients, nonpulsatile continuous-flow ventricular assist devices are gradually replacing pulsatile ones. Their advantages include a smaller pump, fewer moving parts, and lower thrombogenicity. In animal models, nonpulsatile flow has been repeatedly shown to induce or enhance the stress response and to unfavorably alter regional blood flow distribution within organs, such as the kidney and brain. Consequently, assessment of renal and hepatic function over time in patients receiving nonpulsatile flow for many months was appropriate, and the substantial United Network for Organ Sharing (UNOS) database provided this opportunity. These patients do differ from experimental animals in that their baseline pulsatile flow condition involves a low cardiac output, which would be expected to induce organ compromise despite pulsatile flow. As a result, these patients' stress responses may be maximal at the time of nonpulsatile flow initiation. It follows that the liver and kidneys would benefit from enhanced blood flow in the face of increased cardiac output, whether or not that flow is pulsatile. Encouragingly, the authors found no reduction in liver and kidney function among patients in whom those organs had normal function before implanting the assist device (Fig 1 in the orginal article). An accompanying editorial[1] notes that an increased incidence of gastrointestinal bleeding has been associated with nonpulsatile assist devices. This occurrence remains an unsolved mystery that causes unscheduled trips to our operating rooms.

G. P. Gravlee, MD

Reference

1. Miller LW. Is pulsatile blood flow no longer essential? *Circulation*. 2009;120: 2313-2314.

Minimally Invasive, Minimally Reimbursed? Anesthesia for Endoscopic Cardiac Surgery Is Not Reflected Adequately in the German Diagnosis-Related Group System

Kottenberg-Assenmacher E, Merguet P, Kamler M, et al (Universitätsklinikum Essen, Germany)

J Cardiothorac Vasc Anesth 23:142-146, 2009

Objectives.—In the German diagnosis-related group (G-DRG) system, hospital reimbursement for anesthesia is linked to specific surgical procedures, irrespective of case duration. Accordingly, costs of innovative procedures, such as endoscopic cardiac surgery, may be underreimbursed. The authors assessed to what extent anesthesia costs for endoscopic cardiac surgery are reimbursed with the G-DRG system.

Design.—Retrospective analysis.

Setting.—University hospital.

Participants.—Eighty-four patients were studied undergoing general anesthesia for minimally invasive endoscopic port-access intracardiac surgery (n = 42) or conventional "open" surgery (n = 42) for similar indications.

Interventions.—None.

Measurements and Main Results.—The authors measured anesthesia staffing time, costs, and reimbursement for endoscopic cardiac surgery and compared results with data from a matched group undergoing conventional surgery. Endoscopic surgery increased anesthesia staffing time per case by 521 minutes (977 minutes ± 177 *v* 456 ± 92, mean ± standard deviation, $p = 0.0001$) and costs by approximately 200%. Anesthesia duration increased by 152 minutes (503 minutes ± 89 *v* 351 ± 69, $p = 0.0001$). In contrast, staffing reimbursement did not increase at the time of the patient's surgery (€500/case [446-569] *v* 492 [452-508], $p = 0.75$, median [interquartile range]) or with the 2007 G-DRG matrix (€548/case [463-559] *v* 503 [503-568], $p = 0.48$). Cost recovery was only 66% ± 17.4% and 72.7 ± 38.9 in the 2007 G-DRG matrix, respectively.

Conclusions.—It was shown that (1) endoscopic cardiac surgery consumed more anesthesia resources and was underreimbursed both relative to actual costs and to conventional surgery, (2) costs for such anesthesia services were inappropriately reflected in the G-DRG system, and (3) a DRG system's inability to adapt timely to innovative procedures may adversely affect anesthesia departments and medical progress.

▶ This article nicely analyzes resource utilization for endoscopic cardiac surgery and concludes that the German diagnosis-related group (DRG) system has thus far failed to adapt its reimbursement to the anesthesia resources consumed. About 10 years ago I worked in an institution that introduced port-access cardiopulmonary bypass to its practice, whereupon my partners and I quickly learned that this procedure required 2 staff anesthesiologists and a resident or nurse anesthetist for its first 1 to 2 hours. Of course, there was no increase in reimbursement for this commitment of personnel. Since that time, increased reimbursement for off-pump coronary artery bypass grafting (CABG) has successfully been achieved, so there is reason for hope that both government-based and private reimbursement systems will eventually respond to changing needs. Accompanying editorials provide additional perspectives, including recognition that the learning curve associated with new technologies initially prolongs procedures, but eventually can shorten them to the point that they are faster than the one being replaced.[1,2]

G. P. Gravlee, MD

References

1. De Hert SG. A European view managed health care plans: better or cheaper treatment strategies. *J Cardiothorac Vasc Anesth*. 2009;23:137-139.

2. Reich DL, Galati M. An American view American and European anesthesia reimbursement policies' effects on the adoption of novel techniques. *J Cardiothorac Vasc Anesth*. 2009;23:140-141.

Variation in perioperative vasoactive therapy in cardiovascular surgical care: Data from the Society of Thoracic Surgeons

Hernandez AF, Li S, Dokholyan RS, et al (Duke Univ School of Medicine, Durham, NC; et al)

Am Heart J 158:47-52, 2009

Background.—The appropriate use of vasoactive cardiovascular drugs in high-risk coronary artery bypass grafting (CABG) patients has not been well characterized.

Methods.—We performed a detailed chart analysis on 2,390 randomly selected patients undergoing CABG between January 2004 and June 2005 at 55 hospitals participating in the Society of Thoracic Surgeons' National Adult Cardiac Surgery Database. Patients were eligible if they had elective/urgent CABG with an ejection fraction (EF) <40%, or if they had an elective or urgent CABG at ≥65 years with diabetes, or a glomerular filtration rate <60 mL/min per 1.73 m^2. Logistic regression modeling was used to determine predictors of and provide risk-adjusted frequencies of postoperative vasoactive therapies.

Results.—Vasoactive therapy was used in 90% of patients. Inotropes/vasopressors were used in 28% (668), vasodilators in 18% (430), and the combination in 43% (1,037). Predictors of any inotrope use were preoperative atrial fibrillation (odds ratio [OR] 1.48), other arrhythmia (OR 2.09), EF (OR 1.09 per 5-unit decrease), severe mitral regurgitation (OR 2.56), 3-vessel coronary artery disease (OR 1.35), New York Heart Association class IV (1.38), on-pump (OR 1.86), other procedure (OR 2.51), and peripheral vascular disease (OR 1.28) (all OR $P < .05$). Hospital-level risk-adjusted rates of any inotrope use varied significantly from 100% to 35% ($P < .01$) and vasodilator rates varied from 100% to 10% ($P < .01$).

Conclusions.—There is marked hospital variation in the use of vasoactive therapies in high-risk CABG patients in clinical practice, indicating an important area for further research to better clarify best practice.

▶ This study involving 48 cardiac surgical centers in essence measures the popularity of the various vasoactive drugs used during coronary artery bypass grafting (CABG) in patients who have low left ventricular ejection fractions. Unsurprisingly, the presence of substantial variation in vasoactive drug use across institutions despite a fairly homogeneous patient population indicates that physician biases contribute importantly to decisions about vasoactive drug use. Fig 1 in the original article demonstrates the relative frequency of use of these drugs, except that the bar representing nitroprusside is too high by a factor of 10. The presence of severe mitral regurgitation and simultaneous performance of a cardiac operation in addition to CABG were the two strongest predictors of vasoactive drug use. As the authors suggest, prospective comparisons of different vasoactive drug choices are needed, but this is unlikely to transpire in the absence of a new competing drug for which a pharmaceutical company seeks Food and Drug Administration (FDA) approval. In the absence of such prospective comparisons, evidence-based improvement in clinical decision making about the use of these drugs will partly depend upon recording more information about the decisions being made, for example, blood pressure, cardiac output, and left ventricular contractility. Such analyses would be further aided by stratification of vasoactive drug selection decisions into pre-CPB, post-CPB, and postoperative epochs.

G. P. Gravlee, MD

Levosimendan Reduces Cardiac Troponin Release After Cardiac Surgery: A Meta-analysis of Randomized Controlled Studies

Zangrillo A, Biondi-Zoccai G, Mizzi A, et al (Istituto Scientifico San Raffaele, Milan, Italy; Univ of Turin, Italy; et al)
J Cardiothorac Vasc Anesth 23:474-478, 2009

Objectives.—The authors performed a meta-analysis to investigate the effects of levosimendan in cardiac surgery. Inotropic drugs have never shown beneficial effects on outcome in randomized controlled studies, with the possible exception of levosimendan.

Design.—A meta-analysis.

Setting.—Hospitals.

Participants.—A total of 139 patients from 5 randomized controlled studies were included in the analysis.

Interventions.—None.

Measurments and Main Results.—Four investigators independently searched BioMedCentral and PubMed. Inclusion criteria were random allocation to treatment, and comparison of levosimendan versus control performed on cardiac surgery patients. Exclusion criteria were duplicate publications, nonhuman experimental studies, and no outcome data. The endpoint was postoperative cardiac troponin release. Levosimendan was associated with a significant reduction in cardiac troponin peak release (weighted mean difference = 2.5 ng/dL [−3.86, −1.14], $p = 0.0003$) and in time to hospital discharge (weighted mean difference = −1.38 days [−2.78, 0.03], $p = 0.05$). No other relevant outcome (mortality, myocardial infarction, atrial fibrillation, time on mechanical ventilation, and intensive care unit stay) was improved in those patients receiving levosimendan.

Conclusions.—Levosimendan has cardioprotective effects, resulting in reduced postoperative cardiac troponin release.

▶ Levosimendan is a drug that induces increased inotropy and modest vasodilation while increasing the efficiency of myocardial energy use. As suggested by this study, levosimendan also appears to provide myocardial protection. Reports of its use in cardiac surgery have been largely favorable. Unfortunately, an American study in nonsurgical patients with advanced congestive heart failure failed to confirm the improvements in mortality and symptom control that had been observed in European studies. From a drug manufacturer's financial standpoint, daily use of a drug in several million congestive heart failure patients generates substantially more revenue than selective use of the same drug for a day or 2 in several hundred thousand cardiac surgical patients a year. Consequently, interest on the part of pharmaceutical companies in pursuing Food and Drug Administration approval for levosimendan has unfortunately waned. As a result, this helpful drug is available in several European countries, while its fate in the United States remains unclear.

G. P. Gravlee, MD

A Randomized Trial Evaluating Different Modalities of Levosimendan Administration in Cardiac Surgery Patients With Myocardial Dysfunction

De Hert SG, Lorsomradee S, vanden Eede H, et al (Univ of Amsterdam, The Netherlands)

J Cardiothorac Vasc Anesth 22:699-705, 2008

Objective.—To evaluate the effects of 2 different administration modalities of levosimendan (start before cardiopulmonary bypass [CPB] and at the end of CPB) compared with a standard treatment with milrinone started at the end of CPB in cardiac surgery patients with a preoperative ejection fraction <30%.

Design.—A prospective study.

Setting.—A university hospital.

Participants.—Sixty patients undergoing elective cardiac surgery with CPB.

Interventions.—Patients were randomly assigned to 3 different treatment options for weaning from CPB after cardiac surgery. Group A received milrinone, 0.5 µg/kg/min, after the release of the aortic cross-clamp; group B received levosimendan, 0.1 µg/kg/min, after the induction of anesthesia; and in group C, levosimendan, 0.1 µg/kg/min, was started immediately after the release of the aortic cross-clamp. In all patients, additional dobutamine, 5 µg/kg/min, was initiated after the release of the aortic cross-clamp. Norepinephrine maintained mean arterial pressure constant.

Measurements and Main Results.—Stroke volume after surgery was initially higher than at baseline in all groups and highest in group B. Stroke volume declined 12 hours after surgery in group A but not in groups B and C ($p < 0.05$ between groups), despite similar filling pressures. Four patients in group A, none in group B, and 1 in group C died within 30 days of surgery. Postoperative atrial fibrillation was observed in 10 patients in group A, 7 patients in group C, and only 1 in group B ($p < 0.01$). No differences were observed in postoperative troponin I release among groups.

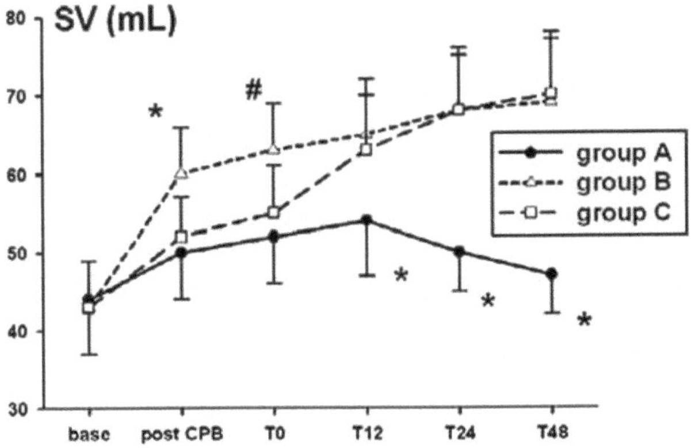

FIGURE 1.—Stroke volume (SV) at the start of surgery (base), 15 minutes after the end of CPB (post-CPB), at arrival in the ICU (T0), and 12 (T12), 24 (T24), and 48 (T48) hours later in the 3 study groups. Data are mean ± standard deviation. *Statistically significant different from both other groups for $p < 0.01$. #Statistically significant difference between groups A and C for $p < 0.01$. For the sake of clarity, standard deviation bars are represented in only 1 direction. (Reprinted from De Hert SG, Lorsomradee S, vanden Eede H, et al. A randomized trial evaluating different modalities of levosimendan administration in cardiac surgery patients with myocardial dysfunction. *J Cardiothorac Vasc Anesth*. 2008;22:699-705.)

TABLE 3.—Inotropic and Vasopressor Medication

	Group A (n = 20)	Group B (n = 20)	Group C (n = 20)
Dobutamine			
Total dose (μg/kg)	12,067 ± 3,299*	2,477 ± 1,567	3,526 ± 2,095
Time (h)	32 ± 13*	15 ± 5	16 ± 5
Norepinephrine			
Total dose (μg)	22,572 ± 8,772*	5,183 ± 4,256	9,241 ± 3,751
Number of patients	20	18	20
Time (h)	36 ± 14*	13 ± 9	19 ± 6
Study medication			
Total dose (μg/kg)	1,387 ± 943	118 ± 33	119 ± 40
Duration (h)	72 ± 41*	22 ± 4	23 ± 3
IABP			
No. of patients	6	6	6
Post-CPB duration (h)	10 ± 84*	45 ± 11	52 ± 20

NOTE. Data are mean ± standard deviation.
Abbreviation: IABP, intra-aortic balloon pump.
*Statistically significant difference compared with the other groups ($p < 0.01$).

Conclusion.—In the conditions of the present study, starting the levosimendan treatment before CPB was associated with a higher initial postoperative stroke volume and a lower incidence of postoperative atrial fibrillation, but had no effect on the extent of postoperative troponin I release (Fig 1, Table 3).

▶ DeHert et al have performed an interesting study comparing 3 different inotropic regimens in patients with severely compromised ventricular function, most of whom were undergoing coronary artery bypass grafting combined with an undisclosed valvular procedure. All patients received dobutamine 5 mcg/kg/min at the time of separation from cardiopulmonary bypass. The difference between the 3 groups was in the use of milrinone alone in 1 group, and 2 different dosing regimens for levosimendan in the other 2 groups. All groups ultimately did well, with a few differences pointed out in the abstract. Table 3 reveals that group A (milrinone and dobutamine) had lower cardiac output, higher systemic vascular resistance, and required substantially higher doses of dobutamine and norepinephrine to achieve the desired mean arterial pressure and cardiac output values. Consequently, it appears that the use of levosimendan 0.1 mcg/kg/min in combination with dobutamine 5 mcg/kg/min produced the desired hemodynamics most of the time without further intervention for and better sustained stroke volume improvement over the entire study period (Fig 1). Although the hemodynamics were slightly more favorable when levosimendan was introduced after induction of anesthesia (group B), the only evidence for a myocardial protective effect was a lower incidence of postoperative atrial fibrillation, hence it would appear reasonable to begin levosimendan before or after CPB. Levosimendan is a very interesting and promising new intropic drug. Its ultimate place in our therapeutic armamentarium remains to be determined. Levosimendan is not yet available in the United States, but clinical trials are underway.

G. P. Gravlee, MD

Ketamine Attenuates Delirium After Cardiac Surgery With Cardiopulmonary Bypass

Hudetz JA, Patterson KM, Iqbal Z, et al (Med College of Wisconsin, Milwaukee; Clement J. Zablocki Veterans Administration Med Ctr, Milwaukee, WI)

J Cardiothorac Vasc Anesth 23:651-657, 2009

Objective.—To determine if ketamine attenuates postoperative delirium concomitant with an anti-inflammatory effect in patients undergoing cardiac surgery using cardiopulmonary bypass.

Design.—A prospective randomized study.

Setting.—A Veterans Affairs medical center.

Participants.—Cardiac surgical patients.

Interventions.—Patients at least 55 years of age randomly received placebo (0.9% saline, n = 29) or an intravenous bolus of ketamine (0.5 mg/kg intravenously, n = 29) during anesthetic induction in the presence of fentanyl and etomidate.

Measurements and Main Results.—Delirium was assessed by using the Intensive Care Delirium Screening Checklist before and after surgery. Serum C-reactive protein concentrations were determined before and 1 day after surgery. The incidence of postoperative delirium was lower ($p = 0.01$, Fisher exact test) in patients receiving ketamine (3%) compared with placebo (31%). Postoperative C-reactive protein concentration was also lower ($p < 0.05$) in the ketamine-treated patients compared with the placebo-treated patients. The odds of developing postoperative delirium were greater for patients receiving placebo compared with ketamine treatment (odds ratio = 12.6; 95% confidence interval, 1.5-107.5; logistic regression).

Conclusions.—After cardiac surgery using cardiopulmonary bypass, ketamine attenuates postoperative delirium concomitant with an anti-inflammatory effect.

▶ Ketamine, an old drug, continues to emerge from relative obscurity with a variety of surprising uses such as postoperative pain pre-emption and treatment, and recently, neuroprotective effects have been demonstrated from this drug that had long been considered a neurologic liability. This study is relatively small, but the results are impressive if taken at face value. However, the study does not paint a clear picture of the severity of the observed dementias. It seems that the dementias observed were not terribly severe because demented patients did not experience prolongations of their stays in the intensive care unit or hospital. Dementias may act like neuropsychologic deficits: if you look hard enough for them, you will find them. Clinical significance is harder to assess.

G. P. Gravlee, MD

Hetastarch increases the risk of bleeding complications in patients after off-pump coronary bypass surgery: A randomized clinical trial

Hecht-Dolnik M, Barkan H, Taharka A, et al (Kaiser Permanente Med Ctr, Oakland, CA; Univ of California, Berkeley)

J Thorac Cardiovasc Surg 138:703-711, 2009

Objective.—Hetastarch is an artificial colloid widely used intraoperatively in fluid-replacement regimens. Previous studies have found that the intraoperative administration of hetastarch may increase the risk of postoperative bleeding in patients who undergo coronary artery bypass graft surgery with cardiopulmonary bypass. Previous published reports have not examined this risk in patients who underwent coronary artery bypass grafting without cardiopulmonary bypass.

Methods.—In a randomized clinical trial, 156 patients undergoing off-pump coronary artery bypass grafting were assigned to receive either 1 liter of hetastarch or 1 liter of albumin as part of intraoperative volume replacement. Sample recruitment was halted in a review per protocol by the study's Data Safety Monitoring Committee. We assessed the rate of postoperative bleeding by monitoring the number of units of blood products transfused in the first 24 postoperative hours in the intensive care unit and the hourly chest tube drainage in the first 12 postoperative hours.

Results.—Intraoperative administration of 1 liter of hetastarch was associated with statistically significant increases in 3 measures: transfusion requirements on postoperative day 1 (red blood cells, 1.14 vs 0.40 units,

$P = .017$; fresh-frozen plasma, 0.57 vs 0.15, $P = .009$; platelets, 0.35 vs 0.10, $P = .013$); the overall likelihood of receiving transfusion on postoperative day 1 (46.2% vs 25.6%, $P = .012$); and the volume of chest tube drainage in the first 12 hours postoperatively (732.0 vs 563.6 mL, $P < .001$).

Conclusion.—In patients undergoing off-pump coronary artery bypass, the intraoperative administration of hetastarch increases the postoperative transfusion requirement and the volume of blood drained postoperatively.

▶ The authors correctly point out that previous studies have associated hetastarch use with increased bleeding and transfusion in patients undergoing operations using cardiopulmonary bypass (CPB). This appears to be the first prospective comparison of hetastarch with albumin in operations performed without CPB. The volume of hetastarch used (1000 mL) has previously been considered insufficient to induce clinically significant impairment in blood clotting, yet chest tube drainage in the first 12 postoperative hours was higher with hetastarch than albumin. Postoperative caregivers were blinded to the intraoperative use of hetastarch versus albumin, but intraoperative caregivers were not blinded, so possibly incomplete blinding could have influenced intraoperative decisions that in turn impacted postoperative transfusion outcomes. However, it appears more likely that volumes of hetastarch, which have been traditionally considered safe, increase bleeding to a clinically significant degree with or without CPB. Newer starches with lower molecular weights and different substitution patterns appear to induce less coagulopathy than hetastarch. At present, it seems reasonable for practitioners to avoid using hetastarch in cardiac surgical patients, and perhaps in all patients.

G. P. Gravlee, MD

Long-term outcomes of percutaneous mitral balloon valvuloplasty versus open cardiac surgery

Song J-K, Kim M-J, Yun S-C, et al (Univ of Ulsan College of Medicine, Seoul, South Korea)

J Thorac Cardiovasc Surg 139:103-110, 2010

Objectives.—We sought to compare long-term outcomes between percutaneous mitral valvuloplasty and open heart surgery.

Methods.—The study evaluated 402 patients who underwent percutaneous mitral valvuloplasty and 159 patients who underwent open heart surgery between January 1, 1995, and December 31, 2000. The rates of cardiovascular death or repeated intervention (redo percutaneous mitral valvuloplasty or open heart surgery) were determined over a median follow-up of 109 months (mean ± SD, 106 ± 27). The therapeutic effects on adverse outcomes were estimated by the Cox proportional hazards model adjusting differences in the severity of illness before intervention.

The effects of the cardiac rhythm and echocardiographic score were also tested.

Results.—The observed (unadjusted) event-free survival was similar for both groups, and the hazard ratio for the clinical events after percutaneous mitral valvuloplasty as compared with after open heart surgery was 1.510 (95% confidence interval, 0.914–2.496; $P = .1079$). However, the adjusted hazard ratio was 3.729 (95% confidence interval, 1.963–7.082; $P < .0001$), showing a higher event-free survival in the open heart surgery group. The adjusted hazard ratio after percutaneous mitral valvuloplasty as compared with after open heart surgery in patients with echocardiographic scores of 8 or more and atrial fibrillation were 5.348 (95% confidence interval, 2.504–11.422; $P < .001$) and 3.440 (95% confidence interval, 1.805–6.555; $P = .0002$), respectively, whereas the hazard ratio in patients with echocardiographic scores less than 8 and normal sinus rhythm did not show differences.

Conclusions.—Open heart surgery was associated with a higher adjusted rate of long-term event-free survival than percutaneous mitral valvuloplasty. Patients with high echocardiographic scores or atrial fibrillation showed better outcomes after open heart surgery.

▶ This study differs from previous comparisons by having larger numbers of patients, but it is similar in being a nonrandomized comparison. It is not surprising that long-term functional outcomes with surgical mitral valve replacement are better than those with percutaneous balloon valvuloplasty, so why would patients select the latter over the former? Perhaps they wish to avoid major surgery with a prolonged recovery in favor of a catheter intervention with no scar, minimal postprocedure pain, and a 24 to 48-hour postprocedure hospital stay. The current data show the expected higher early mortality with surgery, but long-term mortalities are similar, and freedom from reintervention is better with surgery. Because the patients undergoing surgery had higher preprocedure risk profiles, a variety of risk adjustment procedures were applied. These adjustments suggested comparable early risk-adjusted mortality with surgery or percutaneous valvuloplasty. I agree with the authors that a prospective trial is warranted.

G. P. Gravlee, MD

Systematic review of studies of the effect of hyperoxia on coronary blood flow

Farquhar H, Weatherall M, Wijesinghe M, et al (Med Res Inst of New Zealand, Wellington; Univ of Otago, Wellington, New Zealand; et al)

Am Heart J 158:371-377, 2009

Background.—International guidelines recommend the routine use of oxygen in the initial treatment of myocardial infarction, yet it is uncertain what effect this might have on physiologic and clinical outcomes.

Methods.—We undertook a systematic search of Medline, Cochrane Database of Systematic Reviews, EMBASE, and CINHAL using the key words "oxygen," "coronary blood flow," "hyperoxia," and "coronary circulation" to identify human studies involving a measure of coronary blood flow while breathing oxygen and room air. The primary outcome measure was coronary blood flow; secondary outcomes included coronary vascular resistance and myocardial oxygen consumption.

Results.—From 2,072 potential publications, there were 6 studies from 4 publications that met the inclusion criteria, with 6 healthy subjects and 61 subjects with cardiac disease. It was not possible to undertake a meta-analysis due to methodological limitations. In the 6 studies, high-concentration oxygen therapy resulted in hyperoxia, with a range in mean PaO_2 of 273 to 425 mm Hg. Hyperoxia caused a significant reduction in coronary blood flow (mean change −7.9% to −28.9%, n = 6 studies). Hyperoxia caused a significant increase in coronary vascular resistance (mean change 21.5% to 40.9%, n = 4 studies) and a significant reduction in myocardial oxygen consumption (mean change −15.3% to −26.9%, n = 3 studies).

Conclusions.—Hyperoxia from high-concentration oxygen therapy causes a marked reduction in coronary blood flow and myocardial oxygen consumption. These physiologic effects may have the potential to cause harm and are relevant to the use of high-concentration oxygen therapy in the treatment of cardiac and other disorders.

▶ This provocative, focused review suggests that high PaO2 levels may potentially harm patients with acute coronary syndromes by increasing coronary vascular resistance, thereby possibly converting the myocardium from its usual state of lactate consumption to that of lactate production. Of note is the fact that the studies included all used FiO_2s approximating 1.0, hence lower FiO_2s such as those achieved from nasal cannula oxygen administration were not assessed. That the data from the 6 studies did not meet statistical criteria for a meta-analysis merits at least a raised eyebrow. As anesthesiologists, when we have a patient with ischemic heart disease or presumed myocardial ischemia, the chances are good that we will administer a very high FiO_2 under the assumption that more is better when it comes to oxygen and ischemic heart disease. Perhaps not.

G. P. Gravlee, MD

Magnesium supplementation during cardiopulmonary bypass to prevent junctional ectopic tachycardia after pediatric cardiac surgery: A randomized controlled study

Manrique AM, Arroyo M, Lin Y, et al (Children's Hosp of Pittsburgh, PA; Univ of Pittsburgh, PA)

J Thorac Cardiovasc Surg 139:162-169, 2010

Objectives.—We analyzed the role of magnesium sulfate ($MgSO_4$) supplementation during cardiopulmonary bypass in pediatric patients undergoing cardiac surgery, assessing the incidence of hypomagnesemia and the incidence of junctional ectopic tachycardia.

Methods.—We performed a randomized, double-blind, controlled trial in 99 children. $MgSO_4$ or placebo was administered during the rewarming phase of cardiopulmonary bypass: group 1, placebo group (29 patients); group 2, 25 mg/kg of $MgSO_4$ (30 patients); and group 3, 50 mg/kg of $MgSO_4$ (40 patients).

Results.—At the time of admission to the cardiac intensive care unit, groups receiving $MgSO_4$ had significantly greater levels of ionized magnesium (group 1, 0.51 ± 0.07; group 2, 0.57 ± 0.09; group 3, 0.59 ± 0.09). Hypomagnesemia before bypass was common (75%–86.2%) and not significantly different among the groups. The proportion of hypomagnesemia decreased significantly at admission to the cardiac intensive care unit in groups receiving $MgSO_4$ (group 1, 77.8%; group 2, 63%; group 3, 47.4%). Patients receiving placebo (group 1) had a significantly greater occurrence of junctional ectopic tachycardia than groups receiving $MgSO_4$ (group 1, n = 5 [17.9%]; group 2, n = 2 [6.7%]; group 3, n = 0 [0%]). Age (<1 month), Aristotle score (>4), and history of cardiac failure were associated with junctional ectopic tachycardia. None of the patients with those characteristics in group 3 had junctional ectopic tachycardia. No association was found between study groups and the Pediatric Risk of Mortality score or length of stay in the cardiac intensive care unit.

Conclusions.—Supplementation with $MgSO_4$ during cardiopulmonary bypass seems to reduce the incidence of hypomagnesemia and junctional ectopic tachycardia at admission to the cardiac intensive care unit. This effect seems to be dose related.

▶ Postoperative junctional ectopic tachycardia (JET) vexes pediatric cardiac surgery teams, and this prospective study strongly suggests that prophylaxis with magnesium reduces its incidence. Although this information is helpful, many, if not most, centers already use prophylactic magnesium in both adult and pediatric patients undergoing cardiopulmonary bypass (CPB). However, these authors evaluated 2 different dosing levels of magnesium and found that higher doses confer additional benefit in the prevention of JET. It seems plausible that the higher dose group could have experienced more hypotension or an impaired recovery of muscle strength, but these aspects apparently were not assessed. It also seems possible that beneficial effects could be enhanced with sustained administration of magnesium prophylaxis, so there is need for further study. For the present, this study supports the routine use of supplemental magnesium during CPB in children.

G. P. Gravlee, MD

A Randomized Trial Evaluating Amiodarone for Prevention of Atrial Fibrillation After Pulmonary Resection

Tisdale JE, Wroblewski HA, Wall DS, et al (Purdue Univ, Indianapolis, IN; Indiana Univ School of Medicine, Indianapolis; Indiana Univ Hosp of Clarian Health Partners, Indianapolis)

Ann Thorac Surg 88:886-895, 2009

Background.—Atrial fibrillation (AF) occurs commonly after anatomic pulmonary resection. In this study, the efficacy of amiodarone for prevention of post–pulmonary resection AF was investigated.

Methods.—One hundred thirty patients undergoing lobectomy, bilobectomy, or pneumonectomy were randomly assigned prospectively to receive amiodarone (n = 65) or no prophylaxis (control group, n = 65). The amiodarone group received 1,050 mg by continuous intravenous infusion over 24 hours, initiated at the time of anesthesia induction, followed by 400 mg orally twice daily until hospital discharge or for a maximum of 6 days. The primary endpoint was AF requiring treatment during hospitalization. Secondary endpoints included postoperative length of hospital and intensive care unit stays.

Results.—There were no significant differences between the amiodarone and control groups in demographics, comorbid conditions, extent of pulmonary resection, or preoperative or postoperative use of β-blockers or calcium-channel blockers. The incidence of AF was lower in the amiodarone group than in the control group (13.8% versus 32.3%, $p = 0.02$; relative risk reduction = 57%). There was no difference between the amiodarone and control groups in median length of hospital stay (7 versus 8 days, $p = 0.79$), but median length of intensive care unit stay was shorter in the amiodarone group (46 versus 84 hours, $p = 0.03$). There was no significant difference between the amiodarone and control groups in the incidence of pulmonary complications or other adverse effects.

Conclusions.—Amiodarone prophylaxis significantly reduces the incidence of AF after anatomic pulmonary resection, and is associated with a significant reduction in length of intensive care unit stay.

▶ This randomized prospective study used a slow intravenous loading dose of amiodarone (approximately 0.75 mg/minute for 24 hours) beginning at the induction of anesthesia, followed by oral amiodarone for the remainder of hospitalization. This approach reduced the incidence of atrial fibrillation, which has long been associated with prolonged intensive care unit (ICU) or hospital stays in patients undergoing lobectomy or pneumonectomy. In this study, only the duration of ICU stay was reduced by the absence of atrial fibrillation. Presumably, similar results could be obtained if amiodarone prophylaxis was initiated preoperatively, but it generally takes several days of oral amiodarone administration to reach therapeutic plasma concentrations. The "slow intravenous load" approach used in this study is pharmacokinetically elegant because new postoperative atrial fibrillation in this patient population most often occurs 24 hours or more after completion of surgery. In cardiac surgery prophylaxis, using either a beta-adrenergic blocker or amiodarone is effective for reducing the incidence of postoperative atrial fibrillation, but the higher incidence of chronic obstructive pulmonary disease (COPD) in lung resection patients may favor the selection of amiodarone even if β-blockers should prove equally efficacious.

G. P. Gravlee, MD

Anesthetic Management of Percutaneous Aortic Valve Implantation: Focus on Challenges Encountered and Proposed Solutions

Covello RD, Maj G, Landoni G, et al (Università Vita-Salute San Raffaele, Milan, Italy; et al)

J Cardiothorac Vasc Anesth 23:280-285, 2009

Objective.—To describe 6 months of experience in the anesthetic management of percutaneous aortic valve implantation.

Design.—An observational, cohort study.

Setting.—A university hospital.

Participants.—Eighteen high-risk patients with relative contraindications to surgical valve replacement (78 ± 8.7 years, logistic EuroSCORE 26 ± 19.1).

Intervention.—An Edwards/Sapien Aortic Bioprosthesis (Edwards Lifesciences LLC, Irvine, CA) was implanted in patients with severe symptomatic aortic stenosis who underwent percutaneous retrograde aortic valve implantation without cardiopulmonary bypass. The procedure was performed using general anesthesia (15 patients) or sedation (3 patients).

Measurements and Main Results.—The valve was successfully implanted in all patients. One patient had prolonged ventricular fibrillation that required advanced cardiopulmonary resuscitation, endotracheal intubation, and placement of an intra-aortic balloon pump. Six patients had vascular access site complications managed either percutaneously or surgically. Five patients were extubated in the catheterization laboratory. All patients were transferred to the intensive care unit for monitoring, and all but one were discharged to an intermediate care unit within 24 hours. Early postoperative complications included acute renal failure (1 patient), arrhythmias (1 atrial fibrillation and 1 transient heart block), and stroke (1 patient). One patient died 58 days after the procedure for noncardiac reasons.

Conclusions.—Transcatheter aortic valve implantation is possible in selected high-risk patients. Anesthesiologists must be aware of current technology in order to have an active role in patient selection, to develop monitoring and standards of care in the cardiac catheterization laboratory, and to plan postoperative management.

▶ This report basically details observations in a single center that collected 18 percutaneous aortic valve replacements fairly soon after introduction of the technique. It should provide some encouragement to those who believe that the sky is falling on cardiothoracic anesthesiologists in direct proportion to the increasing availability of interventional cardiology procedures for atherosclerotic and valvular heart disease. It appears that most percutaneous valve procedures are being performed under general anesthesia (or as in this study, some with very delicately managed sedation). Monitoring is fairly intense, and typically includes intra-arterial pressure measurement, central venous access, and either transesophageal or transthoracic echocardiography. To me, this sounds more like opportunity knocking than like a bell tolling for cardiothoracic anesthesiologists.

G. P. Gravlee, MD

Hematocrit on Cardiopulmonary Bypass and Outcome After Coronary Surgery in Nontransfused Patients

Ranucci M, Conti D, Castelvecchio S, et al (IRCCS Policlinico S. Donato, Milan, Italy)

Ann Thorac Surg 89:11-18, 2010

Background.—Preoperative anemia and the lowest registered hematocrit value on cardiopulmonary bypass are recognized risk factors for morbidity and mortality after coronary operations. A low hematocrit often results in blood transfusions with all of the associated possible complications. The relative contribution of these three factors to long-term outcome is still not well established. This study aimed to identify the role of preoperative anemia and hemodilution during cardiopulmonary bypass as determinants of morbidity and mortality after coronary operations.

Methods.—A consecutive series of 3,003 patients was analyzed. They had all undergone isolated coronary operations without receiving blood transfusions during their hospital stay. The preoperative hematocrit and the lowest hematocrit on cardiopulmonary bypass were analyzed in a multivariable model as predictors of major morbidity and operative mortality.

Results.—After adjustment for the other explanatory variables, both the preoperative hematocrit and the lowest hematocrit on cardiopulmonary bypass were found to be independent risk factors for major morbidity, but not for operative mortality. However, low values of preoperative hematocrit were not associated with an increased morbidity, provided that the lowest hematocrit on cardiopulmonary bypass was maintained above 28%. Median values of the lowest hematocrit on cardiopulmonary bypass below 25% were associated with an increased major morbidity rate.

Conclusions.—Excessive hemodilution during cardiopulmonary bypass is a risk factor for major morbidity even in the absence of blood transfusions. Techniques that aim to reduce the fall in hematocrit during cardiopulmonary bypass, including blood cardioplegia, may be useful, especially in patients with a low preoperative hematocrit.

▶ Over my span of 30 years as a cardiothoracic anesthesiologist, debate about optimal hematocrit (HCT) management during cardiopulmonary bypass (CPB) has been continuous. Like all human studies on this subject, this one retrospectively analyzes a large database, seeking correlations with adverse outcomes. The unique aspect of this particular study is the preoperative identification of a sizable group of mildly anemic (HCT < 40%) patients undergoing coronary artery bypass grafting (CABG) who did not receive a perioperative blood transfusion. This group was then stratified by lowest CPB HCT for a comparison of outcomes. The use of low CPB circuit priming volumes and hemofiltration during CPB facilitated this effort, which offers the appeal of separating the "chicken from the egg" because previous retrospective studies have been largely unsuccessful in separating out the obvious interaction between low CPB HCT and RBC transfusion. Both low HCT and RBC transfusion have been repeatedly associated with perioperative morbidity. The authors purport to show that if one can take a patient with a preoperative HCT < 40% and keep that patient's minimum CPB HCT above 28%, then this will reduce the incidence of perioperative morbidity (principally duration of ventilation and renal dysfunction). Nevertheless, the differences are small and inconclusive. In particular, the graphic relationship of lowest CPB HCT to major morbidity appears biphasic, suggesting that a minimum CPB HCT of 24% produces almost the same outcome as one of 28%, while a minimum HCT of 25% is worse than one of either 24% or 28%. Debate continues, as it will until someone performs a large prospective human study comparing different HCT levels during CPB.

G. P. Gravlee, MD

A Randomized Clinical Trial Investigating the Relationship Between Aprotinin and Hypercoagulability in Off-Pump Coronary Surgery

Desai PH, Kurian D, Thirumavalavan N, et al (Boston Univ School of Medicine, MA; et al)

Anesth Analg 109:1387-1394, 2009

Background.—Off-pump coronary artery bypass (OPCAB) surgery is associated with a hypercoagulable state in which the platelet thrombin receptor, protease-activated receptor-1 (PAR-1), helps propagate a thrombin burst within saphenous vein grafts. Aprotinin, used in cardiothoracic surgery mainly for its antifibrinolytic properties, also spares platelet PAR-1 activation due to thrombin. We hypothesized that this

PAR-1 antagonistic property provides an antithrombotic benefit during OPCAB surgery.

Methods.—Patients were randomly assigned to receive saline ($n = 38$) or a modified full-dose regimen of aprotinin ($n = 37$) IV during OPCAB surgery. Blood sampled perioperatively from the coronary sinus, skin wounds, and systemic circulation was analyzed to test coagulation and platelet function. Major adverse cardiovascular events were monitored by obtaining troponin I at 24 h (myocardial infarction), predischarge computed tomography angiography (vein graft thrombosis), and by clinical examination for stroke.

Results.—Coronary sinus blood obtained immediately after OPCAB surgery showed significantly less activation in the aprotinin group, as judged by reduced formation of platelet-leukocyte conjugates ($P < 0.02$) and platelet-derived microparticles ($P < 0.05$). The aprotinin group showed inhibition of platelet aggregation induced by thrombin ($P = 0.007$) but not adenosine diphosphate. Thrombin generation, defined by F1.2 levels, was significantly reduced by aprotinin in the coronary sinus but not in skin wound incisions. Major adverse cardiovascular events were significantly reduced in aprotinin-treated patients (5.4% vs 29.7%, $P < 0.05$). Aprotinin also demonstrated antifibrinolytic properties through diminished red blood cell transfusion ($P < 0.04$) and reduced blood loss postoperatively (603 ± 330 vs 810 ± 415 mL, $P < 0.004$).

Conclusion.—This study demonstrates that aprotinin protects patients undergoing OPCAB surgery from a hypercoagulable state by diminishing thrombin-induced platelet activation and thrombin generation within saphenous vein grafts, while maintaining systemic hemostatic and antifibrinolytic benefits. These results support further investigation of aprotinin and other PAR-1 antagonists in OPCAB surgery.

▶ Aprotinin is a fascinating drug that just would not go gracefully into the good night. It is no longer sold in the United States because of its adverse event profile, which has recently been confirmed by a large Canadian trial. This study investigated many process variables in a small population of patients undergoing off-pump coronary artery bypass grafting. Most blood clotting variables showed no difference. The authors included saphenous vein graft occlusion in their major adverse event category, whether or not this was associated with a myocardial infarction or the need for a new coronary intervention. These saphenous vein occlusion differences (6 placebo vs 1 aprotinin) were grouped with myocardial infarctions (4 placebo vs 1 aprotinin) and stroke (1 placebo vs 0 aprotinin) to achieve statistical significance for the different incidences (29.7% placebo vs 5.4% aprotinin) of major adverse cardiovascular events. This post hoc lumping of outcomes arguably constitutes a statistical stretch. Differences in blood loss and transfusion, while statistically significant, were modest. It appears that most patients did not require transfusion. This study will be insufficient to reverse the tide for aprotinin, but the vein graft patency difference merits additional study in a larger patient population.

G. P. Gravlee, MD

5 Pediatric Anesthesia

The Impact of Oral Premedication with Midazolam on Respiratory Function in Children

von Ungern-Sternberg BS, Erb TO, Habre W, et al (Princess Margaret Hosp for Children, Australia; Univ Children's Hosp Basel, Switzerland; Univ Hosp Geneva, Switzerland; et al)
Anesth Analg 108:1771-1776, 2009

Background.—Premedication with midazolam is commonly used in children to reduce anxiety and improve cooperation before anesthesia. However, it has the potential to alter respiratory function because of its muscle relaxant properties. We assessed functional residual capacity (FRC), ventilation homogeneity, using a lung clearance index (LCI), and respiratory mechanics in children awake and 20 min after oral premedication with midazolam (0.3 mg/kg).

Methods.—FRC and LCI were measured using a SF_6 multibreath washout technique while respiratory resistance and elastance were extracted from the input impedance obtained by forced oscillation technique in 18 children (3–8 yr) before and after oral premedication with midazolam.

Results.—Premedication led to a small (6.5%) but statistically significant decrease in group mean FRC from 25.0 (SD 1.4) to 23.4 (1.9) mL/kg and an associated increase in LCI by 7.8% from 6.4 (0.4) to 6.9 (0.4), indicating increased ventilation inhomogeneities. Furthermore, midazolam resulted in a statistically significant increase in respiratory resistance by 7.4% from 3.38 (0.6) to 3.62 (0.6) cm H_2O s/L ($P < 0.001$) and in respiratory elastance by 9.2% from 48.8 to 52.9 cm H_2O s/L ($P < 0.001$). The changes in FRC, LCI, resistance and elastance were significantly correlated ($P < 0.001$).

Conclusions.—In children with normal lungs, premedication with a relatively small-dose of midazolam led to mild changes in respiratory variables shortly after its administration. However, the anesthesiologist should be aware that using midazolam in children at high-risk of respiratory complications under anesthesia might lead to a greater decrease in respiratory function (Table 1).

▶ Midazolam, the most commonly used premedicant in children, has been shown to cause changes in respiratory function that could have potentially deleterious effects. In this prospective trial, respiratory function was assessed before and following anxiolytic doses of midazolam. Statistically significant,

TABLE 1.—Changes in Respiratory Variables Before and After Premedication with Midazolam

	Pre	Post	% Change	*P*
Functional residual capacity (mL/kg)	25.0 (1.4)	23.4 (1.9)	−6.5 (5.0)	<0.001
Lung clearance index	6.40 (0.4)	6.89 (0.4)	7.8 (7.0)	<0.001
Tidal volume (mL/kg)	8.64 (1.4)	8.40 (1.5)	−3.0 (4.9)	0.025
Respiratory rate (per min)	24.6 (3.0)	24.1 (2.9)	−1.7 (5.5)	0.176
Minute ventilation (mL/kg)	213 (47)	202 (46)	−4.7 (6.9)	0.006
Raw (cm H_2O s/L)	3.38 (0.6)	3.62 (0.6)	7.4 (8.8)	<0.001
H (cm H_2O/L)	48.8 (9.7)	52.9 (9.1)	9.2 (8.5)	<0.001

Values are given as mean (SD). Significances as determined with a paired *t*-test.

but small, changes were observed as seen in Table 1 and Fig 1 in the original article. These changes are of questionable clinical significance. However, several factors are important to consider. First, the dose was small and children were not significantly sedated. Second, the post midazolam measurements were taken 20 minutes after an oral dose likely prior to maximal effect. Finally, all children were healthy with no respiratory disease or other comorbidities. The small, but consistent, changes observed in the study setting suggest that larger doses might produce clinically significant deterioration in respiratory function. Likewise, midazolam use in children with compromised respiratory function might also be more likely to cause clinically significant changes in respiratory function.

S. Black, MD

Prediction of Preoperative Anxiety in Children: Who Is Most Accurate?

Maclaren JE, Thompson C, Weinberg M, et al (Univ of California, Irvine; Yale Univ School of Medicine, New Haven, CT; et al)

Anesth Analg 108:1777-1782, 2009

Background.—In this investigation, we sought to assess the ability of pediatric attending anesthesiologists, resident anesthesiologists, and mothers to predict anxiety during induction of anesthesia in 2 to 16-yr-old children ($n = 125$).

Methods.—Anesthesiologists and mothers provided predictions using a visual analog scale and children's anxiety was assessed using a valid behavior observation tool the Modified Yale Preoperative Anxiety Scale. All mothers were present during anesthetic induction and no child received sedative premedication. Correlational analyses were conducted.

Results.—A total of 125 children aged 2–16 yr, their mothers, and their attending pediatric anesthesiologists and resident anesthesiologists were studied. Correlational analyses revealed significant associations between attending predictions and child anxiety at induction ($r_s = 0.38$, $P < 0.001$). Resident anesthesiologist and mother predictions were not significantly related to children's anxiety during induction ($r_s = 0.01$ and 0.001, respectively). In terms of accuracy of prediction, 47.2% of predictions made by attending anesthesiologists were within one standard deviation of the observed anxiety exhibited by the child, and 70.4% of predictions were within two standard deviations.

Conclusions.—We conclude that attending anesthesiologists who practice in pediatric settings are better than mothers in predicting the anxiety of children during induction of anesthesia. Although this finding has significant clinical implications, it is unclear if it can be extended to attending anesthesiologists whose practice is not mostly pediatric anesthesia.

▶ Accurate ability to predict a child's anxiety preoperatively and at induction is an important tool in improving the perioperative experience and outcome for pediatric surgical patients. Perioperative anxiety is an important determinant of a number of negative postoperative events, including increased postoperative pain and increased incidence of maladaptive behaviors postoperatively. Prediction, of which patients would have significant anxiety with induction, would allow interventions to attempt to decrease anxiety before induction and perhaps decreased perioperative problems. This prospective trial looks primarily at the ability of attending pediatric anesthesiologists, anesthesiology residents, and mothers to predict anxiety of pediatric patient with induction of anesthesia. Interestingly, pediatric attending anesthesiologists, but not residents or mothers, were able to predict level of anxiety in the patients at induction. This suggests that experienced pediatric anesthesiologists rather than parents would be the more reliable person to determine whether preoperative sedation should be used. As the authors point out, this study involves anesthesiologists that practice pediatric anesthesiology as their primary clinical activity, and would not necessarily be true of anesthesiologists that care for pediatric patients as a small portion of a general practice.

S. Black, MD

Addition of clonidine or dexmedetomidine to bupivacaine prolongs caudal analgesia in children

El-Hennawy AM, Abd-Elwahab AM, Abd-Elmaksoud AM, et al (Ain-Shams Univ, Cairo, Egypt)
Br J Anaesth 103:268-274, 2009

Background.—Caudal block is a common technique for paediatric analgesia but with the disadvantage of short duration of action after single injection. Caudal dexmedetomidine and clonidine could offer significant analgesic benefits. We compared the analgesic effects and side-effects of dexmedetomidine and clonidine added to bupivacaine in paediatric patients undergoing lower abdominal surgeries.

Methods.—Sixty patients (6 months to 6 yr) were evenly and randomly assigned into three groups in a double-blinded manner. After sevoflurane in oxygen anaesthesia, each patient received a single caudal dose of bupivacaine 0.25% (1 ml kg^{-1}) combined with either dexmedetomidine 2 μg kg^{-1} in normal saline 1 ml, clonidine 2 μg kg^{-1} in normal saline 1 ml, or corresponding volume of normal saline according to group assignment. Haemodynamic variables, end-tidal sevoflurane, and emergence time were monitored. Postoperative analgesia, use of analgesics, and side-effects were assessed during the first 24 h.

Results.—Addition of dexmedetomidine or clonidine to caudal bupivacaine significantly promoted analgesia time [median (95% confidence interval, CI): 16 (14–18) and 12 (3–21) h, respectively] than the use of bupivacaine alone [median (95% CI): 5 (4–6) h] with $P<0.001$. However, there was no statistically significant difference between dexmedetomidine and clonidine as regards the analgesia time ($P=0.796$). No significant difference was observed in incidence of haemodynamic changes or side-effects.

Conclusions.—Addition of dexmedetomidine or clonidine to caudal bupivacaine significantly promoted analgesia in children undergoing

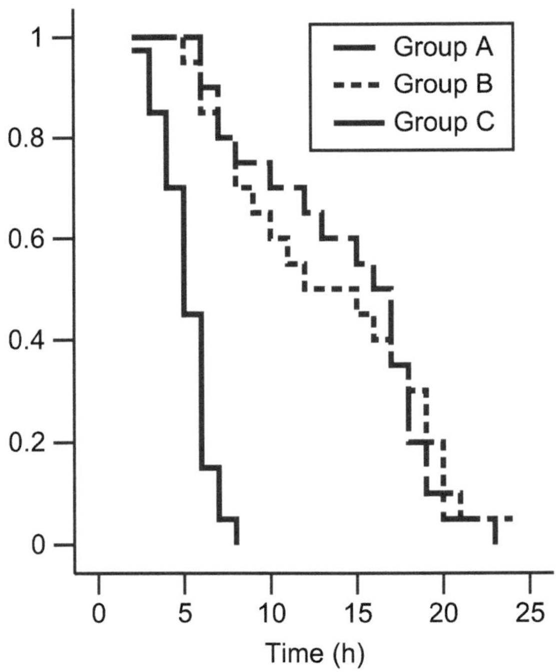

FIGURE 2.—Kaplan–Meier survival curve of time to first analgesic administration. (Reprinted from El-Hennawy AM, Abd-Elwahab AM, Abd-Elmaksoud AM, et al. Addition of clonidine or dexmedetomidine to bupivacaine prolongs caudal analgesia in children. *Br J Anaesth*. 2009;103:268-274, with permission from The Board of Management and Trustees of the British Journal of Anaesthesia, Oxford University Press.)

TABLE 4.—Postoperative Side-Effects and Rehabilitation Data. Values Reported as Mean (SD) or as Frequency (%)

	Group A	Group B	Group C	P-value
PACU duration (min)	68 (14.7)	72 (11.3)	65 (13.1)	0.246
Pruritis	1 (5%)	1 (5%)	2 (10%)	0.765
Diphenhydramine	0 (0%)	1 (5%)	1 (5%)	0.596
PONV (no.)	9 (45%)	8 (40%)	7 (35%)	0.812
Ondansetron	6 (30%)	7 (35%)	5 (25%)	0.788
Time to micturition (h)	8.1 (3.4)	7.6 (2.9)	8.3 (3.1)	0.769
Urinary retention (h)	0 (0%)	0 (0%)	1 (5%)	0.362
Clear liquid intake (h)	4.2 (2.6)	4.9 (2.8)	4.5 (2.8)	0.720
Solid intake (h)	23 (12)	24 (11)	22 (9)	0.841
Discharge home	49 (10)	46 (9)	48 (13)	0.672

lower abdominal surgeries with no significant advantage of dexmedetomidine over clonidine and without an increase in incidence of side-effects (Fig 2, Table 4).

► In a prospective, randomized trial, the authors compared caudal analgesia with 0.25% bupivacaine alone after lower extremity surgery in children with the addition of either dexmedetomidine or clonidine to the caudal. Addition of either agent prolonged the duration of analgesia significantly as seen in Fig 2, but there was no difference between the 2 additives. There was no increase in side effects, delay to micturition, or increased time to discharge in the patients who received either clonidine or dexmedetomidine to the caudal with bupivacaine. The authors note the dexmedetomidine has a number of potential advantages over clonidine. However, none of these were noted in this study suggesting that the less expensive clonidine is the more cost effective choice.

For further reading on this subject I suggest an article by Asano et al.[1]

S. Black, MD

Reference

1. Asano T, Dohi S, Ohata S, Shimonaka H, Idia H. Antinociception by epidural and systemic alpha(2)-adrenoceptor agonists and their binding affinity in rat spinal cord and brain. *Anesth Analg.* 2000;90:400.

Predicting the efficacy of convection warming in anaesthetized children

Stanger R, Colyvas K, Cassey JG, et al (Univ of Newcastle, Australia; John Hunter Hosp, Newcastle, Australia)

Br J Anaesth 103:275-282, 2009

Background.—We previously described a convection warming technique. This study further analyses the children in that original study with three aims: (i) to investigate factors purported to influence children's heating rates, (ii) to describe the most effective usage of this warming technique, and (iii) to understand better the physiology of convection warming.

Methods.—Children having anaesthesia for elective surgery lasting longer than 90 min in ambient temperature 21°C were warmed by a 'Bair Hugger' attached to a custom-built heat dissipation unit. Relationships between child and procedure characteristics and various thermal measures were analysed, and a thermodynamic model was evaluated.

Results.—Thirty-nine children (aged 2 days to 12.5 yr) were studied. There were statistically significant correlations between a number of factors (e.g. height and weight) and heating efficacy. Our model demonstrated the impact of changing patient characteristics on temperature profiles. Neither the morphological characteristics nor our model could predict an individual's T_{core} behaviour.

Conclusions.—(i) Although the effectiveness of this warming technique is influenced by patient/procedure characteristics, these do not predict normothermia (uncertainty ±28 min). Effectiveness is independent of simple thermal measures. (ii) Previously described measures of vasoconstriction are not valid in children. (iii) Our model shows children's thermal properties change with their T_{core}. However, key factors are unknown for an individual and our model does not predict heating efficacy. (iv) To minimize the risk of hyperthermia, we recommend continuous measurement of T_{core} during convection heating. The device air temperature should be turned to medium (38°C) as T_{core} approaches 37°C.

▶ In 39 pediatric patients warmed under general anesthesia with a convection-warming blanket, the authors attempted to identify factors that would effectively predict rate of warming and allow for prediction of time the patient would rewarm to reach normothermia. This would allow for use of convection warming with decreased risk for hyperthermia, which is relatively common in pediatric patients. The authors investigated patient factors, procedure factors, and calculations designed to predict heat deficit at the time warming was initiated. Finally, thermodynamic calculations were evaluated to predict rate of warming. Patient age and size were related to rate of warming with younger smaller patients having a faster rate of warming. Unfortunately, none of the measures investigated allowed accurate prediction of rate of warming. Prediction of time to reach normothermia was no more accurate than ± 28 minutes. The authors concluded the only careful monitoring of core temperature would allow optimal use of convection warming.

S. Black, MD

Medication Overdoses Leading to Emergency Department Visits Among Children

Schillie SF, Shehab N, Thomas KE, et al (CDC, Atlanta, GA)
Am J Prev Med 37:181-187, 2009

Background.—The high prevalence of medication use increases the potential for medication overdoses, especially among children.

Purpose.—This paper describes the burden of unintentional pediatric medication overdoses in order to target new prevention efforts.

Methods.—Data were analyzed in 2007 and 2008 from the National Electronic Injury Surveillance System, collected January 1, 2004, through December 31, 2005, to estimate the number of emergency department visits resulting from unintentional medication overdoses among children aged ≤18 years in the U.S. These data were analyzed by patient demographics, overdose cause, and implicated products, and compared to visits for nonpharmaceutical consumer product poisonings.

Results.—Based on 3034 cases, an estimated 71,224 emergency department visits for medication overdoses were made annually by children aged ≤18 years, representing 68.9% of emergency department visits for unintentional pediatric poisonings. The rate of unintentional poisonings from medications was twice the rate of those from nonpharmaceutical consumer products (9.2 visits per 10,000 individuals per year [95% CI = 7.3, 11.0] vs 4.2 per 10,000 individuals per year [95% CI = 3.3, 5.0]). Four fifths (82.2%) of visits for medication overdoses were from unsupervised ingestions (children accessing medications on their own); medication errors and misuse resulted in 14.3% of visits. Most visits (81.3%) involved children aged ≤5 years, and commonly available over-the-counter medications were implicated in one third (33.9%) of visits.

Conclusions.—Medication overdoses among children, notably unsupervised ingestions, represent a substantial burden in terms of emergency department visits and hospitalizations. New efforts to prevent pediatric medication overdoses are needed.

▶ When you prescribe something for a patient to take home whether for pain therapy or other things, remember to caution the patient. That might be especially true to give written instructions, in that leaving outpatient surgery as the patient and family members may forget about this in an otherwise emotional day. Remember that there are essentially 200 poisonings from accidental childhood ingestions in children mostly under the age of 5 years.

M. F. Roizen, MD

The addition of fentanyl to 1.5 mg/ml ropivacaine has no advantage for paediatric epidural analgesia

Cho JE, Kim JY, Hong JY, et al (Yonsei Univ College of Medicine, Seoul, Korea)

Acta Anaesthesiol Scand 53:1084-1087, 2009

Background.—Epidural opioids are frequently combined with local anaesthetics for an additive antinociceptive effect. We investigated the efficacy of epidural fentanyl to 1.25 or 1.5 mg/ml ropivacaine for post-operative epidural analgesia in children.

Methods.—One hundred and eight children undergoing hypospadias repair were randomized to receive 1.25 mg/ml ropivacaine ($R_{1.25}$ group), 1.25 mg/ml ropivacaine with 0.2 mcg/kg/h of fentanyl ($R_{1.25}F$ group), 1.5 mg/ml ropivacaine ($R_{1.5}$ group) or 1.5 mg/ml ropivacaine with 0.2 mcg/kg/h of fentanyl ($R_{1.5}F$ group) for post-operative epidural analgesia. The epidural catheter was threaded caudally through the L4-5 interspace. The face, legs, activity, cry, consolability (FLACC) score was assessed at every hour and at FLACC score >4, an epidural bolus of 0.5 ml/kg of ropivacaine 1.5 mg/ml was given as the rescue analgesia. The incidence of side effects such as hypoxia, sedation, pruritus, nausea and/or vomiting was recorded.

Results.—The need for rescue analgesia was higher in the $R_{1.25}$ group compared with that in the other three groups (all $P < 0.05$). The incidence of side effects was higher in the $R_{1.5}F$ group compared with that in the $R_{1.25}$ and $R_{1.5}$ groups (both $P = 0.010$).

Conclusion.—The addition of 0.2 mcg/kg/h fentanyl to 1.5 mg/ml ropivacaine increased the incidence of side effects without improvement of analgesia in infants and children undergoing hypospadias repair. The use of plain 1.25 mg/ml ropivacaine increased the need for rescue analgesia and this could be compensated by addition of fentanyl (Table 2).

▶ Addition of narcotic to local anesthetic solutions for epidural infusions for postoperative analgesia has been effective in adult patients. In this randomized

TABLE 2.—Need for Rescue Analgesia and FLACC Score

	Group $R_{1.25}$	Group $R_{1.25}F$	Group $R_{1.5}$	Group $R_{1.5}F$
Need for rescue analgesia	19	5*	8*	5*
FLACC score				
0–6 h	2 (0–8)	2 (0–5)	2 (0–6)	2 (0–6)
6–24 h	0 (0–4)†	0 (0–2)†	0 (0–2)†	0 (0–1)†
24–48 h	0 (0–7)	0 (0–4)†	0 (0–5)†	0 (0–4)†
48–72 h	0 (0–7)	0 (0–4)†	0 (0–2)†	0 (0–5)†

Values are number or median (range).

Group $R_{1.25}$, continuous epidural analgesia with 1.25 mg/ml ropivacaine; Group $R_{1.25}F$, continuous epidural analgesia with 1.25 mg/ml ropivacaine with fentanyl; Group $R_{1.5}$, continuous epidural analgesia with 1.5 mg/ml ropivacaine; Group $R_{1.5}F$, continuous epidural analgesia with 1.5 mg/ml ropivacaine with fentanyl, FLACC, face, legs, activity, cry, consolability.

*$P < 0.05$ compared with Group $R_{1.25}$.

†$P < 0.05$ compared with value during 0–6 h within group.

prospective trial, the efficacy of adding fentanyl to 2 epidural ropivacaine infusions after hypospadias repair was studied. Table 2 shows results related to need for rescue analgesia. The lower dose of ropivacaine was associated with a higher rate of need for rescue analgesia, which was improved with either addition of fentanyl or increasing the dose of ropivacaine. Each maneuver was equally successful. Addition of fentanyl to the higher ropivacaine dose did not improve analgesia but did increase complication rate. The lowest side-effect profile and greatest efficacy for analgesia were seen in the higher dose ropivacaine without fentanyl group. This suggests that in this population, epidural fentanyl has a limited role.

S. Black, MD

Prevention of propofol-induced pain in children: combination of alfentanil and lidocaine *vs* alfentanil or lidocaine alone

Kwak HJ, Min SK, Kim JS, et al (Gachon Univ of Medicine and Science, Incheon, Korea; Ajou Univ School of Medicine, Suwon, Korea)

Br J Anaesth 103:410-412, 2009

Background.—Pain from a propofol injection is a common side-effect in paediatric patients. This prospective, randomized, double-blind study evaluated the efficacy of a combined pretreatment of alfentanil with lidocaine on the incidence and severity of propofol injection pain in children.

Methods.—After obtaining parental consent, 120 paediatric patients were allocated randomly into one of the three groups (n=40, in each). The patients in the alfentanil group received alfentanil 15 $\mu g\,kg^{-1}$ 90 s before the propofol injection. The patients in the lidocaine group received propofol 3 $mg\,kg^{-1}$ premixed with lidocaine 0.1% over a 15 s period. The patients in the combination group received both alfentanil and lidocaine.

Results.—The incidence of propofol injection pain (severity 2 or more) in the combination group (2.6%) was significantly lower than that in the alfentanil and lidocaine groups (30% and 38.5%, respectively) (P=0.001 and <0.001, respectively). No patient in the combination group complained of moderate or severe pain from propofol injection.

Conclusions.—Our study demonstrated that the combination treatment of two different analgesic modalities, alfentanil and lidocaine, could prevent the moderate and severe pain on propofol injection, and reduce the incidence of mild pain compared with each drug alone (Table 2).

▶ In this prospective trial, 120 pediatric patients aged 3 to 10 years undergoing general anesthesia with an intravenous induction without premedication were studied to evaluate efficacy of added anesthetic agents to decrease pain on injection with propofol. Patients received alfentanil, lidocaine mixed with propofol, or both, and pain on injection was assessed. Combination of lidocaine and alfentanil virtually eliminated pain and prevented all but mild pain with injection of propofol as shown in Table 2. It was noted that the use of the alfentanil resulted in decreases in blood pressure; however, there was no significant

TABLE 2.—Incidence and Severity of Pain on the Propofol Injection. Values are Number of Patients (%)

Severity of pain	Alfentanil ($n = 40$)	Lidocaine ($n = 39$)	Combination ($n = 39$)
1 (No pain)	28 (70.0)	24 (61.5)	38 (97.4)*†
2 (Mild pain)	9 (22.5)	10 (25.6)	1 (2.6)*†
3 (Moderate pain)	1 (2.5)	4 (10.3)	0 (0.0)
4 (Severe pain)	2 (5.0)	1 (2.6)	0 (0.0)

*$P<0.05$ compared with the lidocaine group
†$P<0.05$ compared with the alfentanil group

hypotension. The combination of lidocaine and alfentanil was effective in eliminating moderate or severe pain that is otherwise relatively common with propofol injection in children without untoward side effects.

For further reading on this subject I suggest articles by Aouad et al.[1]

S. Black, MD

Reference

1. Aouad MT, Siddik-Sayyid SM, Al-Alami AA, Baraka AS. Multimodal analgesia to prevent propofol-induced pain: pretreatment with remifentanil and lidocaine versus remifentanil or lidocaine alone. *Anesth Analg*. 2007;104:1540-1544.

Monitoring Electrical Skin Conductance: A Tool for the Assessment of Postoperative Pain in Children?

Hullett B, Chambers N, Preuss J, et al (Univ of Western Australia; Princess Margaret Hosp for Children, Western Australia; et al)

Anesthesiology 111:513-517, 2009

Background.—Monitoring changes in electrical skin conductance has been described as a potentially useful tool for the detection of acute pain in adults. The aim of this study was to test the method in pediatric patients.

Methods.—A total of 180 postoperative pediatric patients aged 1–16 yr were included in this prospective, blinded observational study. After arrival in the recovery unit, pain was assessed by standard clinical pain assessment tools (1–3 yr: Face Legs Activity Cry Consolability Scale, 4–7 yr: Revised Faces Scale, 8–16 yr: Visual Analogue Scale) at various time points during their stay in the recovery room. The number of fluctuations in skin conductance per second (NFSC) was recorded simultaneously.

Results.—Data from 165 children were used for statistical analysis, and 15 patients were excluded. The area under the Receiver Operating Characteristic curve for predicting moderate to severe pain from NFSC was 0.82 (95% confidence interval 0.79–0.85). Over all age groups, an NFSC cutoff value of 0.13 was found to distinguish between no or mild

TABLE 1.—Characteristics of the Sample

	Age Group			
	1–3 yrs	4–7 yrs	8–16 yrs	Full Sample
Characteristics of data				
Number of patients	51	54	60	165
Total number of pain assessments	426	377	452	1255
Pain assessments per patient, median (IQR) [minimum–maximum]	8 (6–10) [3–15]	7 (5–8) [4–13]	7 (5–9) [3–18]	7 (6–9) [3–18]
Characteristics of patients				
Age, yrs, mean (SD)	2.3 (0.81)	5.5 (1.21)	12.1 (2.50)	6.9 (4.49)
Anxiety score, mean (SD)	6.9 (3.39)	7.0 (1.61)	6.1 (1.36)	6.7 (2.12)
Operation time, min, mean (SD)	42.1 (36.24)	46.7 (48.79)	60.7 (36.16)	50.4 (41.29)
Body temperature, °C, mean (SD)	36.4 (0.57)	36.2 (0.49)	36.3 (0.48)	36.3 (0.51)
Recovery time, min, mean (SD)	30.9 (7.66)	29.0 (7.79)	28.8 (9.70)	29.5 (8.50)
Characteristics of measurements				
Pain rating category, n (%)				
None (0)	315 (73.9)	310 (82.2)	281 (62.2)	906 (72.2)
Mild (1–3)	30 (7.0)	30 (8.0)	63 (13.9)	123 (9.8)
Moderate (4–5)	38 (8.9)	12 (3.2)	53 (11.7)	103 (8.2)
Severe (6–10)	43 (10.1)	25 (6.6)	55 (12.2)	123 (9.8)
NFSC, median (IQR) [minimum–maximum]	0.13 (0–0.60) [0–2.65]	0 (0–0.13) [0–1.57]	0.07 (0–0.20) [0–2.72]	0.07 (0–0.27) [0–2.72]

IQR = interquartile range; NFSC = number of fluctuations per second; SD = standard deviation.

TABLE 2.—Characteristics of Skin Conductance Test Using the Number of Fluctuations in Skin Conductance per Second (NFSC) of at least 0.13 as a Positive Test Result

Group	Prevalence of Moderate to Severe Pain	Sensitivity (%)	Specificity (%)	PPV	NPV
Whole sample	18.0	90.3	64.0	35.5	96.8
Age 1–3 years	19.1	93.8	52.0	31.5	97.3
Age 4–7 years	9.8	97.3	72.9	28.1	99.6
Age 8–16 years	23.9	85.2	67.1	44.9	93.5

NPV = negative predictive value; PPV = positive predictive value.

versus moderate or severe pain with a sensitivity of 90% and a specificity of 64% (positive predictive value 35%, negative predictive value 97%).

Conclusions.—NFSC accurately predicted the absence of moderate to severe pain in postoperative pediatric patients. The measurement of NFSC may therefore provide an additional tool for pain assessment in this group of patients. However, more research is needed to prospectively investigate the observations made in this study and to determine the clinical applicability of the method (Tables 1 and 2).

► As the authors point out, pain in pediatric patients is a global health issue. This is, in part, due to difficulty in accurately assessing pain in pediatric patients, especially young children. The authors compare a monitor of electrical skin conductance with accepted tools for clinical assessment of pain in children postoperatively. Table 1 shows that severe pain by conventional measures was uncommon. In Table 2, the predictive value of skin conductance measures was compared with the clinical assessment. Using this tool, moderate or severe pain would be effectively recognized but often overdiagnosed. This suggests that this tool, in addition to clinical monitoring, might increase the likelihood that pediatric patients have optimal pain control. However, limitations, such as use of a device on the hands of children recovering from anesthesia, would need to be addressed.

S. Black, MD

A Comparison of High Volume/Low Concentration and Low Volume/High Concentration Ropivacaine in Caudal Analgesia for Pediatric Orchiopexy

Hong J-Y, Han SW, Kim WO, et al (Yonsei Univ College of Medicine, Seoul, Korea)

Anesth Analg 109:1073-1078, 2009

Background.—It is unclear whether the volume or concentration of local anesthetic influences its spread and quality of caudal analgesia when the total drug dose is fixed.

TABLE 2.—Postoperative Data

	LVHC group ($n = 37$)	HVLC group ($n = 36$)	P
Time to recovery (min)			
Oral intake	59.6 ± 26.8	63.6 ± 27.8	0.532
Voiding	138.1 ± 56.8	134.6 ± 51.8	0.788
Discharge	192.4 ± 43.2	191.3 ± 52.0	0.922
Side effects in RR			
Vomiting	2 (5.4%)	3 (8.3%)	0.184
Facial flushing	2 (5.4%)	4 (11.1%)	0.092
Sedation	18 (48.6%)	16 (44.4%)	0.719
Motor weakness	3 (8.1%)	0 (0%)	0.113
Rescue analgesics after discharge			
First acetaminophen time (min)*	363.0 (272.5–420.5)	554.5 (365.0–735.0)	<0.001
Number of patients*	28 (75.7%)	18 (50.0%)	0.030

Data are mean ± SD, number of patients (%), or median (interquartile ranges). Time to recovery is defined as the time from when the patient entered the recovery room to drinking water, self-voiding, and discharge. Rescue analgesic: CHEOPS >4. Sedation: modified Ramsay Sedation Scale >3.

RR = recovery room; LVHC = low volume/high concentration; HVLC = high volume/low concentration.

*$P < 0.05$.

Methods.—We performed this study in a prospective, randomized, observer-blind manner. Children aged 1–5 yr received a constant dose of 2.25 mg/kg of ropivacaine prepared as either 1.0 mL/kg of 0.225% (low volume/high concentration [LVHC], $n = 37$) or 1.5 mL/kg of 0.15% solution (high volume/low concentration [HVLC], $n = 36$). Both solutions contained radiopaque dye.

Results.—The median spread levels with ranges in the HVLC group (confirmed by fluoroscopic examination) were significantly higher (T6, T3-11) than in the LVHC group (T11, T8-L2). There were no significant differences in recovery times, postoperative pain scores, or side effects between the two groups. After discharge, fewer children in the HVLC group required rescue oral acetaminophen compared with the LVHC group (50.0% vs 75.7%). First oral acetaminophen time was found to be significantly longer with HVLC patients than LVHC patients (363.0 min vs 554.5 min).

Conclusions.—We confirmed (with fluoroscopy) that a caudal block with 1 mL/kg ropivacaine spreads to T11 and to T6 with 1.5 mL/kg. If the total dose is fixed, caudal analgesia with a larger volume of diluted ropivacaine (0.15%) provides better quality and longer duration after discharge than a smaller volume of more concentrated ropivacaine (0.225%) in children undergoing day-case orchiopexy. The spread level of ropivacaine correlated significantly with the first oral acetaminophen time after discharge (Table 2).

▶ To help define whether it is primarily drug dose or volume of drug administered for caudal analgesia that determines anesthetic spread and analgesic duration, this prospective randomized, blinded study was carried out. Identical total doses of ropivacaine were given before orchiopexy comparing dilute, high volume with more concentrated, lower total volume preparations with a 50%

difference in volume. Anesthetic spread was significantly greater in the low concentration, high volume group (Fig 2 in the original article). While intraoperative hemodynamics and immediate postoperative pain control were similar (Figs 3 and 4 in the original article), duration of analgesia was longer in the low concentration high volume group. These results suggest that using a dilute solution allows for ideal analgesia while minimizing risk of complications.

For further reading on this subject I suggest articles by Silvani et al,[1] and Verghese et al.[2]

S. Black, MD

References

1. Silvani P, Camporesi A, Agostino MR, Salvo I. Caudal anesthesia in pediatrics: an update. *Minerva Anesthesiol.* 2006;72:453-459.
2. Verghese ST, Hannallah RS, Rice LJ, Belman AB, Patel KM. Caudal anesthesia in children: effect of volume versus concentration of bupivacaine on blocking spermatic cord traction response during orchidopexy. *Anesth Analg.* 2002;95: 1219-1223.

The Risk Factors for Hypoxemia in Children Younger than 5 Years Old Undergoing Rigid Bronchoscopy for Foreign Body Removal

Chen L-H, Zhang X, Li S-Q, et al (Fudan Univ, Shanghai, China; et al)
Anesth Analg 109:1079-1084, 2009

Background.—Removal of an airway foreign body (FB) is usually performed by rigid bronchoscopy under general anesthesia, but the choice of anesthesia and ventilation techniques varies greatly among anesthesiologists and institutions. Hypoxemia is the most commonly observed adverse event during rigid bronchoscopy. It is influenced by a variety of factors including the patient's medical condition, the type of surgical procedure, and the anesthetic technique. In the current study, we investigated risk factors that statistically correlate with intraoperative or postoperative hypoxemia in young patients undergoing rigid bronchoscopy.

Methods.—From January 2007 to December 2008, 384 children younger than 5-yr-of-age subjected to rigid bronchoscopy for FB removal were included in the study. The detailed clinical information and perioperative adverse events were recorded. Surgical outcomes and incidence of perioperative adverse events were compared among different ventilation modes (spontaneous ventilation, manual intermittent positive pressure ventilation, and manual jet ventilation) and different anesthetic techniques (total IV anesthesia and inhaled anesthesia). An amalgamated dataset was used for the analysis of factors that correlated with perioperative hypoxemia.

Results.—In children who received total IV anesthesia with spontaneous ventilation during rigid bronchoscopy, we observed more intraoperative body movement and breath holding, significantly longer duration of emergence from anesthesia, lower percentage of successful FB removal, and

TABLE 3.—Adverse Events in Different Ventilation and Anesthetic Technique Groups

	Controlled Ventilation (CV)		Spontaneous Ventilation (SV)	
	MPPV	MJV	TIVA	SIHA
Body movement (%)	2.2	1.2	11.8*	3.2
Hypoxemia (%)	23.4	9.2*	25.5	16.7
Breath-holding (%)	0	0	13*	3.7
Laryngospasm (%)	7.1	3.1	14.5*	6.7
Postoperative airway obstruction (%)	6	4.1	8.2	7.1
Pneumothorax (case)	3	4	2	0
Reintubation (%)	5	0	8	4
Change of ventilation (%)	0	0	10	3

The data are represented as percentage or number of cases.
MPPV = manual intermittent positive pressure ventilation; MJV = manual jet ventilation; TIVA = total intravenous anesthesia; SIHA = sevoflurane inhaled anesthesia.
*$P < 0.05$ compared with the other three groups.

TABLE 4.—Logistic Regression Model for the Occurrence of Intraoperative Hypoxemia

	B	*P*	OR	95% CI for OR Lower	95% CI for OR Upper
Age	−0.403	0.048	0.668	0.448	0.996
Type of FB	0.976	0.027	2.654	1.118	6.298
Duration of operation	0.139	0.000	1.150	1.094	1.208
Pneumonia	1.345	0.003	3.837	1.602	9.193
Ventilation mode		0.000			
Spontaneous ventilation	1.148	0.035	3.152	1.087	9.140
Jet ventilation	−1.827	0.000	0.161	0.058	0.447

B = coefficient; OR = odds ratio; 95% CI for OR = 95% confidence interval for odds ratio; FB = foreign body.

TABLE 5.—Logistic Regression Model for the Occurrence of Postoperative Hypoxemia

	B	*P*	OR	95% CI for OR Lower	95% CI for OR Upper
Type of FB	1.190	0.036	3.289	1.081	10.000
Duration of emergence from anesthesia	0.152	0.000	1.164	1.097	1.236

B = coefficient; OR = odds ratio; 95% CI for OR = 95% confidence interval for odds ratio; FB = foreign body.

more postoperative laryngospasm. Children in the manual jet ventilation group had the least occurrence of intraoperative hypoxemia. Five factors strongly correlated with intraoperative hypoxemia. Younger age, plant seed as the type of FB, longer surgical duration, pneumonia before the procedure, and spontaneous ventilation mode significantly increased the risk of intraoperative hypoxemia, whereas manual jet ventilation mode decreased it. Two factors were associated with postoperative hypoxemia: plant seed as a FB and prolonged duration of emergence from anesthesia.

Conclusion.—We identified risk factors associated with intraoperative or with postoperative hypoxemia in rigid bronchoscopy which included patient age, type of FB, duration of surgical procedure, pneumonia before the procedure, ventilation mode, and duration of emergence from anesthesia. These results provide evidence that will help clinicians to reduce the incidence of hypoxemia in high-risk children (Tables 3-5).

▶ This large, prospective, observational study presents some interesting findings. First, it is important to note that this study was conducted at a center that has a great deal of experience with these procedures, as evidenced by the fact that 384 patients were included in the study in an 18-month period of time. The authors divided patients by intraoperative ventilation mode (spontaneous or controlled) and intraoperative anesthetic type. In addition, patient demographics, complications related to the presence of a foreign body in particular pneumonia, and the type of foreign body were noted. Tables 3-5 reveal the authors findings regarding risk factors for intraoperative and postoperative complications. Hypoxemia was the most common. Patients who had spontaneous ventilation had a higher incidence of hypoxemia, and total intravenous anesthesia for spontaneous ventilation was associated with a higher incidence of intraoperative movement and delayed emergence. Jet ventilation resulted in the lowest incidence of hypoxemia. These findings suggest that the historical preference for spontaneous ventilation in these cases may no longer be the optimal approach.

S. Black, MD

Children's Desire for Perioperative Information

Fortier MA, Chorney JM, Rony RYZ, et al (Univ of California, Irvine; Univ of Wisconsin, Madison; et al)

Anesth Analg 109:1085-1090, 2009

Background.—The purpose of this investigation was to identify what perioperative information children want to receive from the medical staff.

Methods.—As a first step, we developed an instrument based on a qualitative study conducted with children in Great Britain, input from a focus group, and input from school children. On the day of surgery, 143 children aged 7–17 yr completed a 40-item assessment of desired surgical information and a measure of anxiety (State-Trait Anxiety Inventory for Children). Parents completed a measure assessing their child's temperament (Emotionality, Activity, Sociability, and Impulsivity Survey) and a measure of their own anxiety (State-Trait Anxiety Inventory).

TABLE 2.—Children's Desire for Information (CDI) Frequencies—"I Really Have to Know"

Percentage Endorsed	Content of Question
22.6	1. When I am awake will you tell me what happens next the whole time?
36.5	2. Will the doctor come and see me before the operation?
51.8	3. Will the doctor tell me about the operation and what it will be like when I go home?
54.0	4. When will I get to go home?
43.1	5. What is going to happen?
43.8	6. What are they going to do?
51.8	7. What am I allowed to eat before the operation? After the operation?
37.5	8. What will they do to me?
36.8	9. Will I get a needle?
38.2	10. What will happen afterward?
14.0	11. Will I lie down?
56.6	12. When will I eat after the operation?
29.6	13. When will I go back to school?
39.3	14. Will I have to come back?
33.3	15. Will I go back to the hospital?
47.8	16. How long will I be asleep for?
44.0	17. How will they put me to sleep?
41.0	18. How do you get put to sleep?
61.9	19. Will I wake up in the middle of the surgery?
46.3	20. How long will the operation take?
40.3	21. How long will I be in the operating room?
52.3	22. Will I stay overnight?
42.4	23. How long will I be in the hospital?
35.1	24. How long will I be away from school after the operation?
28.2	25. What does the operating room look like?
26.0	26. What does the recovery room look like?
24.4	27. Are you allowed to use game boys?
58.0	28. Will my mom and dad be there when I wake up?
51.1	29. When you are asleep will you feel it?
63.1	30. Will the operation hurt?
71.5	31. Will there be pain? If so how bad will it be?
66.2	32. Will I feel any pain?
67.7	33. How long will I be in pain after the operation?
53.1	34. How is it going to feel?
51.5	35. Will I feel sick or drowsy after the operation?
57.7	36. Will I be alright?
53.1	37. Can this problem I have come back?
40.0	38. Will I have scars?
36.9	39. What will the cut be like?
23.1	40. Who will mind my pet?

Results.—Results indicated that the vast majority of children had a desire for comprehensive information about their surgery, including information about pain and anesthesia, and procedural information and information about potential complications. The most highly endorsed items by children involved information about pain. Children who were more anxious endorsed a stronger desire for pain information and lesser tendency to avoid information. Younger children wanted to know what the perioperative environment would look like more than adolescent children.

TABLE 3.—Five Most Highly Endorsed Items by Children in Information Desired and Information Avoidance Category

Percentage Endorsed	
I really have to know + I might want to know	
91.5	How long will I be in pain after the operation?
89.3	Will I feel any pain?
88.4	Will there be pain? If so, how bad will it be?
87.7	Will the operation hurt?
86.2	Will I be alright?
I don't want to know	
19.1	Will I get a needle?
13.1	What are they going to do?
12.6	Will I have to come back?
12.5	What will they do to me?
12.3	What will the cut be like?

Conclusions.—We conclude that the majority of children aged 7–17 yr who undergo surgery want to be given comprehensive perioperative information and health care providers should ensure adequate information regarding postoperative pain is provided (Tables 2 and 3).

▶ In this very interesting and well-conducted study, the authors investigated the types of information that children aged 7 years to 17 years wanted to know or desired not to know before elective surgical procedures. The authors recognized the limitation in using parents as proxies for children to determine what information should be discussed preoperatively. Tables 2 and 3 indicate the percentage of children who wanted to know information contained in 40 questions and what information was most desired most commonly and avoided most commonly. It is interesting that most children desired answers to most questions posed, in particular related to pain, eating, and expectations for going home. Also interesting is that the more anxious the child, the more information was desired. What is not evaluated in this study is the impact of providing the information that the pediatric patients in this study indicated they wanted to know. Fig 1 in the original article shows suggested information to discuss with pediatric patients. The next phase would be to compare anxiety and perioperative behavior between pediatric patients who have a structured approach to providing information based on these results with those who do not.

S. Black, MD

Effect of prophylactic paracetamol administration at time of vaccination on febrile reactions and antibody responses in children: two open-label, randomised controlled trials

Prymula R, Siegrist C-A, Chlibek R, et al (Univ of Defence, Hradec Kralove, Czech Republic; Univ of Geneva, Switzerland)

Lancet 374:1339-1350, 2009

Background.—Although fever is part of the normal inflammatory process after immunisation, prophylactic antipyretic drugs are sometimes recommended to allay concerns of high fever and febrile convulsion. We assessed the effect of prophylactic administration of paracetamol at vaccination on infant febrile reaction rates and vaccine responses.

Methods.—In two consecutive (primary and booster) randomised, controlled, open-label vaccination studies, 459 healthy infants were enrolled from ten centres in the Czech Republic. Infants were randomly assigned with a computer-generated randomisation list to receive three prophylactic paracetamol doses every 6–8 h in the first 24 h (n = 226) or no prophylactic paracetamol (n = 233) after each vaccination with a ten-valent pneumococcal non-typeable *Haemophilus influenzae* protein D-conjugate vaccine (PHiD-CV) co-administered with the hexavalent diphtheria-tetanus-3-component acellular pertussis-hepatitis B-inactivated poliovirus types 1, 2, and 3-H *influenzae* type b (DTPa-HBV-IPV/Hib) and oral human rotavirus vaccines. The primary objective in both studies was the reduction in febrile reactions of 38·0°C or greater in the total vaccinated cohort. The second objective was assessment of immunogenicity in the according-to-protocol cohort. These studies are registered with ClinicalTrials.gov, numbers NCT00370318 and NCT00496015.

Findings.—Fever greater than 39·5°C was uncommon in both groups (after primary: one of 226 participants [<1%] in prophylactic paracetamol group *vs* three of 233 [1%] in no prophylactic paracetamol group; after booster: three of 178 [2%] *vs* two of 172 [1%]). The percentage of children with temperature of 38°C or greater after at least one dose was significantly lower in the prophylactic paracetamol group (94/226 [42%] after primary vaccination and 64/178 [36%] after booster vaccination) than in the no prophylactic paracetamol group (154/233 [66%] after primary vaccination and 100/172 [58%] after booster vaccination). Antibody geometric mean concentrations (GMCs) were significantly lower in the prophylactic paracetamol group than in the no prophylactic paracetamol group after primary vaccination for all ten pneumococcal vaccine serotypes, protein D, antipolyribosyl-ribitol phosphate, antidiphtheria, antitetanus, and antipertactin. After boosting, lower antibody GMCs persisted in the prophylactic paracetamol group for antitetanus, protein D, and all pneumococcal serotypes apart from 19F.

Interpretation.—Although febrile reactions significantly decreased, prophylactic administration of antipyretic drugs at the time of vaccination should not be routinely recommended since antibody responses to several vaccine antigens were reduced.

▶ One of the reasons for prophylactic acetaminophen is that a large percentage of kids get febrile reaction after immunization. It is thought that you prevent some of the adverse effects of immunization by preventing the febrile reactions. One of the adverse effects of febrile reactions is that those vulnerable to mitochondrial disorders can have them provoked by febrile reactions—as is one of the rare forms of autism provoked by febrile reactions. That is, one of the very rare and very few associations we know of vaccinations and autism that is in people who have the risk of autism from mitochondrial disease beforehand and would get it with another febrile reaction, get it after a febrile reaction to immunization.

While prophylactic administration of Tylenol or other drugs that decrease febrile reactions seems like a good idea, such administration of Tylenol decreases successful antibodies generation significantly. Thus, the best prophylaxis against the febrile reaction is hydration beforehand, and aggressively preventing and treating such febrile reactions with more hydration afterwards.

M. F. Roizen, MD

The Effects of Propofol Infusion on Hepatic and Pancreatic Function and Acid-Base Status in Children Undergoing Craniotomy and Receiving Phenytoin

Türe H, Mercan A, Koner O, et al (Yeditepe Univ School of Medicine, Istanbul, Turkey)

Anesth Analg 109:366-371, 2009

Background.—In this study, we investigated the effects of propofol infusion on hepatic and pancreatic enzymes and acid-base status compared with baseline values in children undergoing craniotomy who were receiving phenytoin for antiepileptic prophylaxis.

Methods.—In this prospective clinical study, we measured the serum aspartate aminotransferase (AST), alanine aminotransferase (ALT), γ-glutamyl transpeptidase (GGT), alkaline phosphatase (ALP), pancreatic amylase, lipase, and triglyceride levels of 30 children ranging from 4 to 12 yr. All children received propofol anesthesia and were taking phenytoin for antiepileptic prophylaxis. Patients already receiving phenytoin were continued on their medication. Peroral 5 mg $\cdot$ kg^{-1} $\cdot$ d^{-1} phenytoin was started in patients who were not receiving phenytoin. Serum AST, ALT, GGT, ALP, bilirubin, pancreatic amylase, lipase, and triglyceride levels were studied on admission to the hospital, 1 day before surgery, and on postoperative Days 1, 3, 5, and 7. Arterial blood gas samplings were taken after tracheal intubation, during the operation (2nd and 4th h), just after extubation, and 1, 2, 6, and 12 h after extubation.

TABLE 3.—The Percentage of Patients with Elevated Enzymes Levels

Variables (Normal Range)	% (*n*)
AST (<38 U/L)	17 (5)
ALT (<49 U/L)	71 (21)
GGT (<24 U/L)	80 (24)
ALP (<300 U/L)	37 (11)
Pancreatic amylase (35–120 U/L)	27 (8)
Lipase (15–45 U/L)	13 (7)
Triglyceride (<190 mg/dL)	37 (11)

AST = aminotransferase; ALT = alanine aminotransferase; GGT = γ-glutamyl transpeptidase; ALP = alkaline phosphatase.

Results.—Serum AST, ALT, GGT, ALP, pancreatic amylase, lipase, and triglyceride levels were increased significantly in the postoperative period compared with baseline with a peak value on postoperative Day 1 and returned to normal values within a week. Base excess levels after extubation were significantly decreased compared with baseline. They were in the normal range, however, and returned to baseline values by 6 h after surgery. There were no clinical signs of hepatitis or pancreatitis. Bilirubin levels were normal. None of the children developed complications related to the liver or pancreas during the 4–6 mo after surgery.

Conclusions.—Despite the slightly increased pancreatic and hepatic enzyme levels during the postoperative period, anesthesia maintenance with propofol in children undergoing craniotomy had no significant clinical effect on the acid-base status or pancreas or liver enzymes (Table 3).

▶ In this prospective study, the impact of short term propofol infusion in children receiving phenytoin was investigated on liver and pancreatic enzymes, acid-base status, and triglyceride levels were studied. Transient elevations in liver and pancreatic enzymes as well as triglycerides were noted. However, on average these levels remained within normal ranges as seen in Figs 1, 2 and 3 in the original article. Table 3 reports the percentage of patients with elevated enzymes postoperatively, but most had retuned to normal levels at hospital discharge. Results of this small study suggest that short term propofol infusions in children, even those receiving other drugs known to impact liver function, are safe.

S. Black, MD

A comparison of the laryngeal mask airway with the facemask and oropharyngeal airway for manual ventilation by first responders in children

Blevin AE, McDouall SF, Rechner JA, et al (John Radcliffe Hosp, Oxford, UK; Royal Berkshire Hosp, Reading, UK)

Anaesthesia 64:1312-1316, 2009

In adults, first responders to a cardiopulmonary arrest provide better ventilation using a laryngeal mask airway than a facemask. It is unclear if the same is true in children. We investigated this by comparing the ability of 36 paediatric ward nurses to ventilate the lungs of 99 anaesthetised children (a model for cardiopulmonary arrest) using a laryngeal mask airway and using a facemask with an oropharyngeal airway. Anteroposterior chest wall displacement was measured using an ultrasonic detector. Nurses achieved successful ventilation in 74 (75%) of cases with the laryngeal mask airway and 76 (77%) with facemask and oropharyngeal airway ($p = 0.89$). Median (IQR [range]) time to first breath was longer for the laryngeal mask airway (48 (39–65 [8–149])) s than the facemask/airway (35 (25–53 [14–120]) s; $p < 0.0001$). In 10 cases (10%) the lungs were ventilated using the laryngeal mask airway but not using the facemask/ oropharyngeal airway. We conclude that ventilation is achieved rapidly using a facemask and oropharyngeal airway, and that the laryngeal

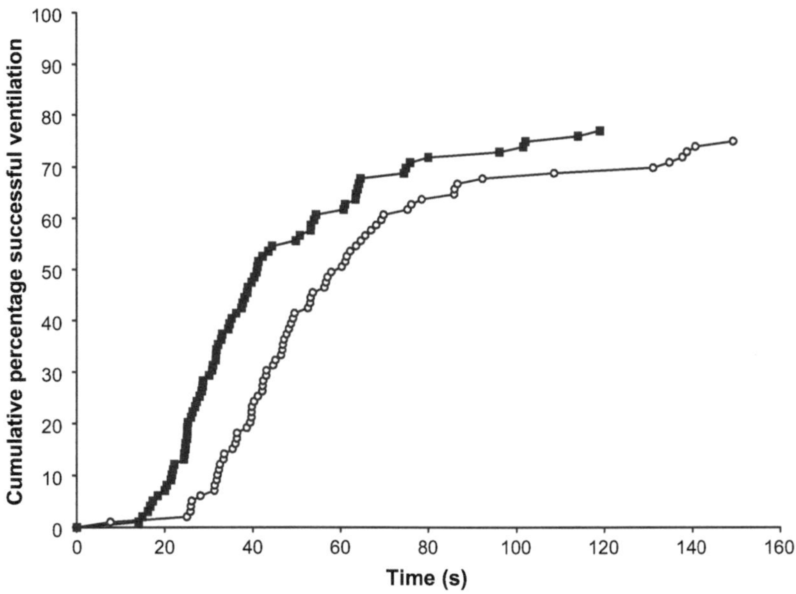

FIGURE 2.—Cumulative frequency plot showing time to first successful ventilation by paediatric ward nurses for both the laryngeal mask airway (open circles) and facemask with oropharyngeal airway (filled squares). (Reprinted from Blevin AE, McDouall SF, Rechner JA, et al. A comparison of the laryngeal mask airway with the facemask and oropharyngeal airway for manual ventilation by first responders in children. *Anaesthesia*. 2009;64:1312-1316, with permission from John Wiley & Sons, Inc.)

TABLE 1.—Number of Attempts Required for Successful Placement of the Laryngeal Mask Airway (LMA) or Facemask and to Achieve 60% or More of the Reference Standard* Anteroposterior Chest Expansion. Values Are Number (Proportion).

	LMA (*n* = 99)	Facemask (*n* = 99)	p value
First attempt	67 (68%)	76 (77%)	
Second attempt	6 (6%)	0	
Third attempt	1 (1%)	0	
Total successful ventilation	74 (75%)	76 (77%)	0.868

*Defined as the average chest displacement achieved by the senior anaesthetist over five breaths using facemask ventilation.

mask airway may represent a useful second line option for first responders (Fig 2, Table 1).

▶ Laryngeal mask airway (LMA) has been suggested to be an appropriate early tool for use by first responders to cardiopulmonary arrest who are not experienced in advanced airway techniques. In this study, the success rate and time to success in ventilation of anesthetized pediatric patients by pediatric ward nurses was studied to determine the efficacy of LMA compared with ventilation with a mask and oral airway in pediatric patients. Fig 2 in the original article reveals that time to initial breath was slightly longer for LMA use. In Table 1, success rates were similar between the two tools. The nurses had not had previous significant experience with the LMA. A significant limitation is that the appropriate size LMA and oral airway were chosen by an experienced anesthetist. The authors conclude that an LMA is an appropriate device for first responders in pediatric arrest situations.

S. Black, MD

Prospective randomized controlled multi-centre trial of cuffed or uncuffed endotracheal tubes in small children

Weiss M, Dullenkopf A, Fischer JE, et al (Univ Children's Hosp Zurich, Switzerland; Univ of Heidelberg, Germany; et al)
Br J Anaesth 103:867-873, 2009

Background.—The use of cuffed tracheal tubes (TTs) in small children is still controversial. The aim of this study was to compare post-extubation morbidity and TT exchange rates when using cuffed *vs* uncuffed tubes in small children.

Methods.—Patients aged from birth to 5 yr requiring general anaesthesia with TT intubation were included in 24 European paediatric anaesthesia centres. Patients were prospectively randomized into a cuffed TT group (Microcuff® PET) and an uncuffed TT group (Mallinckrodt®, Portex®, Rüsch®, Sheridan®). Endpoints were incidence of post-extubation stridor and the number of TT exchanges to find an appropriate-sized tube. For cuffed TTs, minimal cuff pressure required to seal the airway was noted; maximal cuff pressure was limited at 20 cm H_2O with a pressure release valve. Data are mean (SD).

Results.—A total of 2246 children were studied (1119/1127 cuffed/uncuffed). The age was 1.93 (1.48) yr in the cuffed and 1.87 (1.45) yr in the uncuffed groups. Post-extubation stridor was noted in 4.4% of patients with cuffed and in 4.7% with uncuffed TTs (P=0.543). TT exchange rate was 2.1% in the cuffed and 30.8% in the uncuffed groups (P<0.0001). Minimal cuff pressure required to seal the trachea was 10.6 (4.3) cm H_2O.

Conclusions.—The use of cuffed TTs in small children provides a reliably sealed airway at cuff pressures of ≤20 cm H_2O, reduces the need for TT exchanges, and does not increase the risk for post-extubation stridor compared with uncuffed TTs (Tables 5-7).

▶ In this large, prospective trial, use of cuffed versus uncuffed endotracheal tubes was compared in young children under the age of 5. When the properly

TABLE 5.—Primary Outcomes: Post-Extubation Morbidity and Therapy

	Cuffed Tubes Final After Exchanges (n = 1197)	Uncuffed Tubes Final After Exchanges (n = 1049)	Cuffed Tubes Initial without Exchange (n = 1095)	Uncuffed Tubes Initial Without Exchange (n = 780)
Duration of tracheal intubation (min) [mean (SD)]	107.5 (79.9)	99.0 (72.8)**	103.0 (76.6)	93.8 (71.7)**
Extubation (awake/asleep)	49.0%/51.0%	46.7%/51.4%	48.2%/51.8%	43.6%/56.4%
Laryngospasm	4.5%	3.5%	4.6%	3.4%
Time from extubation to assessment (min) [mean (SD)]	30.4 (27.6)	27.6 (24.4)*	30.6 (27.7)	26.4 (23.3)*
Inspiratory stridor: all	4.4%	4.7%	4.3%	4.4%
Inspiratory stridor: with signs of severe dyspnoea	0.33%	0.29%	0.37%	0.26%
Epinephrine nebulizer (% patients with stridor/% all patients)	18.9/0.84	30.6/1.44	15.1/0.73	22.4/1.40
NSAID (% patients with stridor/% all patients)	30.2/1.38	36.7/1.72	30.2/1.47	30.6/2.1
Systemic steroids (% patients with stridor/% all patients)	20.8/0.92	22.4/1.05	15.1/0.73	18.4/1.15
Unplanned ICU-admission (% patients with stridor/% all patients)	5.6/0.25	2.1/0.10	5.7/0.27	2.04/1.13
Need for re-intubation (% patients with stridor /% all patients)	3.8/0.18	2.1/0.10	3.8/0.18	2.04/1.13

*P < 0.05
**P < 0.01

TABLE 6.—Stridor Rates PER Age Group. NS, Not Significant

Age Groups	Cuffed Tubes (final) (n)	Stridor (n)	Uncuffed Tubes (Final) (n)	Stridor (n)
All (A–D)	1197	53 (4.4%)	1049	49 (4.7%)^{NS}
A: 0 to <8 months	326	9 (2.8%)	298	14 (4.7%)^{NS}
B: 8 to <18 months	247	15 (6.1%)	234	8 (3.4%)^{NS}
C: 18 to <36 months	311	15 (4.8%)	266	17 (6.4%)^{NS}
D: 36 to <60 months	313	14 (4.8%)	251	10 (4.0%)^{NS}

TABLE 7.—Reasons for Tube Exchange and Incidence; Data Expressed as Number of Incidents or as Indicated

	Cuffed Tubes Initial ($n=1119$)	Uncuffed Tubes Initial ($n=1127$)
Tube passage		
Resistance to pass into the trachea	7	46***
Leakage (n tested)	1112	1081
>20 cm H_2O inflation pressure for air leak	10	112***
Sealing (n tested)	1102	969
Peak inspiratory pressure used (cm H_2O) [mean (SD)]	17.3 (3.4)	16.3 (3.2)***
No audible air leak	1018	398
Acceptable air leak	78	383
Excessive air leak	6	188
Minimal cuff pressure for sealing cm H_2O [mean (SD)]	10.6 (4.3)	—
Tube exchange		
Tube exchange	24 (2.1%)	347 (30.8%)****
Reason for tube exchange		
Resistance to pass the tube	7	46***
No air leak at 20 cm H_2O	10	112***
Excessive air leak at IPPV	6	188***
Others (too long preformed tube)	1	1
Patients with more than one tube exchange	5	87***
Total number of tube exchanges	29	434***
Throat pack used	2.7%	10.0%**

**$P=0.01$
***$P<0.001$
****$P<0.0001$

chosen size cuffed tube, there was no increase in postoperative stridor associated with use of cuffed tubes in any age group as shown in Tables 5 and 6. The incidence of multiple intubations was significantly greater in the uncuffed group as shown in Table 7, and the incidence of successful capnography was higher with use of properly placed cuffed endotracheal tubes. Clearly, appropriately sized and positioned cuffed endotracheal tubes with cuff inflated to minimal levels can be used safely in children of all ages and may have benefits.

S. Black, MD

Healthcare Provider and Parent Behavior and Children's Coping and Distress at Anesthesia Induction

Chorney JM, Torrey C, Blount R, et al (Dalhousie Univ, Nova Scotia, Canada; Univ of California, Irvine; Univ of Georgia, Athens; et al)

Anesthesiology 111:1290-1296, 2009

Background.—To date, no study has evaluated the impact of specific healthcare provider and parent behaviors on children's distress and coping during anesthesia induction.

Method.—Extensive digital video data were collected on 293 two-to ten-yr-old children undergoing anesthesia induction with a parent present. Anesthesiologist, nurse, and parent behavior and children's distress and coping were coded using the Revised Preoperative Child–Adult Medical Procedure Interaction Scale administered using specialized coding software.

Results.—Anesthesiologists and parents engaged in higher rates of most behaviors than nurses. Overall, adult emotion-focused behavior such as empathy and reassurance was significantly positively related to children's distress and negatively related to children's coping behaviors. Adult distracting behavior such as humor and distracting talk showed the opposite pattern. Medical reinterpretation by anesthesiologists was significantly positively related to children's coping behaviors, but the same behavior by parents was significantly positively related to children's distress.

TABLE 1.—Rates of Adult Behaviors during Anesthesia Induction

	Anesthesiologists	Nurses	Parents	Friedman Statistic
Reassurance				
Mean (SD)	0.74 (0.73)[a]	0.14 (0.34)[b]	0.81 (1.27)[a]	195.8*
Median (IQR)	0.55 (0.76)	0.00 (0.13)	0.30 (1.03)	
Empathy				
Mean (SD)	0.04 (0.18)[a]	0.01 (0.05)[b]	0.02 (0.16)[a,b]	15.41*
Median (IQR)	0.00 (0.00)	0.00 (0.00)	0.00 (0.00)	
Nonprocedural talk				
Mean (SD)	0.67 (0.93)[a]	0.07 (0.22)[c]	0.35 (0.63)[b]	156.6*
Median (IQR)	0.33 (0.94)	0.00 (0.00)	0.00 (0.48)	
Humor				
Mean (SD)	0.75 (0.72)[a]	0.23 (0.46)[b]	0.67 (0.77)[a]	161.8*
Median (IQR)	0.57 (0.84)	0.00 (0.27)	0.44 (0.98)	
Reinterpretation				
Mean (SD)	2.74 (2.05)[a]	0.39 (0.57)[c]	0.98 (1.17)[b]	284.3*
Median (IQR)	0.24 (0.53)	0.63 (1.52)		
Empathic touch				
Mean (SD)	0.11 (0.16)[b]	0.04 (0.10)[c]	0.52 (0.31)[a]	322.5*
Median (IQR)	0.03 (0.15)	0.00 (0.02)	0.56 (0.48)	

Different superscript letters denote differences between adults at $P < 0.001$ (*e.g.*, values in a row with superscript a are not significantly different, but are significantly higher than those with superscript b).

IQR = interquartile range.

*$P < 0.001$.

TABLE 2.—Correlations among Adult Behaviors during Anesthesia Induction

	Anesthesiologist–Parent	Nurse–Parent	Anesthesiologist–Nurse
Reassurance	0.358*	0.216*	0.13
Empathy	0.126	0.072	0.026
Nonprocedural talk	0.432*	0.194*	0.056
Humor	0.327*	0.199*	0.200*
Reinterpretation	0.133	0.079	−0.083
Empathic touch	−0.064	0.042	0.039

Spearman rank order correlations.
*$P < 0.001$.

TABLE 3.—Relations between Adults Behavior and Children's Distress and Regulating Behaviors

	Child Distress Behavior	Child Regulating Behavior
Emotion-focused behavior (all adults)	0.575*	−0.269*
Distracting behavior (all adults)	−0.210*	0.286*
Reinterpretation		
Anesthesiologist	−0.077	0.370*
Parent	0.202*	0.042
Nurse	−0.020	0.023

Emotion-focused behavior includes reassurance, empathy, and empathic touch; distracting behavior includes nonprocedural talk and humor. Spearman rank order correlations reported.
*$P < 0.001$.

Conclusions.—The data presented here provide evidence for a relation between adult behaviors and children's distress and coping at anesthesia induction. These behaviors are trainable, and hence it is possible to test whether modifying physician behavior can influence child behavior in future studies (Tables 1-3).

► Distress during induction of anesthesia in pediatric patients is a common problem and may be correlated with postoperative problems, such as increased pain and maladaptive behavior. In this observational trial, the impact of adult behavior on the pediatric patient's distress or coping mechanisms was investigated. Adult behaviors were defined as emotion focused (empathy, reassurance, empathetic touch), distracting (talk about nonmedical topics, humor), and reinterpretation (describing medical devices and procedures as something else—mask induction as astronaut game, for example). Table 1 shows the rates of each type of behavior by adults, Table 2 shows the correlation between behavior of the adults in the operating room, and Table 3 shows the impact of adult behavior on the child's behavior. There are 2 particularly interesting points. First, emotion-focused behavior that intuitively would seem to be helpful actually increased distress and decreased coping in the child. Similar findings have been seen in office procedures. In addition, adult behaviors were linked, suggesting that adults take cues for behavior from each other. These results suggest, as the authors note, that training anesthesiologists and nurses to use distress-reducing, distracting behaviors could influence parents to do the same, which would, overall, decrease distress behavior in the patient. This is a potential low risk intervention to improve the perioperative experience for pediatric patients.

For further reading on this subject I suggest an article by Manimala et al.[1]

S. Black, MD

Reference

1. Manimala M, Blount R, Cohen L. The effects of parental reassurance versus distraction on child distress and coping during immunizations. *Child Health Care*. 2000;29:161-177.

The Incidence of Intraoperative Awareness in Children: Childhood Awareness and Recall Evaluation

Malviya S, Galinkin JL, Bannister CF, et al (Univ of Michigan Health Systems, Ann Arbor; Univ of Colorado, Denver, CO; Emory Univ, Atlanta, GA)

Anesth Analg 109:1421-1427, 2009

Background.—There is a considerable discrepancy between the reported incidences of awareness under anesthesia in children (0.2%–2.7%). In this prospective, observational, cohort study we evaluated 1) the incidence of awareness during general anesthesia in children across three settings, 2) factors contributing to awareness, and 3) short-term psychological effects of awareness.

Methods.—Children (aged 5–15 yr) who underwent general anesthesia were included, and all perioperative data including anesthetic drugs were collected prospectively. Children were interviewed three times postoperatively using a semistructured questionnaire. All cases of possible or probable awareness were discussed with the child's care providers to confirm or refute the memories. Internal consensus among investigators across sites was reached, and these cases and a random selection of others were reviewed by three external reviewers. For the purpose of this study, possible/probable awareness was defined as cases with agreement between the internal consensus and at least two of the three external reviewers.

Results.—One thousand seven hundred eighty-four children completed at least one interview. Thirty-two cases were coded as possible or probable awareness by at least one entity (i.e., either the internal consensus or one of the external reviewers). Fourteen of these cases met the definition for possible/probable awareness, making the incidence of awareness 0.8%. Six of the 14 children with awareness (43%) remembered feeling scared during their surgery and three (21%) reported hurting. Two children in this group (14%) said they would feel worse if they had to have surgery again, which was not significantly different from reports of children with no recall (15%). None of the children with awareness required

TABLE 4.—Relationship Between Demographics, Perioperative Factors, and Awareness

	No Awareness ($n = 1770$)	Possible/Probable Awareness ($n = 14$)
Age	10 ± 3.2	10.5 ± 2.4
Male gender	961 (54%)	9 (64%)
ASA I–II	1648 (93%)	13 (93%)
ASA III-IV	122 (7%)	1 (7%)
Surgical procedure		
Endoscopic procedure	194 (11%)	5 (36%)*
Cardiac[a]	8 (<1%)	0
Otorhinolaryngology	413 (23%)	3 (21%)
Orthopedic	382 (22%)	2 (14%)
Urologic	219 (12%)	2 (14%)
Ophthalmologic	146 (8%)	0
General surgery[b]	330 (19%)	2 (14%)
Diagnostic procedures[c]	53 (3%)	0
Other[d]	25 (1%)	0
Perioperative medications		
Benzodiazepine	654 (37%)	7 (50%)
Opiate	1543 (87%)	12 (86%)
Propofol	1225 (69%)	9 (64%)
Sevoflurane	1542 (87%)	13 (93%)
Nitrous oxide	1616 (91%)	14 (100%)
Isoflurane	1039 (59%)	9 (64%)
Neuromuscular blockade	370 (21%)	3 (21%)
Airway management		
Endotracheal intubation	1210 (69%)	12 (86%)
Laryngeal mask	515 (29%)	2 (14%)
Face mask	34 (2%)	0
>1 intubation attempts	95 (5%)	1 (7%)
Anesthesia duration (min)	87.7 ± 71.6	75.7 ± 68.6

[a]Includes seven cardiopulmonary bypass cases and one nonpump.
[b]Includes abdominal, gynecologic, peripheral, plastics, thoracic (noncardiac).
[c]Includes radiologic imaging, cardiac catheterization.
[d]Includes neurologic, renal, vascular.
*$P = 0.014$ versus all other procedures (relative risk = 4.5 [1.5–13.6]).

psychological follow-up. Endoscopic procedures were associated with a higher risk for awareness (relative risk = 4.5 [confidence interval 1.5–13.6]).

Conclusions.—Although 0.8% of children experienced possible/probable awareness in this study, none experienced short-term psychological distress (Table 4).

▶ The authors studied over 1 700 pediatric patients prospectively at 3 institutions to access incidence of recall in children. The incidence of 0.8% is slightly higher than that reported in adults. Table 4 includes factors evaluated and their relationship to awareness in this study. Interestingly, anesthetic technique did not influence risk—including the use of benzodiazepines or muscle relaxants. Unlike adults, children did not appear to have short-term psychological consequences related to their awareness experience even though many felt fear and/or pain. The authors review potential reasons for these differences.

S. Black, MD

Intraocular pressures after ketamine and sevoflurane in children with glaucoma undergoing examination under anaesthesia

Jones L, Sung V, Lascaratos G, et al (City Hosp, Birmingham, UK; et al)

Br J Ophthalmol 94:33-35, 2010

Aim.—For accurate intraocular pressure (IOP) measurement in very young children examination under anaesthesia (EUA) may be necessary. Most anaesthetic agents used for EUA have some effect on IOP. We compared IOPs in children after ketamine and sevoflurane anaesthesia.

Methods.—Consecutive patients with definite or suspected glaucoma, uncooperative for reliable IOP measurement in clinic and requiring EUA, were included in this study. IOPs were measured after intramuscular injection (5 mg/kg) or intravenous injection (2 mg/kg) of ketamine using a Perkins applanation tonometer. Three measurements were taken from each eye. The IOPs were rechecked after sevoflurane, given for maintenance anaesthesia. Mean IOPs were used for analysis. Paired t test was used to assess the differences in IOPs for the whole group and one-way ANOVA for the three subgroups (ketamine IOP <20, 20–30, >30 mmHg).

Results.—The records of eight patients (16 eyes) were available for review. The mean age was 55.42 (SD 25, range 26–89) months. Seventy data-points from both eyes (35 EUAs) were used for the analysis. The mean IOP after sevoflurane (17 (SD 10) mmHg) was statistically lower than after ketamine (24.4 (SD 12.7) mmHg, p<0.001). The percentage difference was 28.5 (SD 20.8; 95% CI 23.5 to 33.4)). The difference between the subgroups was not statistically significant (p = 0.192).

Conclusion.—Sevoflurane lowers the IOP significantly compared with the IOP measured after ketamine. This difference is independent of the IOP level. It may be important to use ketamine as the induction anaesthetic agent when accurate IOP measurement is necessary during EUA for children (Table 3).

▶ The authors measured intraocular pressure (IOP) in pediatric glaucoma patients first with ketamine intramuscular (IM) or intravenous (IV) and then with addition of sevoflurane. Time between the sevoflurane measurements

TABLE 3.—Variation of Sevoflurane Intraocular Pressure in the Three Subgroups of Ketamine Intraocular Pressure

Variable	Mean Ket–Sev (mmHg)*	Data Points (n)	Mean Reduction (%)	SD	95% CI	p Value
Ketamine IOP (mmHg)						
<20	2.83	26	22.75	25.12	12.60 to 32.90	<0.001
20–30	8.28	21	33.25	19.17	24.52 to 41.98	<0.001
>30	11.72	23	30.59	15.45	23.91 to 37.27	<0.001

IOP, intraocular pressure; Ket, ketamine; Sev, sevoflurane.
*Difference between ketamine and sevoflurane measurements.

and the initial administration of ketamine was not noted. The authors found that addition of sevoflurane after ketamine sedation resulted in decreases in IOP. Data was subdivided to determine if initial IOP influenced the decrease seen with addition of sevoflurane. These results are presented in Table 3. Similar decreases in IOP were seen regardless of initial level. The authors concluded that to avoid underestimation of true IOP, ketamine should be used. Ketamine IOP is felt by ophthalmologists to reflect awake IOP.

S. Black, MD

Continuous peripheral nerve blocks for postoperative analgesia in children: feasibility and side effects in a cohort study of 339 catheters

Dadure C, Bringuier S, Raux O, et al (Lapeyronie Univ Hosp, Montpellier, France)

Can J Anaesth 56:843-850, 2009

Introduction.—Perioperative continuous peripheral nerve blocks (CPNB) are increasingly being used in children. Only one previous study has reported adverse events of CPNB in a high number of pediatric cases. We evaluated the indications, block efficacy, and adverse events related to CPNB in children.

Methods.—All CPNBs that were performed in children for postoperative analgesia over a 5-year period at the Montpellier University Hospital in France were included in this study. The first bolus dose and the continuous doses of local anesthetic were not standardized. In the postoperative period, demographic data, quality of analgesia, amount of rescue analgesic medication, child/parent satisfaction, and adverse events were recorded in our Departmental Regional Anesthesia registry.

Results.—A total of 339 catheters were evaluated in 292 children ASA physical status I to III. The median age was 8 yr (0.6–17 yr) and the median weight was 28 kg (7–116 kg). The main surgical indications were hip, femoral, or tibial osteotomies (44.5%) and club foot repair (27.4%). The local anesthetics used were either bupivacaine or ropivacaine. The mean volume of the local anesthetic bolus dose was 0.49 ± 0.16 mL · kg^{-1}, and the mean regimen of local anesthetic continuous infusion was 0.11 ± 0.04 mL · kg^{-1} · hr^{-1}. The median duration of CPNB was 61.6 hr (range 0–264 hr). Pain relief, which was evaluated with the children at rest, was considered optimal in the majority of patients throughout the study period. The Children and Infants Postoperative Pain Scale (CHIPPS) was used in children age 0–6 yr and the Visual Analog Pain Scale (VAS) was used in children 7 yr and older. There were no major adverse events. There were 211 minor adverse events recorded in 153 CPNBs (45.1%). The most frequently reported complication (20.1%) involved mechanical problems with the catheter, followed by nausea and vomiting (14.7%).

Conclusion.—CPNBs are indicated after orthopedic surgery in children. Our results demonstrate that CPNBs are feasible in the pediatric setting,

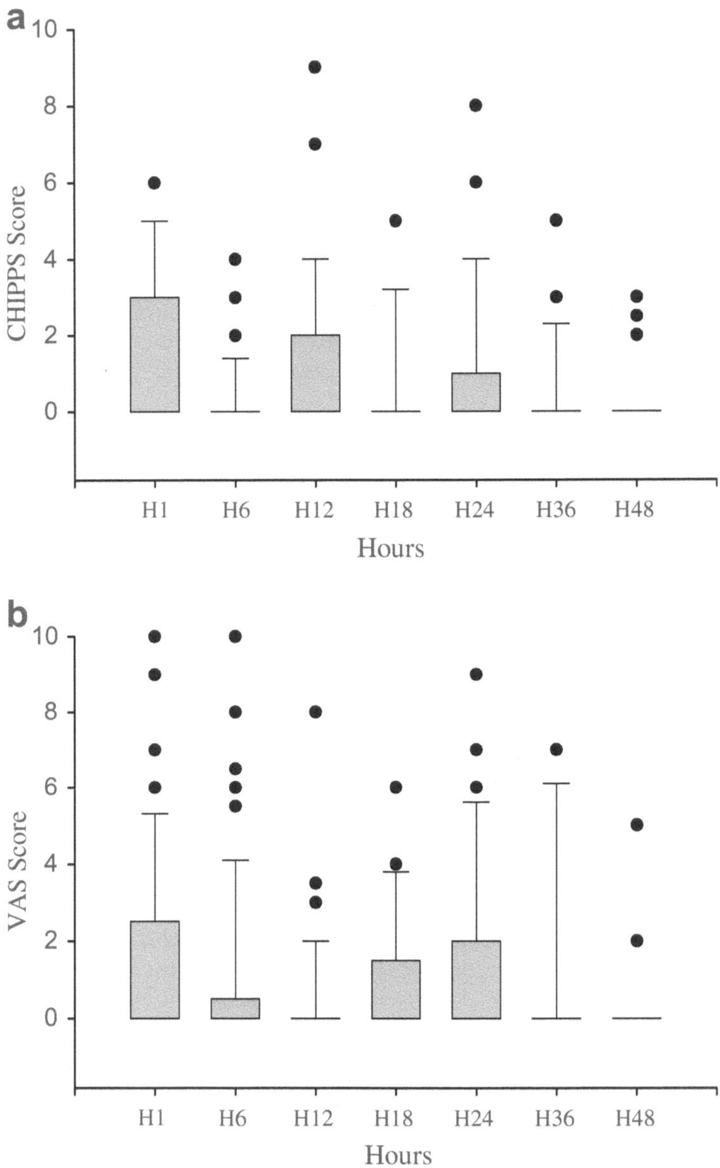

FIGURE 1.—a Children and Infants Postoperative Pain Scale (CHIPPS) scores in the youngest children (6 mth to 6 yr) during the first postoperative 48 hr. The box represents the 25th to 75th percentiles; the dark line is the median. The extended bars represent the 10th to 90th percentiles, and the dark circles represent values outside this range. The median pain score was zero during the first 48 hr postoperatively. **b** VAS scores in the oldest children (7–17 yr) during the first 48 hr postoperatively. The box represents the 25th to 75th percentiles; the dark line represents the median. The extended bars represent the 10th to 90th percentiles, and the dark circles represent values outside this range. Note that the median pain score was zero during the first 48 hr postoperatively. (Reprinted from Dadure C, Bringuier S, Raux O, et al. Continuous peripheral nerve blocks for postoperative analgesia in children: feasibility and side effects in a cohort study of 339 catheters. *Can J Anaesth*. 2009;56:843-850.)

TABLE 1.—Demographic Data and Surgical Indications Expressed as the Median (Extremes) or Number of Cases (Percent)

Age (yr)	8 (0.6–17)
Age range (%)	
0–6 yr	43.73
7–17 yr	56.27
Sex ratio (male/female)	0.55/0.45
Weight (kg)	28 (7–116)
Catheter duration (hr)	61.6 (0–264)
Surgical indications, no. of cases (%)	
Osteotomies	151 (44.5)
Club foot repair	93 (27.4)
Analgesia	20 (6)
Hallux valgus repair	14 (4.1)
Knee ligamentoplasty	13 (3.8)
Ankle arthrodesis	9 (2.7)
Plastic surgery	7 (2.1)
Others	32 (9.4)

and in skilled hands, they promote prolonged analgesia in the majority of patients without major adverse events. The most common minor adverse events are catheter-related mechanical problems and postoperative nausea and vomiting (Fig 1, Tables 1 and 2).

► Continuous peripheral nerve blocks with an indwelling catheter have been used successfully in adult patients and are well studied. In this retrospective review, efficacy for prolonged analgesia and complications of continuous peripheral nerve blocks in pediatric patients was reviewed. Over 300 catheters were placed in just under 300 patients under general anesthesia or sedation using a nerve stimulator technique under sterile technique. Children ranged in age from under 1 year to 17 years old. Procedures were lower extremity orthopedic procedures associated with significant pain postoperatively. (Table 1) Fig 1 demonstrates the excellent analgesia for the first 48 hours postoperatively, achieved with continuous peripheral blocks. Adverse events are reported in Table 2. Nausea and vomiting were the most common adverse event behind mechanical difficulties with the catheter. No infections or neurologic injuries occurred. These results suggest that continuous peripheral nerve blocks have similar efficacy in pediatric patients as in adults.

S. Black, MD

TABLE 2.—Adverse Events by Catheter Location Among the Total Adverse Events ($n = 211$)

	Mechanical Complications	PONV	Urinary Retention	Pruritus	Persistent Motor Block	Paresthesia	Inflammatory Local Signs	Adverse Events (%)
Axillary	6	4	0	0	6	2	0	18 (8.5)
Infraclavicular	7	1	0	0	2	3	1	14 (6.6)
Interscalene	0	1	0	0	0	1	0	2 (0.9)
Femoral	14	5	2	1	2	3	0	27 (12.8)
PCB	17	24*	1	2	2	2	0	48 (22.8)
Popliteal	24	15	2	0	49*	11	1	102 (48.4)
Total, *n* (%)	68 (32.2)	50 (23.8)	5 (2.4)	3 (1.4)	61 (28.9)	22 (10.4)	2 (0.9)	211 (100)

PCB psoas compartment block; *PONV* postoperative nausea and vomiting.
$^{*}P<0.05$

Agrichemicals in surface water and birth defects in the United States
Winchester PD, Huskins J, Ying J (Indiana Univ School of Medicine, Indianapolis; Univ of Cincinnati, OH)
Acta Pædiatr 98:664-669, 2009

Objectives.—To investigate if live births conceived in months when surface water agrichemicals are highest are at greater risk for birth defects.

Methods.—Monthly concentrations during 1996–2002 of nitrates, atrazine and other pesticides were calculated using United States Geological Survey's National Water Quality Assessment data. Monthly United States birth defect rates were calculated for live births from 1996 to 2002 using United States Centers for Disease Control and Prevention natality data sets. Birth defect rates by month of last menstrual period (LMP) were then compared to pesticide/nitrate means using logistical regression models.

Results.—Mean concentrations of agrichemicals were highest in April–July. Total birth defects, and eleven of 22 birth defect subcategories, were more likely to occur in live births with LMPs between April and July. A significant association was found between the season of elevated agrichemicals and birth defects.

Conclusion.—Elevated concentrations of agrichemicals in surface water in April–July coincided with higher risk of birth defects in live births with LMPs April–July. While a causal link between agrichemicals and birth defects cannot be proven from this study an association might provide clues to common factors shared by both variables.

▶ This study is probably one of the most disturbing of 2009 because it implies that the agrichemicals and pesticides used may well have profound effects on our unborn children. And clearly, there is also early indication that these pesticides contribute to diseases later in life, the highest incidence of which belongs to farmers who use their own well water. How much is the epidemic of autism due to the agrichemical industry? We don't know the answer to this, but this article and many like it indicate that this is a field that is ripe for research, and the good news is that such research seems to be on the way.

M. F. Roizen, MD

Does higher quality early child care promote low-income children's math and reading achievement in middle childhood?
Dearing E, McCartney K, Taylor BA (Boston College, Chestnut Hill, MA)
Child Dev 80:1329-1349, 2009

Higher quality child care during infancy and early childhood (6-54 months of age) was examined as a moderator of associations between family economic status and children's (N = 1,364) math and reading achievement in middle childhood (4.5-11 years of age). Low income was less strongly predictive of underachievement for children who had been in higher quality care than for those who had not. Consistent with a cognitive advantage hypothesis, higher quality care appeared to promote achievement indirectly via early school readiness skills. Family characteristics associated with selection into child care also appeared to promote the achievement of low-income children, but the moderating effect of higher quality care per se remained evident when controlling for selection using covariates and propensity scores.

▶ Why am I reviewing this article? Especially in an anesthesia area? It is because child care has become so important to so many of our own staff and physicians and CRNAs. The choice seems so important for Childhood Development. The real reason for this article is to show you that childcare matters and its quality matters a great deal, and that there is a technique—the observation record of care giving environment (see page 1334 of this article) that talks about how you can evaluate (by observation) the quality of child care your child might receive.

M. F. Roizen, MD

Early Exposure to Anesthesia and Learning Disabilities in a Population-based Birth Cohort

Wilder RT, Flick RP, Sprung J, et al (Mayo Clinic, Rochester, MN)
Anesthesiology 110:796-804, 2009

Background.—Anesthetic drugs administered to immature animals may cause neurohistopathologic changes and alterations in behavior. The authors studied association between anesthetic exposure before age 4 yr and the development of reading, written language, and math learning disabilities (LD).

Methods.—This was a population-based, retrospective birth cohort study. The educational and medical records of all children born to mothers residing in five townships of Olmsted County, Minnesota, from 1976 to 1982 and who remained in the community at 5 yr of age were reviewed to identify children with LD. Cox proportional hazards regression was used to calculate hazard ratios for anesthetic exposure as a predictor of LD, adjusting for gestational age at birth, sex, and birth weight.

Results.—Of the 5,357 children in this cohort, 593 received general anesthesia before age 4 yr. Compared with those not receiving anesthesia (n = 4,764), a single exposure to anesthesia (n = 449) was not associated with an increased risk of LD (hazard ratio = 1.0; 95% confidence interval, 0.79–1.27). However, children receiving two anesthetics (n = 100) or three or more anesthetics (n = 44) were at increased risk for LD (hazard ratio = 1.59; 95% confidence interval, 1.06–2.37, and hazard ratio = 2.60; 95% confidence interval, 1.60–4.24, respectively). The risk for LD increased with longer cumulative duration of anesthesia exposure (expressed as a continuous variable) ($P = 0.016$).

Conclusion.—Exposure to anesthesia was a significant risk factor for the later development of LD in children receiving multiple, but not single anesthetics. These data cannot reveal whether anesthesia itself may contribute to LD or whether the need for anesthesia is a marker for other unidentified factors that contribute to LD.

► This article by Wilder et al is perhaps one of the most important for our specialty. This article approaches what happens to the developing brain with exposure, and even what happens to the elderly brain with exposure to anesthetics. This carefully done article from the Mayo Clinic shows that repeated anesthetic exposures greatly increase the risk of learning disabilities, and those disabilities correlate with duration of anesthesia exposure. What we don't know is whether it was the disease the person is being anesthetized to or concomitants of that which causes the learning disabilities, or whether it is something relating to the anesthetic on the immature brain. But also importantly, what happens to the elderly brain with clear evidence of postoperative delirium and neurocognitive dysfunction after surgery? Unfortunately this study, like many excellent studies, leaves us with more questions than answers. It will be a fertile field to investigate for many years to come, and may help us better understand what memory and consciousness really are.

M. F. Roizen, MD

6 Head Injury and Neuroanesthesia

Neurocognitive Performance in Hypertensive Patients after Spine Surgery

Yocum GT, Gaudet JG, Teverbaugh LA, et al (Columbia Univ, NY)

Anesthesiology 110:254-261, 2009

Background.—Cognitive dysfunction is fairly common after noncardiac surgery and may be related to intraoperative blood pressure management. The authors present an analysis of risk factors for cognitive deterioration after spine surgery in older patients, with particular emphasis on intraoperative blood pressure in normotensive and hypertensive patients.

Methods.—This is a *post hoc* cohort analysis of 45 patients enrolled before undergoing lumbar laminectomy or microdiscectomy. The patients underwent a battery of 5 neuropsychometric tests preoperatively, and 1 day and 1 month postoperatively. Computerized anesthesia records were used to obtain intraoperative mean arterial pressure (MAP) data. Simple linear regressions between intraoperative MAP and postoperative cognitive performance were performed, and multivariate linear regression models of postoperative cognitive performance were constructed to analyze potential risk factors for cognitive decline after surgery.

Results.—Twenty-one normotensive patients (mean age, 62.4 yr) and 24 hypertensive patients (mean age, 67.9 yr) were included in this analysis. There was a significant positive relationship between minimum intraoperative MAP values and 1-day cognitive performance by simple linear regression in hypertensive ($P = 0.003$), but not normotensive, patients. In multivariate linear regression analysis of cognitive performance, there was a significant interaction between hypertension and minimum intraoperative MAP at 1 day and 1 month.

Conclusions.—In hypertensive patients, there was a significant relationship between minimum intraoperative MAP and decline in cognitive function 1 day and 1 month after surgery. A prospective controlled trial of intraoperative blood pressure control, especially during induction of anesthesia when MAP values typically drop, is needed to confirm these findings (Tables 3 and 4).

▶ Early postoperative cognitive dysfunction is often troubling to the patient and family. While most often patients with early postoperative cognitive dysfunction recover fully, it has been associated with poorer long-term

TABLE 3.—Multivariate Linear Regression Analyses of Composite Z Scores at 1 Day and 1 Month after Reverse Elimination

Test	1 Day Coefficient (SE)	*P*	1 Month Coefficient (SE)	*P*
Age	—	—	—	—
Hypertension	−0.13 (0.07)	0.06	−0.07 (0.08)	0.42
Previous CVA	—	—	—	—
Years of education	—	—	—	—
Duration of surgery	—	—	−0.005 (0.002)	0.02*
Minimum MAP (% baseline)	0.24 (0.48)	0.61	−0.30 (0.69)	0.67
Wong/Baker FACES rating				
—Baseline	—	—	—	—
—1 Day	−0.08 (0.03)	0.01*	—	—
Hypertension*Minimum MAP	1.56 (0.45)	0.001*	1.75 (0.69)	0.02*

Data presented only for variables included in the final models. — indicates variable was initially included in the model but was removed during reverse elimination.

CVA = cerebrovascular accident; MAP = mean arterial pressure; SE = standard error of independent variable in final multivariate model.

*Statistically significant with *P* values as indicated.

TABLE 4.—Intraoperative Vasopressor Medication Use

	Normotensive	Hypertensive
Ephedrine		
Patients administered (%)	8/21 (38.1%)	11/24 (45.8%)
Mean total dose (mg)	8.13 ± 2.59	18.64 ± 12.87
Phenylephrine		
Patients administered (%)	5/21 (23.8%)	6/24 (25.0%)
Mean total dose (mcg)	256.0 ± 156.5	120.0 ± 121.3

Doses are presented as means ± SD of only those patients who received the respective medication.

outcome. In this study, the authors evaluate several variables in a group of patients undergoing spine surgery who received perioperative cognitive function testing when they served as a control group for a study investigating cognitive dysfunction after carotid endarterectomy. The authors found that duration of surgery was associated with increased risk for cognitive dysfunction in the early postoperative period. They in particular investigated in relationship of intraoperative blood pressure and cognitive function. In hypertensive and normotensive patients average stable blood pressure as compared with baseline was not different between groups and did not correlate with postoperative cognitive function (Fig 2 in the original article). In hypertensive but not normotensive patients, lowest intraoperative blood pressure did correlate with postoperative cognitive dysfunction (Fig 3 in the original article, Table 3). Other studies have not found a relationship between intraoperative blood pressure and cognitive function. However, in this small trial the authors confirmed that hypertensive patients are at greater risk for transient hypotension, required more vasopressor treatment (Table 4), and that this transient hypotension in hypertensive patients was associated with decreased cognitive function in the early postoperative period. It is interesting that blood pressures were similar during most of the procedure, and was significantly different only transiently. This suggests that perhaps even greater attention should be paid to brief and often anticipated periods of hypotension, such as in the post induction and positioning periods.

For further reading on this subject I suggest an article by Moller et al.[1]

S. Black, MD

Reference

1. Moller JT, Cluitmans P, Rasmussen LS, et al. Long-term postoperative cognitive dysfunction in the elderly ISPOCD1 study. ISPOCD investigators. International Study of Post-Operative Cognitive Dysfunction. *Lancet.* 1998;351:857-861.

Intraoperative Fraction of Inspired Oxygen Is a Modifiable Risk Factor for Surgical Site Infection after Spinal Surgery

Maragakis LL, Cosgrove SE, Martinez EA, et al (Johns Hopkins Univ School of Medicine, Baltimore, MD)

Anesthesiology 110:556-562, 2009

Background.—Surgical site infections (SSI) after spinal surgery increase morbidity, mortality, length of hospital stay, and costs. Most previously identified risk factors for these infections, such as severity of illness and procedure duration, are not amenable to intervention. This study sought to identify modifiable risk factors associated with SSI after spinal surgery.

Methods.—This is a case-control study including case identification and review of medical records. A total of 104 patients with SSI after spinal surgery were compared to 104 randomly selected control patients without SSI after spinal surgery in a 926-bed tertiary care hospital in Baltimore, Maryland, between April 1, 2001 and December 31, 2004.

Results.—Multivariate analysis identified independent risk factors for SSI after spinal surgery including prolonged procedure duration (odds ratio [OR], 4.7; 95% confidence interval [95% CI], 1.6–14; $P < 0.001$), American Society of Anesthesiologists score of 3 or greater (OR, 9.7; 95% CI, 3.7–25; $P < 0.001$), lumbar-sacral operative level (OR, 2.9; 95% CI, 1.2–7.1; $P = 0.02$), posterior approach (OR, 3.5; 95% CI, 1.2–9.7; $P = 0.02$), instrumentation (OR, 2.5; 95% CI, 1.1–6.0; $P = 0.03$), obesity (OR, 4.0; 94% CI, 1.6–10; $P < 0.01$), razor shaving before surgery (OR, 3.6; 95% CI, 1.2–11; $P = 0.02$), and intraoperative administered fraction of inspired oxygen of less than 50% (OR, 12; 94% CI, 4.5–33; $P < 0.001$).

Conclusions.—In addition to previously reported risk factors, this study identified intraoperative administered fraction of inspired oxygen of less than 50% as an independent, modifiable risk factor for SSI after spinal surgery. Intraoperative administration of at least 50% fraction of inspired oxygen should be tested prospectively as an intervention to prevent SSI after spinal surgery (Tables 1 and 2).

▶ Postoperative surgical site infections remain an important cause of morbidity and of increased cost. In this case-controlled, retrospective study, the authors attempted to identify modifiable risk factors in the perioperative period that influence risk for surgical site infections. Alteration of these risk factors would potentially improve outcome and reduce cost. Over approximately three and a half years just under 4000 laminectomies and fusions were performed with 104 surgical site infections identified. The authors used clear guidelines for

TABLE 1.—Selected Unadjusted Risk Factors for SSI after Spinal Surgery

Patient Characteristic/ Risk Factor	Cases (n = 104)*	Controls (n = 104)*	Unadjusted OR (95% CI)	*P* Value
Median age, years (SD)	59.4 (15.8)	50.6 (14.0)		0.04
Female gender	53 (51%)	54 (52%)	0.96 (0.56–1.7)	0.89
European descent	90 (87%)	80 (77%)	1.9 (0.93–4.0)	0.08
Smoking	21/101 (21%)	25 (24%)	0.84 (0.41–1.7)	0.63
Diabetes	17 (16%)	11 (11%)	1.7 (0.73–3.7)	0.23
Cardiac disease	29 (28%)	13 (13%)	2.7 (1.3–5.6)	<0.01
Obesity	46 (44%)	18 (17%)	3.8 (2.0–7.2)	<0.001
ASA score ≥3	75 (72%)	31 (30%)	6.0 (3.3–11)	<0.001
Karnofsky score ≤60	49 (47%)	26 (25%)	2.6 (1.4–4.9)	<0.01
Previous spinal surgery	72 (69%)	46 (44%)	2.8 (1.6–5.0)	<0.001
Emergent/urgent surgery	10 (10%)	1 (1%)	11 (1.4–87)	0.02
Razor shaving before surgery	27 (26%)	14 (13%)	2.3 (1.1–4.6)	0.03
Antimicrobial prophylaxis within 1 h before surgery	87 (84%)	75 (72%)	0.45 (0.11–1.7)	0.25
Intraoperative nitrous oxide administration†	61/99 (62%)	78/99 (79%)	0.88 (0.49–1.6)	0.66
FIO_2 <50%†	70 (68%)	35 (34%)	4.1 (2.3–7.4)	<0.001
Perioperative glucose >126 mg/dl	82/98 (84%)	58/94 (62%)	3.2 (1.6–6.3)	0.001
Mean lowest intraoperative temperature, °C (SD) [range]	35.5 (0.75) [34.0–38.5]	35.4 (0.77) [33.1–37.1]		0.33
Mean intraoperative infusion rate, ml/min (SD) [range]	14.3 (6.5) [–4.3 to 41.5]	13.6 (5.5) [1.1–33.8]		0.37
Procedure duration >75th percentile‡	40 (38%)	13 (13%)	4.4 (2.2–8.8)	<0.001
Instrumentation	79 (76%)	55 (53%)	2.8 (1.6–5.1)	0.001
Lumbar-sacral level of surgery	79 (76%)	56 (54%)	2.6 (1.4–4.9)	<0.001
Posterior surgical approach	87 (87%)	62 (62%)	4.1 (2.0–8.3)	<0.001
Dural tear	22 (21%)	11 (11%)	2.3 (1.0–5.0)	0.04
Postoperative CSF leak	12 (12%)	3 (3%)	4.4 (1.2–16)	0.03
Transfusion§	67 (64%)	22 (21%)	6.7 (3.6–13)	<0.001

ASA = American Society of Anesthesiologists; CI = confidence interval; CSF = cerebral spinal fluid; FIO_2 = fraction of inspired oxygen; OR = odds ratio; SD = standard deviation.

*Denominator is 104 patients unless another value is noted within the table.

†Administered for the majority of the intraoperative period.

‡75th percentile duration of procedure for the study patients was 352 minutes.

§Transfusion given preoperatively, intraoperatively, or postoperatively.

TABLE 2.—Multivariable Analysis: Adjusted Risk Factors for SSI after Spinal Surgery

Risk Factor	OR (95% CI)*	*P* Value
Procedure duration >75th percentile*	4.7 (1.6–14)	<0.001
ASA score ≥3	9.7 (3.7–25)	<0.001
Lumbar-sacral level of surgery	2.9 (1.2–7.1)	0.02
Posterior surgical approach	3.5 (1.2–9.7)	0.02
Instrumentation	2.5 (1.1–6.0)	0.03
Obesity	4.0 (1.6–10)	<0.01
Razor shaving before surgery	3.6 (1.2–11)	0.02
FIO_2 <50%	12 (4.5–33)	< 0.001

ASA = American Society of Anesthesiologists; CI = confidence interval; FIO_2 = fraction of inspired oxygen; OR = odds ratio.

*75th percentile duration of procedure for the study patients was 352 minutes.

defining surgical site infections. Table 1 reveals impact of potential risk factors on infection rate. Antibiotic administration and temperature were not different between the patients with infections and the case controls. Several factors associated with risk for infection were further submitted to multivariate analysis with results shown in Table 2. Intraoperative FiO_2 administration below 50% was the single greatest risk factor identified. Fig 1 in the original article depicts intraoperative FiO_2 in patients with surgical site infections and controls. Two easily altered risk factors—administering at least 50% FiO_2 and avoidance of shaving the site with a razor—were identified. Given the low cost both in dollars and risks associated with their use, these interventions should be considered for spine surgery patients.

For further reading on this subject I suggest an article by Greif et al.[1]

S. Black, MD

Reference

1. Greif R, Akca O, Horn EP, Kurz A, Sessler DI. Supplemental perioperative oxygen to reduce the incidence of surgical-wound infection. Outcomes Research Group. *N Engl J Med.* 2000;342:161-167.

The Effect of Sedation on Intracranial Pressure in Patients with an Intracranial Space-Occupying Lesion: Remifentanil Versus Propofol

Girard F, Moumdjian R, Boudreault D, et al (Centre Hospitalier de l'Université de Montréal, Canada)

Anesth Analg 109:194-198, 2009

Background.—In this study, we compared the effect of light sedation with remifentanil versus propofol on intracranial (ICP) and cerebral perfusion pressure (CPP) of patients undergoing stereotactic brain tumor biopsy under regional anesthesia.

Methods.—This was a prospective, open-label, randomized, and controlled study. Forty patients undergoing stereotactic brain tumor biopsy under regional anesthesia were randomized into two groups to receive remifentanil or propofol titrated to a level of four on the modified Assessment of Alertness/Sedation Scale. ICP was measured via the biopsy needle.

Results.—At the targeted level of sedation, the rates of infusion for remifentanil and propofol were, respectively, 4.2 ± 1.8 μg · $kg^{-1} \cdot h^{-1}$ and 4.3 ± 2.5 mg · $kg^{-1} \cdot h^{-1}$. At the time of ICP measurement, patients in the remifentanil group had a slower respiratory rate (11/min ± 3 vs 15 per min ± 3, $P = 0.0001$) and a higher Pco_2 (48.3 ± 6.2 mm Hg vs 43.1 ± 5.5 mm Hg, $P = 0.009$) than patients in the propofol group. The mean was similar for both groups, 19.0 ± 11.9 mm Hg vs 16.4 ± 11.1 mm Hg for remifentanil and propofol, respectively ($P = 0.48$). Higher mean arterial blood pressure in the remifentanil group (101.1 ± 13.7 mm Hg vs 85.8 ± 12.7 mm Hg, $P = 0.0008$) resulted in a higher CPP than the propofol group: 82.0 ± 19.0 mm Hg vs 69.5 ± 17.0 ± 19.0 mm Hg ($P = 0.03$).

Conclusion.—Light sedation with remifentanil does not result in a higher ICP than propofol in patients undergoing stereotactic brain tumor biopsy. CPP might be better preserved with remifentanil (Table 3).

▶ Using a prospective, randomized, open label trial, the authors evaluated the impact of sedation with propofol or remifentanil on intracranial pressure (ICP) in patents with intracranial tumors undergoing stereotactic biopsy. The authors had previously compared ICP in patients with and without propofol sedation and found no increase in ICP. Table 3 contains the intraoperative results. In

TABLE 3.—Intraoperative Data Obtained During Intracranial Pressure Measurement[a]

	Group Remifentanil ($n = 20$)	Group Propofol ($n = 20$)	P
Rate of infusion at the targeted level of sedation	4.2 ± 1.8 μg · $kg^{-1} \cdot h^{-1}$	4.3 ± 2.5 mg · $kg^{-1} \cdot h^{-1}$	
Total dosage at the end of ICP measurement	224 ± 114 μg	208 ± 78 mg	
MOAAS score median (range)	4 (4–4)	14 (3–4)	ns
Heart rate (bpm)	75 ± 13	77 ± 12	
Pulse oximetry (%)	98 ± 1	98 ± 2	
Respiratory rate (breath/min)	11 ± 3	15 ± 3	0.0001
Arterial blood gas			
pH	7.34 ± 0.04	7.38 ± 0.04	0.007
Pco_2 (mm Hg)	48.3 ± 6.2	43.1 ± 5.5	0.009
Po_2 (mm Hg)	127 ± 34	147 ± 39	0.008
HCO_3 ($mEq \cdot L^{-1}$)	26 ± 2	25 ± 2	
Angle from the operating table (degrees)	29 ± 15	26 ± 12	
Intracranial pressure (mm Hg)	19.0 ± 11.9	16.4 ± 11.1	0.48
Mean arterial pressure (mm Hg)	101.1 ± 13.7	85.8 ± 12.7	0.0008
Cerebral perfusion pressure (mm Hg)	82.0 ± 19.0	69.5 ± 17.0	0.03

Values are mean ± standard deviation.
MOAAS = modified observer's assessment of alertness/sedation; ICP = intracranial pressure; ns = nonsignificant.
[a]All values were obtained at the end of the 1 min stabilization period for intracranial pressure measurement.

spite of the expected decrease in respiratory rate and increase in CO_2 with remifentanil, there was no increase in ICP compared to sedation with propofol. Similar depths of sedation were obtained. In addition, whereas propofol sedation led to consistent decreases in arterial pressure(about 15% below baseline), there was no consistent decrease in blood pressure with remifentanil sedation. As a result, cerebral perfusion pressure was better maintained. The authors did not report any cases of chest wall rigidity with remifentanil. However, occurrence of chest wall rigidity remains relatively common with remifentanil and could result in significant difficulties during sedation for stereotactic brain biopsy.[1]

S. Black, MD

Reference

1. Girard F, Moumdjian R, Boudreault D, et al. The effect of propofol sedation on intracranial pressure of patients with an intracranial space-occupying lesion. *Anesth Analg*. 2004;99:573-577.

Anesthesia for Carotid Endarterectomy: The Third Option. Patient Cooperation During General Anesthesia

Bevilacqua S, Romagnoli S, Ciappi F, et al (Azienda Ospedaliera Universitaria Careggi, Firenze, Italy)
Anesth Analg 108:1929-1936, 2009

Background.—Carotid endarterectomy is typically performed using either regional or general anesthesia techniques, which exhibit several differences, especially regarding the intraoperative neurological monitoring of patients. In this study, we introduce a technique of general anesthesia (cooperative patient general anesthesia), which allows neurological monitoring of the awake patient during surgery.

Methods.—We prospectively enrolled 181 consecutive adult patients scheduled for carotid endarterectomy. Patients were anesthetized with a total IV anesthesia technique. During carotid clamping, anesthesia was reduced and maintained only with high-dose remifentanil, such that the patient was able to respond to verbal statements and neurological monitoring could be performed. The technique is described in detail. Patient neurological and cardiac outcomes were investigated. Patient and surgeon satisfaction with the technique were also evaluated.

Results.—General anesthesia with a cooperative patient was achieved in 179 patients. No postoperative neurological events were observed. Two (1.1%) nonfatal myocardial infarctions occurred in the early postoperative period in two patients. Eighty-one percent of patients described the operation duration as brief, whereas 19.3% accurately perceived the time they were conscious. Both patients and surgeons were highly satisfied with the technique.

TABLE 3.—Characteristics of the Surgical Procedures ($n = 181$)

Duration of anesthesia, mean (SD), min	107 (21.3)
Duration of surgery, mean (SD), min	85 (14.7)
Carotid clamping time, mean (SD), min	32 (8.7)
Shunt insertion, *n* (%)	22 (12.15)
Repair with patch, *n* (%)	163 (90.05)
Conversion to general anesthesia (due to):	
Patient discomfort, *n* (%)	2 (1.1)
Neurological symptoms, *n* (%)	4 (2.21)
Hemodynamics during carotid clamping:	
Heart rate, mean (SD), bpm	48 (21)
Mean arterial blood pressure, mean (SD), mm Hg	98 (12)

TABLE 4.—Outcome and Acceptance of the Technique ($n = 181$)

Neurological complications within 30 d:	
Any stroke, *n* (%)	0
Neuropsychological injury, *n* (%)	0
Death, *n* (%)	0
Cardiac complications within 30 days:	
Myocardial infarction, *n* (%)	2 (1.1)
Arrhythmias, *n* (%)	2 (1.1)[a]
Death, *n* (%)	0
Questionnaire on awareness:	
Auditory recalls, *n* (%)	172 (95.02)
Visual recalls, *n* (%)	3 (1.66)
Tactile recalls, *n* (%)	173 (95.58)
Recall of muscular paralysis, *n* (%)	0
Recall of vocal cord paralysis, *n* (%)	139 (76.79)
Any recall of pain, *n* (%)	1 (0.55)
Any recall of bad feelings, *n* (%)	2 (1.1)
Perception of real length of surgery, *n* (%)	35 (19.34)
Experienced as a dream, *n* (%)	106 (58.56)
Patients' satisfaction score, *n* (%):	
Very satisfied	112 (61.87)
Satisfied	67 (37.01)
Unsatisfied	2 (1.1)
Very unsatisfied	0
Surgeons' satisfaction score, *n* (%):	
Very satisfied	170 (93.92)
Satisfied	11 (6.08)
Unsatisfied	0
Very unsatisfied	0

[a]Atrial fibrillation.

Conclusions.—In our series, cooperative patient general anesthesia proved to be a safe and satisfactory anesthetic technique for both the patient and surgeon. The technique was characterized by hemodynamic stability, excellent control of ventilatory pattern, continuous neurological monitoring, and immediate and safe conversion to general anesthesia whenever required. Further studies are needed to highlight the advantages of this technique compared with standard general and local anesthesia (Tables 3 and 4).

▶ This is a fascinating description of the application of a novel anesthetic technique to a relatively large number of patients. One hundred and eighty-one patients underwent carotid endarterectomy under general anesthesia with intubation, had the anesthetic depth lightened to allow for gross neurologic exam — of major motor movement on command — during a critical portion of the procedure(carotid cross clamping), and then had the anesthetic depth again increased to a conventional general anesthetic. The airway remained intubated throughout. The described technique bears some similarities to the awake/asleep/awake approach to craniotomies that require intraoperative mapping of eloquent cortex. In these cases, patients undergo the initial period of the craniotomy under conventional general anesthesia and are then emerged and usually extubated during the procedure to allow functional mapping and then have general anesthesia reinduced or the procedure is continued with heavy sedation. These procedures require careful patient selection and surgeon cooperation. While that is not addressed in this study, it seems likely that patient selection and education are important components of successful use of the described technique. In Table 3, operative characteristics are described and carotid cross clamp time averaged about 20 minutes. Table 4 records operative outcome indicating very low complication rates, high intraoperative recall, as you would expect, and high patient satisfaction. While intraoperative neurologic events remote from the period of carotid cross clamping are uncommon, they do occur and can lead to neurologic injury, which would go undetected by this technique.

S. Black, MD

A Comparison of Three Methods of Pain Control for Posterior Spinal Fusions in Adolescent Idiopathic Scoliosis

Milbrandt TA, Singhal M, Minter C, et al (Shriners Hosp for Children, Lexington, KY; Univ of Kentucky, Lexington, Univ of North Carolina, Durham; et al)

Spine 34:1499-1503, 2009

Study Design.—Retrospective cohort study.

Objective.—To compare the efficacy of patient-controlled analgesia (PCA) with morphine alone, a single preoperative intrathecal morphine injection and PCA (IT/PCA), and epidural catheter infusion without PCA (EPI) for postoperative pain control after posterior spinal fusion (PSF) and segmental spinal instrumentation (SSI) in adolescent idiopathic scoliosis (AIS).

Summary of Background Data.—Postoperative pain control after PSF and SSI in AIS can be managed in different ways. EPI provides for a longer

TABLE 3.—Return of Bowel Function Amongst All Groups

	IT/PCA	PCA	EPI
Eating solid (d)	2.6*	3.22	2.036*
BM (d)	3.35	3.73	3.4

*Denotes statistically significant differences ($P < 0.05$).

TABLE 4.—Rate of Minor Complications Amongst All Groups

	IT/PCA (N = 42)	PCA (N = 41)	EPI (N = 55)
Nausea	20 (47%)	13 (31%)	22 (40%)
Vomiting	17 (40%)	17 (41%)	9 (16%)*
Itching	19 (45%)	7 (17%)	27 (49%)*

*Denotes statistically significant differences ($P < 0.05$).

period of pain relief but is reliant on the correct placement and maintenance of the catheter in the epidural space. A single preoperative intrathecal morphine injection also provides for long acting analgesia. No direct comparison of these 3 methods of postoperative pain control has been reported.

Methods.—An IRB-approved retrospective chart review was performed at 2 institutions from 1997 to 2005. The medical record was reviewed to determine pain scores after surgery at multiple time periods. The 3 groups were compared using Student t test and χ^2 and significance was defined as $P < 0.05$.

Results.—There was no statistical difference in the gender, age, magnitude of curve, or number of levels fused in the IT/PCA (N = 42), PCA (N = 41), or EPI (N = 55) groups. Postoperative pain scores were lowest in the IT/PCA group in the first 8 hours ($P < 0.05$) but the pain scores in the EPI group were then lower through 24 hours ($P < 0.05$). Total morphine use (mg/kg) was lower in the IT/PCA group compared with the PCA group at 12 hours and 24 hours ($P = 0.0001$). Return to solid food ingestion was quickest in the EPI group (2.0 days) followed by the IT/PCA (2.6 days) and PCA alone (3.2 days) ($P < 0.002$). Respiratory depression and transient neurologic change occurred most frequently in the EPI group (EPI 11/55 pts vs. 1/42 IT/PCA vs. 0/41 PCA $P < 0.001$). Pruritis was greatest in the epidural group (11/55 $P < 0.05$). There were no intraoperative somatosensory-evoked potential changes or permanent neurologic injury recorded in any group.

Conclusion.—An EPI controls postoperative pain for the longest period of time and allows for a quicker return to consumption of solid foods. However, a single preoperative intrathecal morphine injection controls the pain equally for the first 24 hours with less pruritis and with less adverse events thus requiring less nursing and physician intervention after PSF and SSI in AIS. All methods were safe with no neurologic injury recorded (Tables 3 and 4).

► This excellent retrospective review evaluates pain control and complications after major spine procedures using PCA, single shot intrathecal duramorph and PCA, and epidural narcotic/local anesthetic infusions. In Fig 1 in the original article it is clear that some central neuraxial approach improves pain control. Table 3 reveals different complication profiles related to each pain management strategy. Epidural infusions provided the greatest benefit in terms of long-term pain control, but required more intensive monitoring and more interventions related to complications, none of which led to morbidity. This study suggests that either intrathecal narcotics or epidural infusions provide potential benefits to patients and possibly cost savings related to more prompt recovery (Table 4). Which technique is ideal in a given clinical situation would depend on available resources for management of postoperative complications.

S. Black, MD

A Comparison Between Sevoflurane and Desflurane Anesthesia in Patients Undergoing Craniotomy for Supratentorial Intracranial Surgery

Magni G, Rosa IL, Melillo G, et al (La Sapienza Univ, Rome, Italy; Istituto Dermopatico dell'Immacolata, Rome, Italy)

Anesth Analg 109:567-571, 2009

Background.—Desflurane in neurosurgery may be beneficial because it facilitates postoperative early neurologic evaluation. However, its use has been debated because of its capacity to promote cerebral vasodilatation. Sevoflurane has been extensively used in neurosurgical patients. In this prospective clinical trial, we compared early postoperative recovery and cognitive function in patients undergoing craniotomy for supratentorial expanding lesions and receiving sevoflurane or desflurane anesthesia.

Methods.—One hundred twenty patients, ASA physical status I–III (66 men), Glascow Coma Scale 15, undergoing craniotomy for supratentorial expanding lesions were enrolled in the study. Patients were randomly allocated to two anesthetic regimens. In Group S (60 patients, 52 ± 16 yr), anesthesia was maintained using sevoflurane with end-tidal of 1.5%–2% and was age adjusted to obtain approximately 1.2 minimum alveolar anesthetic concentration. In Group D (60 patients, 60 ± 14 yr), anesthesia was maintained using desflurane with end-tidal of 6%–7% and was age adjusted to obtain approximately 1.2 minimum alveolar concentration. Emergence time was measured as the time from drug discontinuation to the time at which patients opened their eyes; tracheal extubation time was measured as the time from anesthetic discontinuation and tracheal extubation. Recovery time was measured as the time elapsing from discontinuation of anesthetic and the time when patients were able to recall their name and date of birth. Cognitive behavior was evaluated with

TABLE 1.—Anesthetic Requirements in the Two Experimental Groups

	Sevoflurane ($n = 60$)	Desflurane ($n = 60$)
Age (yr)	62.4 ± 16.2	60.4 ± 13.6
ASA physical status (I/II/III)	30/22/8	26/32/2
Anesthesia time (min)	341.2 ± 64.7	363.0 ± 113.4
Surgery time (min)	271.8 ± 68.5	263 ± 113.4
Volatile anesthetic (MAC hour)*	4.9 ± 0.5	4.5 ± 0.9
Fentanyl dosage (μg)	374 ± 100	355 ± 110
Mean midline shift (mm)	4.5 ± 7.1	4.9 ± 5.8

Values are expressed as mean ± SD or percentages.
MAC = minimum alveolar concentration.
*$P = 0.003$.

TABLE 2.—Emergence and Recovery Times in the Two Anesthetic Groups

	Sevoflurane ($n = 60$)	Desflurane ($n = 60$)	P
Emergence	12.2 ± 4.9	10.8 ± 7.2	0.21
Extubation	15.2 ± 3.0	11.3 ± 3.9	<0.0001
Recovery	18.2 ± 2.3	12.4 ± 7.7	<0.0001

All times are expressed in minutes (mean ± SD).
Emergence = time to eye opening; extubation = time to tracheal extubation; recovery = time to orientation.

the Short Orientation Memory Concentration Test. In the postanesthesia care unit, a blinded observer monitored the patients for 3 h; the incidence of hemodynamic events, pain, nausea, and shivering requiring rescue medication was recorded.

Results.—The mean emergence time (12.2 ± 4.9 min in Group S vs 10.8 ± 7.2 min in Group D; $P = \text{ns}$) was similar in the two groups, whereas the mean extubation time and recovery time were longer in Group S (15.2 ± 3.0 min in Group S vs 11.3 ± 3.9 min in Group D and 18.2 ± 2.3 min in Group S vs 12.4 ± 7.7 min in Group D, respectively; $P < 0.001$). The Short Orientation Memory Concentration Test score differed between the two groups only at the earliest assessment (15 min after extubation). No difference between the two groups was found in pain, shivering, nausea, vomiting, and incidence of postoperative hemodynamic events.

Conclusion.—Patients who received desflurane had a shorter extubation and recovery time but similar intraoperative and postoperative incidence of complications compared with those who received sevoflurane (Tables 1 and 2).

▶ In this prospective randomized trial the authors compare emergence and recovery criteria in patients with intracranial tumors anesthetized via a primarily volatile anesthetic technique using desflurane compared with sevoflurane. In addition, they compared intraoperative conditions between these agents. The goal was to determine if superior emergence characteristics anticipated with desflurane would be realized without an untoward increase in intraoperative or postoperative neurologic or hemodynamic events. They found faster extubation and recovery with desflurane as seen in Table 2, and similar but very minimal narcotic use in both as seen in Table 1. Intraoperative brain conditions and perioperative hemodynamics were similar. It would be interesting to see the comparison in use of vasoactive agents between the 2 groups. While the recovery times were statistically different, there is only a few minutes difference in these times that are of questionable clinical significance. As in other articles, it appears that many agents can be used effectively in neurosurgical patients and that no single best approach exists.

For further reading on this subject I suggest articles by Todd et al,[1] and Magni et al.[2]

S. Black, MD

References

1. Todd MM, Warner DS, Sokoll MD, et al. A prospective, comparative trial of three anesthetics for elective supratentorial craniotomy. Propofol/ fentanyl, isoflurane/ nitrous oxide, and fentanyl/nitrous oxide. *Anesthesiology.* 1993;78:1005-1020.
2. Magni G, Baisi F, La Rosa I, et al. No difference in emergence time and early cognitive function between sevoflurane-fentanyl and propofol-remifentanil in patients undergoing craniotomy for supratento-rial intracranial surgery. *J Neurosurg Anesthesiol.* 2005;17:134-138.

The Analgesic Effect of Gabapentin as a Prophylactic Anticonvulsant Drug on Postcraniotomy Pain: A Prospective Randomized Study

Türe H, Sayin M, Karlikaya G, et al (Yeditepe Univ School of Medicine, Istanbul, Turkey)

Anesth Analg 109:1625-1631, 2009

Background.—Gabapentin is an anticonvulsant drug that has analgesic properties for acute postoperative pain. However, the analgesic effect of gabapentin as an antiepileptic prophylactic drug on patients undergoing craniotomy is unclear. In this study, we evaluated the postoperative effectiveness of gabapentin on acute postoperative pain when it is used for antiepileptic prophylaxis in patients undergoing craniotomy for supratentorial tumor resection.

Methods.—Eighty patients undergoing craniotomy for supratentorial tumor resection were randomly assigned into two groups. Patients in Group G ($n = 40$) received oral gabapentin (3×400 mg), and patients in Group P ($n = 40$) received oral phenytoin (3×100 mg) for 7 days before the operation and postoperatively. An identical anesthesia protocol was performed for both the groups. Anesthesia was maintained with propofol and remifentanil infusion. Patient-controlled analgesia with morphine was used, and pain levels were measured. The antiepileptic-related side effects, anesthetic consumption, duration of anesthesia and surgery, tracheal

TABLE 1.—Antiepileptic-Related Side Effects According to Group, *n* (%)

	Gabapentin ($n = 37$)	Phenytoin ($n = 38$)
Fatigue	7 (18.9)	0
Drowsiness	2 (5.4)	0
Dizziness	5 (13.5)	0
Ataxia	2 (5.4)	0
Myalgia	1 (2.7)	1 (2.7)
Antiemetic requirement (*n*)	9 (24.3)	17 (44.7)

TABLE 2.—Characteristics of the Study Groups

	Gabapentin ($n = 37$)	Phenytoin ($n = 38$)	*P*
Female/male (*n*)	20/17	19/19	0.09
Age (yr)	45 ± 14	49 ± 11	0.15
Weight (kg)	71 ± 14	69 ± 16	0.63
ASA status (I/II)	28/9	25/13	0.49
Pathology (*n*)			
Meningioma/glioma/metastases	15/22/0	17/20/1	0.97
Surgical route, *n* (%)			0.95
Frontal	9 (24)	8 (21)	
Parietal	3 (8)	3 (8)	
Temporal	2 (6)	2 (5)	
Pterional	23 (62)	25 (66)	
Duration of surgery (min)	315 ± 65	297 ± 67	0.27
Duration of surgical closure (min)	63 ± 13	66 ± 12	0.66
Duration of anesthesia (min)	353 ± 55	346 ± 68	0.66
Total propofol dose (mg)	1847 ± 548	2293 ± 580	0.01
Total remifentanil dose (μg)	3034 ± 1334	4287 ± 1282	0.01
Tracheal extubation time (min)	16.6 ± 22	4.5 ± 2	<0.001

extubation time, postoperative pain scores, morphine consumption, and sedation scores were recorded.

Results.—Thirty-seven patients in Group G and 38 patients in Group P completed the study. During the preoperative period in Group G, one patient had severe fatigue, one had severe dizziness, and one patient's surgical procedure was changed. The median plasma levels of gabapentin were 34 μmol/mL (range, 23–51 μmol/mL) in 34 patients. In Group P, one patient withdrew from the study preoperatively and one developed transient neurological symptoms postoperatively.

The demographic data and mean duration of anesthesia and surgery were similar in both the groups. The total propofol and remifentanil consumption in Group G (1847 ± 548 mg/3034 ± 1334 μg) was significantly less than that of Group P (2293 ± 580 mg/4287 ± 1282 μg) ($P = 0.01$). However, tracheal extubation could be done earlier in Group P (4.5 ± 2 min) than in Group G (16.6 ± 22 min) ($P < 0.001$). Pain scores were significantly higher in Group P at 15 min, 30 min, and 1 h ($P < 0.001$). The total morphine consumption was also significantly higher in Group P (33 ± 17 mg vs 24 ± 19 mg) ($P = 0.01$). The postoperative sedation scores were significantly higher in Group G at 15 min, 30 min, 1 h, and 2 h ($P < 0.001$).

Conclusions.—The administration of gabapentin to patients undergoing craniotomy for supratentorial tumor resection was effective for acute postoperative pain. It also decreased analgesic consumption after surgery. However, it may lead to side effects such as delayed tracheal extubation and increased sedation postoperatively (Tables 1 and 2).

▶ Prophylaxis for seizures remains a common practice perioperatively for patients undergoing craniotomy for resection of supratentorial tumors. In a prospective randomized trial, use of gabapentin was compared with phenytoin to evaluate the analgesic effect of the gabapentin and to compare the side effect profile of the 2 antiepileptic drugs. All patients had a total intravenous anesthetic technique titrated with BIS and hemodynamic monitoring. Table 1 reports side effects preoperatively and postoperatively. During the 7-day period preoperative during which patients received either gabapentin or phenytoin, the patients receiving gabapentin had significantly more side effects. In contrast, gabapentin provided benefits postoperatively in terms of less need for antiemetic agents. Table 2 reports patient, surgical, and anesthetic characteristics, and reveals a decreased anesthetic requirement in the gabapentin patients. Gabapentin had analgesic effects that are demonstrated by lower pain scores (Fig 1 in the original article) and lower narcotic requirements, (Fig 2 in the original article) as well a sedative effect postoperatively, indicated by longer emergence times and greater sedation scores in the early postoperative period (Fig 3 in the original article). The authors conclude that gabapentin has benefits in terms of analgesia, but acknowledge the increased side effect rate and postoperative sedation. These benefits, combined with the greater cost of gabapentin compared with phenytoin, may limit the routine use of gabapentin as a "combined analgesic/antiepileptic agent" perioperatively in patients undergoing resection of brain tumors.

S. Black, MD

7 Critical Care Medicine

Adult Critical Care

Transcranial Duplex Sonography for Monitoring Hyperacute Intracerebral Hemorrhage

Pérez ES, Delgado-Mederos R, Rubiera M, et al (Hospital Vall d'Hebron, Barcelona, Spain)
Stroke 40:987-990, 2009

Background and Purpose.—Early hematoma growth is one of the main determinants of mortality in patients with intracranial hemorrhage (ICH). Transcranial duplex sonography (TDS) might represent a useful tool for the bedside monitoring of early ICH enlargement. We aimed to correlate ICH volumes measured by TDS and CT scan in patients with ICH evaluated <3 hours of symptom onset.

Methods.—We prospectively studied 34 patients with supratentorial ICH evaluated <3 hours of onset. All patients underwent emergent CT scan and TDS examination on admission and at 6 hours. Major longitudinal, sagittal, and coronal hematoma diameters were measured on CT scan by a neuroradiologist and on TDS by a blinded operator with a time delay <30 minutes between both techniques. Total hematoma volume was determined using the formula for irregular volumes (longitudinal×sagittal×coronal)/2. Early hematoma growth was defined as an increase >20% in the hematoma volume at 6 hours.

Results.—ICH was identified on TDS as an hyperechogenic mass located in the basal ganglia in 28 patients and in the lobar position in 6. Mean hematoma volume at baseline was 86±4 5 mL. At 6 hours, early hematoma growth was seen in 9 (26%) patients. An excellent correlation was found between TDS and CT measurements for all diameters: longitudinal (r=0.91, P<0.001), sagittal (r=0.85, P=0.002), coronal (r=0.79, P=0.022) and for total hematoma volume (r=0.82, P=0.001). When all obtained measures were matched, the intraclass correlation coefficient was 0.888 (95% CI, 0.8 to 0.937).

Conclusion.—TDS showed an excellent correlation with CT in measuring the extent of bleeding in patients with hyperacute ICH. TDS

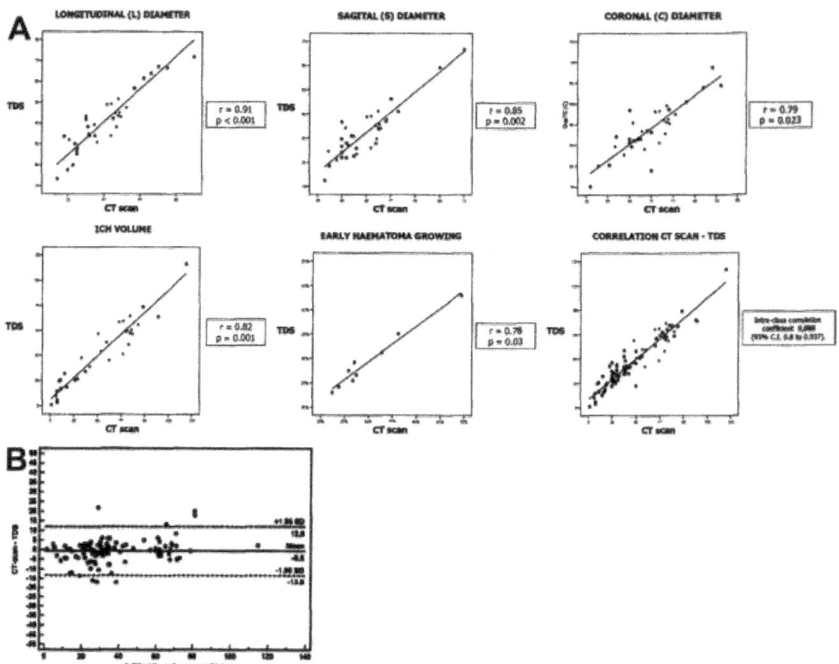

FIGURE 2.—Comparison between both techniques: (A) correlations using Pearson's correlation coefficient, Spearman's (early hematoma growth), and the intraclass correlation coefficient; (B) Bland-Altman test to assess all diameter in both techniques. (Reprinted from Pérez ES, Delgado-Mederos R, Rubiera M, et al. Transcranial duplex sonography for monitoring hyperacute intracerebral hemorrhage. *Stroke.* 2009;40:987-990.)

may represent a reliable useful tool for monitoring ICH noninvasively at the patient's bedside (Fig 2).

► Intracerebral hemorrhage (ICH) is associated with high morbidity and mortality. Several factors determine the negative outcome following ICH, including initial volume of hematoma, decreased level of consciousness, and the growth of the hematoma in the first few hours of ICH. CT and MRI scans are considered to be the gold standard for the evaluation of hematoma. However, both CT and MRI require transporting critically ill, brain-injured patients, and more frequent examination is not possible. The recently refined transcranial duplex sonography (TDS) is a noninvasive technique that allows 2-dimensional imaging of the brain parenchyma and visualization of acute ICH as a hypercore mass. TDS allows examining not only hematoma growth, but also allows assessment of brain hemodynamics and presence of ventricular invasion. This study compared the ICH volume measured by TCD and CT scan in the first 3 hours after the onset of ICH. The authors demonstrate that TCD is a useful bedside technique to identify the extent of ICH < 3 hours after stroke onset, and there was an impressive correlation with CT scan. Although their findings are impressive, it is important to be aware that the hematoma is echogenic and well demarcated from the surrounding brain tissue only in the first few days of the occurrence of ICH. Therefore, TCD cannot reach the sensitivity of CT scan in the detection and follow-up ICH. Furthermore, TCD is operator dependent and infratentorial bleeding may be missed by TCD in a significant number of patients. Although there was an excellent correlation and agreement between all measures (diameter, volume, and volume growth), the study is limited by its sample size. Future studies with a larger number of patients with ICH are needed to confirm their results.

M. Mathru, MD, FCCP

A high ratio of plasma and platelets to packed red blood cells in the first 6 hours of massive transfusion improves outcomes in a large multicenter study

Zink KA, Sambasivan CN, Holcomb JB, et al (Oregon Health and Science Univ, Portland)

Am J Surg 197:565-570, 2009

Background.—In trauma, most hemorrhagic deaths occur within the first 6 hours. This study examined the effect on survival of high ratios of fresh frozen plasma (FFP) and platelets (PLTs) to packed red blood cells (PRBCs) in the first 6 hours.

Methods.—Records of 466 massive transfusion trauma patients (≥10 U of PRBCs in 24 hours) at 16 level 1 trauma centers were reviewed. Transfusion ratios in the first 6 hours were correlated with outcome.

Results.—All groups had similar baseline characteristics. Higher 6-hour ratios of FFP:PRBCs and PLTs:PRBCs lead to improved 6-hour mortality (from 37.3 [in the lowest ratio group] to 15.7 [in the middle ratio group] to 2.0% [in the highest ratio group] and 22.8% to 19.0% to 3.2%, respectively) and in-hospital mortality (from 54.9 to 41.1 to 25.5% and 43.7% to 46.8% to 27.4%, respectively). Initial higher ratios of FFP:PRBCs and PLTs:PRBCs decreased overall PRBC transfusion.

Conclusions.—The early administration of high ratios of FFP and platelets improves survival and decreases overall PRBC need in massively transfused patients. The largest difference in mortality occurs during the first 6 hours after admission, suggesting that the early administration of FFP and platelets is critical (Figs 1 and 2).

▶ Massive transfusion protocols have been established and are strongly suggested by the American College of Surgeons Committee on Trauma. When instituted, these protocols vary widely by institution with regard to the ratios of individual component therapy. The "10 unit" rule of packed red blood cells constituting massive transfusion seems to be widely accepted. Zink and colleagues have retrospectively reviewed the records of 466 patients at 16 level 1 trauma centers comparing component ratios in the first 6 hours of resuscitation. Those patients receiving either higher ratios of fresh frozen plasma (FFP):packed red blood cells (PRBCs) (1:4 or 1:1) or platelet (PLT):PRBCs

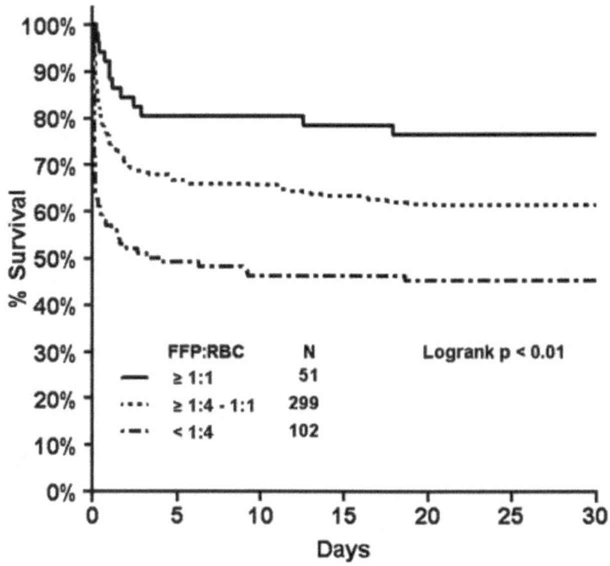

FIGURE 1.—Survival by FFP:red blood cell ratio. (Reprinted from Zink KA, Sambasivan CN, Holcomb JB, et al. A high ratio of plasma and platelets to packed red blood cells in the first 6 hours of massive transfusion improves outcomes in a large multicenter study. *Am J Surg*. 2009;197:565-570, with permission from Elsevier Inc.)

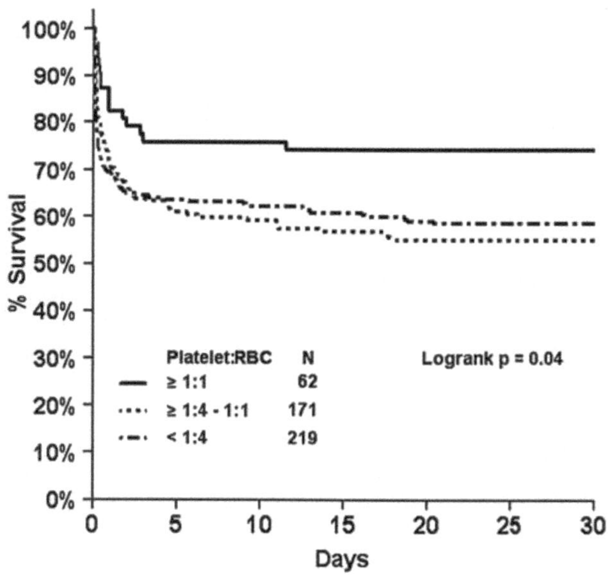

FIGURE 2.—Survival by PLT:red blood cell ratio. (Reprinted from Zink KA, Sambasivan CN, Holcomb JB, et al. A high ratio of plasma and platelets to packed red blood cells in the first 6 hours of massive transfusion improves outcomes in a large multicenter study. *Am J Surg*. 2009;197:565-570, with permission from Elsevier Inc.)

had lower 6 hour mortality and overall lower in-patient mortality than those receiving standard resuscitation protocols basing FFP and platelet therapy upon laboratory values. As further data emerge from massive transfusion protocol data, perhaps the underlying mechanism of mortality in the severely traumatized patient is an undertreated or unrecognized coagulopathy until it is too late. Further research in this area needs to be performed as it may lead to better use of blood products in the ongoing massive resuscitation of the severely injured patient.

M. Mathru, MD, FCCP

A Clinicopathological Confrontation

de Hemptinne Q, Remmelink M, Brimioulle S, et al (Université Libre de Bruxelles, Brussels, Belgium)
Chest 135:944-949, 2009

Background.—The heterogeneity of populations meeting criteria for ARDS may explain in part why no specific treatment has yet been shown to decrease mortality. To define the pathologic alterations associated with the syndrome, particularly the typical pattern of diffuse alveolar damage (DAD), and to evaluate whether etiologies or precipitating factors were missed, we evaluated patients who died with a clinical diagnosis of ARDS and who had a postmortem examination.

Methods.—We conducted a 3-year (2002 to 2004) review of all patients with ARDS (using the American-European Consensus Conference criteria) who died in our ICU and had a postmortem examination. Discrepancies between antemortem and postmortem diagnoses were classified as major and minor using the Goldman classification.

Results.—Of 9,184 hospital admissions, 376 patients had a clinical diagnosis of ARDS. Of these, 169 died; 69 had a postmortem examination, and 64 of these had complete data for analysis. The main cause of death was multiple organ failure (27 of 64 patients). Postmortem examination revealed DAD in 32 patients (50%), pneumonia without DAD in 16 patients (25%), and invasive pulmonary aspergillosis in 8 patients (12.5%). Major unexpected findings were found in 15 patients (23%): 7 Goldman class I (including 4 cases of invasive pulmonary aspergillosis and 1 of disseminated tuberculosis) and 8 Goldman class II.

Conclusions.—In this study, ARDS remains a heterogeneous syndrome because only half of patients with ARDS had typical DAD. Open lung biopsy, if performed, might have led to appropriate therapy and potentially better outcome in five of the patients (Table 1).

▶ Acute respiratory distress syndrome (ARDS) remains a major clinical entity in ICU, and the mortality remains high at 40% to 60%. The purpose of this study is to retrospectively review the clinical-pathological correlates in patients, who died from ARDS and underwent an autopsy, to define the pathological alterations associated with the syndrome with particular reference to the typical

TABLE 1.—Demographic Data and Characteristics of the Study Population ($n = 64$)*

Variables	Values
Age, yr	62 ± 18
Male gender	38 (59)
ICU length of stay, d	11 (2–135)
Pao_2/Fio_2 measured at ARDS diagnosis, mm Hg	128 ± 36
Pao_2/Fio_2 before death, mm Hg	126 ± 54
Severe hypoxemia	20 (31)
Reason for ICU admission	
Medical	43 (67)
Pulmonary	19 (30)
Digestive	10 (16)
Infectious (other than pulmonary)	8 (13)
Cardiovascular	3 (5)
Neurologic	3 (5)
Surgical	21 (33)
Cardiovascular	9 (14)
Digestive	6 (9)
Thoracic	3 (5)
Trauma	2 (3)
Neurologic	1 (2)
ARDS etiology (supposed)	
Pulmonary (primary)	34 (53)
Infectious	26 (41)
Inhalation	2 (3)
Contusion	1 (2)
Other	6 (9)
Extrapulmonary (secondary)	30 (47)
Sepsis	23 (36)
Pancreatitis	4 (7)
Multiple transfusions (TRALI)	2 (3)
Other	1 (2)
Interval between ARDS diagnosis and death, d	6 (0–48)
Primary cause of death (clinically determined)	
Multiple organ failure	27 (42)
Refractory shock	20 (31)
Refractory hypoxemia	9 (14)
Brain death	5 (8)
Other	2 (3)
Therapeutic withholding/withdrawing	32 (50)

TRALI = transfusion-related acute lung injury. Severe hypoxemia was defined as a PAO_2/FIO_2 ratio < 100 mm Hg and/or administration of inhaled nitric oxide. Refractory hypoxemia was defined as an impossibility to maintain $Pao_2 > 60$ mm Hg.
*Values are given as mean ±/SD, No. (%), or median (range).

pattern of diffuse alveolar damage (DAD) and to evaluate whether undiagnosed causal or aggravating factors were missed. The most surprising finding of this retrospective review was that only 50% of patients with ARDS diagnosed using traditional clinical criteria actually had DAD lesions. Their findings were similar to 2 other previous studies. In addition, this series of patients who missed diagnosis include invasive pulmonary aspergillosis (4 patients) and 1 case of disseminated tuberculosis. Untreated, both of these entities carry a very high mortality. If biopsy had been performed (premortem) in these patients, they could have benefited from appropriate antimicrobial therapy. In a previous study, Papazian and coworkers showed that pulmonary biopsies performed in selected patients could result in a change in therapy in 78 of 100 cases. The results of this study also suggest that the concept of ARDS as a syndrome is not a very useful entity, and perhaps it is time for other approaches to be introduced that can better characterize these patients.

M. Mathru, MD, FCCP

Acquired hypernatraemia is an independent predictor of mortality in critically ill patients

O'Donoghue SD, Dulhunty JM, Bandeshe HK, et al (Royal Brisbane and Women's Hosp, Queensland, Australia)

Anaesthesia 64:514-520, 2009

This study reports the incidence and associated mortality of acquired hypernatraemia (Na > 150 mmol.l^{-1}) in a general medical/surgical intensive care unit. Patients admitted over a 5-year period with normal sodium values were eligible for inclusion; exclusions were made for burn/neurosurgical diagnoses and for hypertonic saline therapy. From 3475 admissions (3317 patients), 266 (7.7%) episodes of hypernatraemia were observed. Hospital mortality was 33.5% in the hypernatraemic group and 7.7% in the normonatraemic group ($p < 0.001$). Acquired hypernatraemia was an independent risk factor for in-hospital mortality (OR 1.97, 95% CI

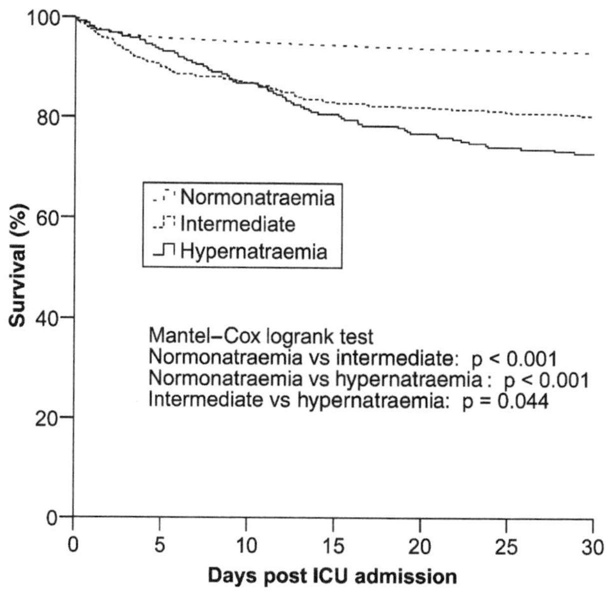

FIGURE 1.—Kaplan–Meier curve of ICU survival to 30 days by sodium group. (Reprinted from O'Donoghue SD, Dulhunty JM, Bandeshe HK, et al. Acquired hypernatraemia is an independent predictor of mortality in critically ill patients. *Anaesthesia*. 2009;64:514-520, with permission from John Wiley & Sons, Inc.)

1.37–2.82, $p < 0.001$). Intermediate sodium levels (145–150 $mmol.l^{-1}$) were associated with increased mortality (OR 1.42, 95% CI 1.02–1.98). Uncorrected sodium at discharge ($p = 0.001$) and peak sodium ($p = 0.001$) were better predictors of mortality than time to onset ($p = 0.71$) and duration of hypernatraemia ($p = 1.0$). Hypernatraemia avoidance is justified, but determinants of hypernatraemia and benefits of targeted treatment strategies require further elucidation (Fig 1).

▶ This is the largest retrospective study to date to investigate the incidence and clinical outcomes of hypernatremia acquired in general medical and surgical ICU. The authors found an incidence of ICU-acquired hypernatremia of 7.7% with an associated mortality of 33.5%. Hypernatremia was also shown to be an independendent predictor of mortality after controlling for age, acute physiology and chronic health evaluation (APACHE) II score, admission category, and comorbid status. The high mortality associated with hypernatremia found in this study during their ICU admission appears to be similar to previous studies, although in-hospital mortality was only previously reported in one other study. Previous studies have shown that in ICU-acquired hypernatremia, fluid balance was negative in two thirds of patients but was positive in one-third of patients. In addition, positive solute balance was found in nearly 40% of patients.[1] Calculation of tonicity balance, and not electrolyte-free water calculations, will guide clinicians to correct sodium in acute dysnatremias.[2]

M. Mathru, MD, FCCP

References

1. Lindner G, Kneidinger N, Holzinger U, Druml W, Schwarz C. Tonicity balance in patients with hypernatremia acquired in the intensive care unit. *Am J kidney Dis.* 2009;54:674-679.
2. Carlotti AP, Bohn D, Mallie JP, Halperin ML. Tonicity balance, and not electrolyte-free water calculations, more accurately guides therapy for acute changes in natremia. *Intensive Care Med.* 2001;27:921-924.

Assessment of Left Ventricular Function by Intensivists Using Hand-Held Echocardiography

Melamed R, Sprenkle MD, Ulstad VK, et al (Hennepin County Med Ctr, Minneapolis, MN)

Chest 135:1416-1420, 2009

Background.—Bedside transthoracic echocardiography (TTE) provides rapid and noninvasive hemodynamic assessment of critically ill patients but is limited by the immediate availability of experienced sonographers and cardiologists.

Methods.—Forty-four patients in the medical ICU underwent near-simultaneous limited TTE performed by intensivists with minimal training in echocardiography, and a formal TTE that was performed by certified

TABLE 1.—Normal vs Abnormal LV Function

Limited TTE by Intensivist	Formal TTE by Echocardiographer Normal Findings	Abnormal Findings
Normal findings	22	4
Abnormal findings	2	16

TABLE 2.—LV Function by Category

Limited TTE by Intensivist	Category 1	Formal TTE by Echocardiographer Category 2	Category 3
Category 1	22	4	0
Category 2	2	9	2
Category 3	0	0	5

sonographers and was interpreted by experienced echocardiographers. Intensivists, blinded to the patient's diagnosis and the results of the formal TTE, were asked to determine whether left ventricular (LV) function was grossly normal or abnormal and to place LV function into one of the following three categories: 1, normal; 2, mildly to moderately decreased; and 3, severely decreased.

Results.—Using the formal TTE as the "gold standard," intensivists correctly identified normal LV function in 22 of 24 cases (92%) and abnormal LV function in 16 of 20 cases (80%). The κ statistic for the agreement between intensivist and echocardiographer for any abnormality in LV function was 0.72 (95% confidence interval [CI], 0.52 to 0.93; $p < 0.001$). Intensivists correctly placed LV function into one of three categories in 36 of 44 cases (82%); in 6 of the 8 cases that were misclassified, the error involved an overestimation of LV function. The κ statistic for agreement between the intensivist and echocardiographer with regard to placement into one of three categories of LV function was 0.68 (95% CI, 0.48 to 0.88; $p < 0.001$).

Conclusions.—Intensivists were able to estimate LV function with reasonable accuracy using a hand-held unit in the ICU, despite having undergone minimal training in image acquisition and interpretation (Tables 1 and 2).

► Transthoracic echocardiography (TTE) is being increasingly used in the intensive care arena to assess hemodynamic function. This evaluation helps to determine the need of inotropes, vasopressors, and preload augmentation. This study examined the ability of the intensivists with minimal training and experience in echocardiography to accurately assess left ventricular (LV) systolic function using a hand-held unit with the interpretation of simultaneously performed comprehensive TTE by an experienced echocardiographer, the reference standard. The observational study found that the inexperienced intensivists were able to differentiate normal and abnormal LV function correctly in 86% of cases; in 82% of cases the intensivists correctly classified LV function as normal, mildly to moderately impaired. When mistakes were made, intensivists most often overestimated LV function. Their results suggest that minimally-trained intensivists using a hand-held unit can make a reasonably accurate assessment of LV function in critically ill patients. The results of this study are similar to the 3 previous studies. This study is limited by small sample size and failure to evaluate diastolic function because diastolic abnormalities are not uncommon in critically ill medical ICU patients. Furthermore, limited TTE performed by minimally trained individuals could fail to identify other important cardiac causes of hemodynamic perturbations such as cor pulmonale, acute valvular abnormalities, and intracardiac shunts.

M. Mathru, MD, FCCP

Brain Hyperthermia After Traumatic Brain Injury Does Not Reduce Brain Oxygen

Spiotta AM, Stiefel MF, Heuer GG, et al (Univ of Pennsylvania School of Medicine, Philadelphia)

Neurosurgery 62:864-872, 2008

Objective.—Hyperthermia can exacerbate outcome after traumatic brain injury (TBI). In this study, we examined the relationship between brain temperature (BT) and core body temperature and the relationship between BT and brain tissue oxygen (BtO_2) to determine whether hyperthermia adversely affects BtO_2.

Methods.—Seventy-two patients (mean age, 41 ± 19 years) admitted to a Level I trauma center after TBI were retrospectively identified from a prospective observational database. Intracranial pressure (ICP), BT, and BtO_2 were recorded continuously. Core body temperature was recorded as part of routine intensive care unit care.

Results.—BT is strongly correlated with core body temperature (correlation coefficient, $r = 0.92$) over a wide range. In addition, BT was correlated with body temperature during periods of normal ICP (IC $P \leq 20$ mmHg; $r = 0.87$) and transiently elevated ICP (ICP range 21–63 mmHg; $r = 0.94$). During periods of brain normothermia (BT < 38.1°C), the average BtO_2 was 36.3 ± 22.9 mmHg. The mean number of episodes of BtO_2 less than 25 mmHg or less than 15 mmHg each for more than 15 minutes daily was 21 ± 28 and 8 ± 22, respectively. The mean BtO_2 (37.2 ± 16.0 mmHg) was similar during periods of brain normothermia and hyperthermia (BT ≥ 38.1°C). When the periods of brain tissue hyperthermia were further categorized into BT ≥ 38.6°C or BT ≥ 39.2°C, mean daily BtO_2 was similar in all of the groups. When BT was 38.1°C or greater, there were fewer episodes of BtO_2 less than 25 mmHg (13.5 ± 24.6; $P < 0.05$) and of BtO_2 less than

15 mmHg (3.3 ± 11.9; $P < 0.05$) than observed during brain normothermia. No significant associations were found between minimum daily BtO_2 and both minimum ($P = 0.81$) and maximum ($P = 0.19$) daily BT or between maximum daily BtO_2 and both minimum ($P = 0.62$) and maximum ($P = 0.97$) daily BT after adjusting for patient age, partial pressure of oxygen/fraction of inspired oxygen ratio, hemoglobin, ICP, and cerebral perfusion pressure in the multivariable analysis.

Conclusion.—In this clinical study, hyperthermia does not seem to reduce BtO_2 or increase the number of episodes of brain tissue hypoxia in patients with severe TBI. These results suggest that hyperthermia may worsen outcome after TBI through mechanisms that may be separate from compromised brain oxygen.

► The investigators in a retrospective fashion examined whether hyperthermia has an adverse effect on brain oxygenation and outcome. Le Roux et al provide compelling evidence that hyperthermia had no effect on brain tissue oxygen partial pressure and there was no relationship demonstrated between hyperthermia and intracranial pressure (ICP). Their findings are contrary to the conventional wisdom that hyperthermia will have a negative outcome on brain-injured patients and that elevated temperature is associated with increased ICP. The precise reason elevation in temperature did not have any negative effect on brain tissue oxygen pressure is not elucidated in this study. In a seminal study Obrist et al demonstrated that brain blood flow and metabolism are markedly reduced in comatosed, brain-injured patients. Based on this finding it is tempting to speculate that temperature may not have the same effect on the cerebral metabolic rate of oxygen in the injured brain as it does in the normal brain, and this may in part explain the finding of this study. The results of this study also raise concerns about therapeutic rationale for hypothermia.

M. Mathru, MD, FCCP

A mitochondria-targeted *S*-nitrosothiol modulates respiration, nitrosates thiols, and protects against ischemia-reperfusion injury

Prime TA, Blaikie FH, Evans C, et al (MRC Mitochondrial Biology Unit, Cambridge, UK; Univ of Otago, Dunedin, New Zealand; et al)

Proc Natl Acad Sci U S A 106:10764-10769, 2009

Nitric oxide ($NO^{\bullet}$) competitively inhibits oxygen consumption by mitochondria at cytochrome *c* oxidase and *S*-nitrosates thiol proteins. We developed mitochondria-targeted *S*-nitrosothiols (MitoSNOs) that selectively modulate and protect mitochondrial function. The exemplar MitoSNO1, produced by covalently linking an *S*-nitrosothiol to the lipophilic triphenylphosphonium cation, was rapidly and extensively accumulated within mitochondria, driven by the membrane potential, where it generated $NO^{\bullet}$ and *S*-nitrosated thiol proteins. MitoSNO1-induced $NO^{\bullet}$

production reversibly inhibited respiration at cytochrome *c* oxidase and increased extracellular oxygen concentration under hypoxic conditions. MitoSNO1 also caused vasorelaxation due to its NO˙ generation. Infusion of MitoSNO1 during reperfusion was protective against heart ischemia-reperfusion injury, consistent with a functional modification of

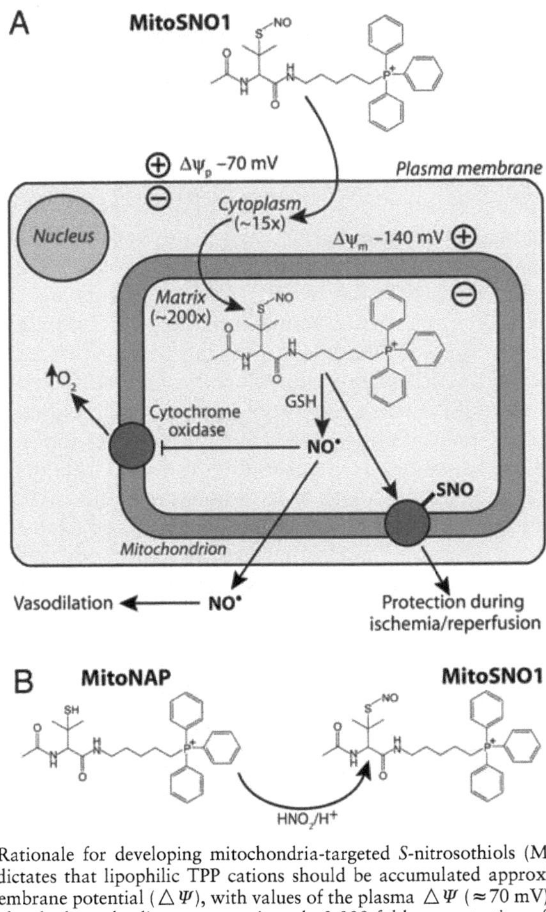

FIGURE 1.—Rationale for developing mitochondria-targeted *S*-nitrosothiols (MitoSNOs). (*A*) The Nernst equation dictates that lipophilic TPP cations should be accumulated approximately 10-fold for every 60 mV of membrane potential ($\Delta\Psi$), with values of the plasma $\Delta\Psi$ ($\approx$70 mV) and mitochondrial $\Delta\Psi$ ($\approx$140 mV) for the heart leading to approximately 3,000-fold concentration of MitoSNO1 within mitochondria. In the oxidizing extracellular environment, MitoSNO1 should be relatively stable. In contrast, glutathione (GSH) within mitochondria should release NO˙ from MitoSNO1, mainly by by transnitrosation to GSNO followed by reduction to release NO˙ by mechanisms that are currently uncertain. The high concentration of NO˙ generated will compete with O_2 for the active site of cytochrome *c* oxidase, particularly when the O_2 concentration is low, and slow respiration while elevating the cytosolic concentration of O_2. MitoSNO1 will also *S*-nitrosate mitochondrial thiol proteins by transferring a nitrosonium group (NO^+) to protein thiolates, modifying their function and may lead to protection during ischemia-reperfusion injury. (*B*) The structure and synthesis of MitoSNO1 by the *S*-nitrosation of the free thiol precursor MitoNAP. (Reprinted from Prime TA, Blaikie FH, Evans C, et al. A mitochondria-targeted S-nitrosothiol modulates respiration, nitrosates thiols, and protects against ischemia-reperfusion injury. *Proc Natl Acad Sci U S A*. 2009;106:10764-10769, with permission from the National Academy of Sciences.)

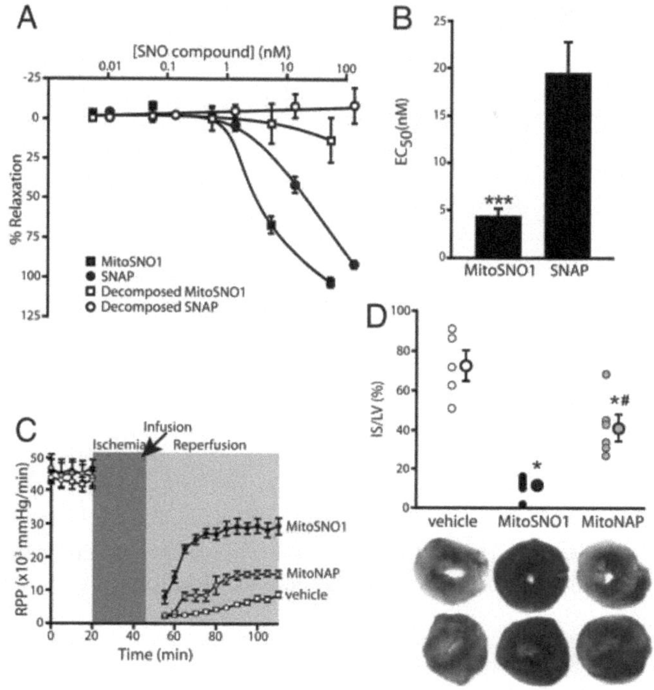

FIGURE 7.—Vasodilatory and tissue protective effects of MitoSNO1. (*A*) Dose-response curves for the effect of MitoSNO1 and related compounds on blood vessel relaxation. Data are means ± SEM, $n = 8$ (MitoSNO1) or $n = 4$ (decomposed MitoSNO1 and SNAP). (*B*) EC_{50} for the effect of MitoSNO1 and SNAP on blood vessel relaxation from (*A*) above. ***, $P < 0.001$ by Student's unpaired *t* test. (*C* and *D*) MitoSNO1 protects against I/R injury in Langendorff-perfused mouse hearts. Hearts were subjected to 25 min of ischemia followed by 1 h of reperfusion. MitoSNO1 or MitoNAP (100 nM final), or vehicle carrier, was added during reperfusion. Hearts were then stained with 2,3,5-triphenyltetrazolium chloride (TTC) to visualize infarct. (*C*) Protection of heart function by MitoSNO1 during I/R injury. Data show rate pressure product (RRP). The arrow indicates where infusion with MitoSNO1 or MitoNAP was initiated. Data are means ± SEM, $n = 6$–7. (*D*) Decreased cardiac infarct size following infusion with MitoSNO1. Upper panel shows typical heart staining. Pale white staining is necrotic infarct, while live tissue stains deep red. Lower panel shows quantitation of infarct size versus area at risk. Data are means ± SEM, $n = 6$–7. *, $P < 0.05$ versus vehicle control group; #, $P < 0.05$ versus vehicle control group (ANOVA). (Reprinted from Prime TA, Blaikie FH, Evans C, et al. A mitochondria-targeted S-nitrosothiol modulates respiration, nitrosates thiols, and protects against ischemia-reperfusion injury. *Proc Natl Acad Sci U S A*. 2009;106:10764-10769, with permission from the National Academy of Sciences.)

mitochondrial proteins, such as complex I, following *S*-nitrosation. These results support the idea that selectively targeting $NO^{\bullet}$ donors to mitochondria is an effective strategy to reversibly modulate respiration and to protect mitochondria against ischemia-reperfusion injury (Figs 1 and 7).

► In this elegant study the investigators describe a molecular approach to selectively generate nitric oxide (NO) and *S*-nitrosothiols within the mitochondria using mitochondria-targeted *S*-nitrsothiols (SNOs). SNOs release NO slowly under oxidizing conditions, but can also release NO rapidly within mitochondria, following transnitrosolation of glutathione (GSH). The exact mechanism by which NO is released is not elucidated in this study. The mitochondria-targeted SNO1 was tested in a rat heart ischemia reperfusion model. MitoSNO1 protected the heart against ischemia-reperfusion injury. The precise mechanism behind this protection is not clear. The most likely mechanism is due to the persistent S-nitrosation of complex I and other mitochondrial proteins, a modification that is also seen during ischemic preconditioning (IPC). Mito SNO1 also caused vasorelaxation due to the release of NO generation. The most significant finding of this study was MitoSNO1, which was most protective when administered during reperfusion unlike the other cardioprotective agents that have to be administered before ischemia-reperfusion injury. The development of mitochondria-targeted NO donors reported here adds to the growing pool of mitochondria-targeted molecules that can be used to manipulate mitochondrial function in global and regional ischemia reperfusion.

M. Mathru, MD, FCCP

Effective Glycemic Control With Aggressive Hyperglycemia Management Is Associated With Improved Outcome in Aneurysmal Subarachnoid Hemorrhage

Latorre JGS, Chou SH-Y, Nogueira RG, et al (SUNY Upstate Med Univ, Syracuse, NY; Brigham and Women's Hosp, Boston, MA; Massachusetts General Hosp, Boston)
Stroke 40:1644-1652, 2009

Background and Purpose.—Hyperglycemia strongly predicts poor outcome in patients with aneurysmal subarachnoid hemorrhage, but the effect of hyperglycemia management on outcome is unclear. We studied the impact of glycemic control on outcome of patients with aneurysmal subarachnoid hemorrhage.

Methods.—A prospective intensive care unit database was used to identify 332 patients with hyperglycemic aneurysmal subarachnoid hemorrhage admitted between January 2000 and December 2006. Patients treated with an aggressive hyperglycemia management (AHM) protocol after 2003 (N = 166) were compared with 166 patients treated using a standard hyperglycemia management before 2003. Within the AHM group, outcome was compared between patients who achieved good (mean glucose burden <1.1 mmol/L) and poor (mean glucose burden ≥1.1 mmol/L) glycemic control. Poor outcome was defined as modified Rankin scale ≥4 at 3 to 6 months. Multivariable logistic regression models correcting for temporal trend were used to quantify the effect of AHM on poor outcome.

Results.—Poor outcome in AHM-treated patients was lower (28.31% versus 40.36%) but was not statistically significant after correcting for temporal trend. However, good glycemic control significantly reduced the incidence of poor outcome (OR, 0.25; 95% CI, 0.08 to 0.80; $P = 0.02$) compared with patients with poor glycemic control within the

TABLE 6.—Glycemic Control and Outcome Within the AHM Group

Variable	Good Control (N = 133)	Poor Control (N = 33)	Adjusted OR (95% CI)	*P**
Primary outcome				
Poor outcome defined as mRS ≥4, N (%)	32 (24.06)	15 (45.45)	0.25 (0.08–0.80)	0.02
Secondary outcome				
Symptomatic vasospasm, N (%)	46 (34.59)	15 (45.45)	0.75 (0.33–1.71)	0.49
DINDs, N (%)	72 (54.14)	23 (69.70)	0.73 (0.31–1.72)	0.48
Complication rates				
Rebleed, N (%)	11 (8.27)	2 (6.06)	1.85 (0.34–10.06)	0.47
Intracranial hypertension, N (%)	59 (44.36)	15 (45.45)	1.10 (0.47–2.57)	0.83
Intracranial hemorrhage, N (%)	21 (15.79)	6 (18.18)	1.16 (0.40–3.40)	0.79
DVT/PE, N (%)	14 (10.53)	8 (24.24)	0.49 (0.17–1.43)	0.19
Cardiac dysfunction, N (%)	38 (28.57)	14 (42.42)	0.55 (0.23–1.32)	0.18
Seizure, N (%)	5 (3.76)	3 (9.09)	0.35 (0.07–1.81)	0.21
Infection, N (%)	62 (46.62)	18 (54.55)	1.00 (0.42–2.40)	0.99
Respiratory failure, N (%)	71 (53.38)	24 (72.73)	0.39 (0.12–1.22)	0.11
Renal failure, N (%)	6 (4.51)	4 (12.12)	0.50 (0.11–2.35)	0.38
Length of stays				
Hospital LOS, median (25%, 75%)	17 (13, 25)	21 (12, 28)	−2.93 (2.28)†	0.20‡
ICU LOS, median (25%, 75%)	13 (10, 16)	14 (9, 18)	0.78 (1.14)†	0.49‡

mRS indicates modified Rankin scale; DINDs, delayed ischemic neurologic deficits; DVT, deep venous thrombosis; PE, pulmonary embolism; LOS, length of stay.
**P* values from logistic regression except Hospital LOS and ICU LOS.
†Parameter estimate (SE).
‡*P* value from linear regression model.

AHM group. No difference in the rate of clinical vasospasm or the development of delayed ischemic neurological deficit was seen before and after AHM protocol implementation.

Conclusion.—AHM results in good glucose control and significantly reduces the odds for poor outcome after aneurysmal subarachnoid hemorrhage in glucose-controlled patients. Further studies are needed to confirm these results (Table 6).

▶ Several lines of experimental and clinical evidence demonstrate a significant association between persistent hyperglycemia and negative outcome in different acute medical and surgical patients. In aneurysmal subarachnoid hemorrhage (aSAH) hyperglycemia is linked to cerebral vasospasm and poor outcome. Intensive insulin therapy is currently advocated for use in critically ill patients without neurological disease. The first study conducted in surgical ICU patients showed significant reduction in morbidity and mortality. However, a recent study in medical ICU patients did not show any effect on morbidity or mortality. The results of these studies suggest that there may be a differential effect of insulin therapy among various types of patients, including those with acute brain injuries. This study examined the impact of aggressive blood sugar control on patient outcome after SAH. This study shows that aggressive hyperglycemia management was independently associated with good outcome. However, no difference in the rate of clinical vasospasm or the development of delayed neurological deficit was seen before and after the implementation of aggressive hyperglycemia management. A word of caution to clinicians when treating brain injured patients with aggressive blood sugar control protocol: The human brain is an obligate glucose consumer, and neuronal tissue is not sensitive to insulin. Therefore, cerebral glucose uptake and metabolism are supply driven. Experimental and clinical evidence suggest that lowering blood glucose concentration reduces brain tissue glucose concentration. Furthermore, persistent hypoglycemia has been associated with peri-ischemic cortical depolarization and poor neurologic outcome. Future studies should determine optimal glucose target in brain-injured patients.

M. Mathru, MD, FCCP

Defining Vasospasm After Subarachnoid Hemorrhage: What Is the Most Clinically Relevant Definition?

Frontera JA, Fernandez A, Schmidt JM, et al (Mount Sinai School of Medicine, NY; Columbia Univ College of Physicians and Surgeons, NY)

Stroke 40:1963-1968, 2009

Background and Purpose.—Vasospasm is an important complication of subarachnoid hemorrhage, but is variably defined in the literature.

Methods.—We studied 580 patients with subarachnoid hemorrhage and identified those with: (1) symptomatic vasospasm, defined as clinical deterioration deemed secondary to vasospasm after other causes were eliminated; (2) delayed cerebral ischemia (DCI), defined as symptomatic vasospasm, or infarction on CT attributable to vasospasm; (3) angiographic spasm, as seen on digital subtraction angiography; and (4) transcranial Doppler (TCD) spasm, defined as any mean flow velocity >120 cm/sec. Logistic regression analysis was performed to test the association of each definition of vasospasm with various hospital complications, and 3-month quality of life (sickness impact profile), cognitive status (telephone interview of cognitive status), instrumental activities of daily living (Lawton score), and death or severe disability at 3 months (modified Rankin scale score 4–6), after adjustment for covariates.

Results.—Symptomatic vasospasm occurred in 16%, DCI in 21%, angiographic vasospasm in 31%, and TCD spasm in 45% of patients. DCI was statistically associated with more hospital complications (N = 7; all $P < 0.05$) than symptomatic spasm (N = 4), angiographic spasm (N = 1), or TCD vasospasm (N = 1). Angiographic and TCD vasospasm were not related to any aspect of clinical outcome. Both symptomatic vasospasm and DCI were related to reduced instrumental activities of daily living, cognitive impairment, and poor quality of life (all $P < 0.05$). However, only DCI was associated with death or severe disability at 3 months (adjusted OR, 2.2; 95% CI, 1.2–3.9; $P = 0.007$).

Conclusions.—DCI is a more clinically meaningful definition than either symptomatic deterioration alone or the presence of arterial spasm by angiography or TCD.

► Vasospasm following subarachnoid hemorrhage (SAH) carries a high morbidity and mortality. This study examined the clinical relevance in various definitions of vasospasm, including symptomatic vasospasm, delayed cerebral ischemia (DCI), transcranial Doppler (TCD)vasospasm, and angiographic vasospasm. This study convincingly demonstrated that DCI, a definition that incorporates both symptomatic worsening and cerebral infarction, is the most clinically relevant definition of vasospasm because it has the strongest association with overall poor outcome, cognitive impairment, and reduced quality of life. Furthermore those who met the criteria of DCI had a more complicated hospital course than other definitions of vasospasm. Symptomatic vasospasm was also associated with cognitive dysfunction and poor quality of life in this study, but not with death or disability. The arterial vasospasm diagnosed by angiography or TCD had no consistent relationship with 3-month outcome. Accordingly, DCI appears to be both most inclusive and a clinically-meaningful definition for capturing the adverse effects of vasospasm after SAH.

M. Mathru, MD, FCCP

Dynamic preload indicators fail to predict fluid responsiveness in open-chest conditions

de Waal EEC, Rex S, Kruitwagen CLJJ, et al (Univ Med Ctr, Utrecht, The Netherlands; Univ Hosp, Germany)

Crit Care Med 37:510-515, 2009

Objective.—Dynamic preload indicators like pulse pressure variation (PPV) and stroke volume variation (SVV) are increasingly being used for optimizing cardiac preload since they have been demonstrated to predict fluid responsiveness in a variety of perioperative settings. However, in open-chest conditions, the value of these indices has not been systematically examined yet. We, therefore, evaluated the ability of PPV and SVV to predict fluid responsiveness under open- and closed-chest conditions.

Design.—Prospective, controlled, clinical study.

Setting.—University hospital.

Patients.—Twenty-two patients scheduled for elective coronary artery bypass graft surgery.

Interventions.—Defined volume loads (VL) (10 mL kg^{-1} hydroxy-ethyl starch 6%) intra- and postoperatively.

Measurements and Main Results.—Stroke volume index was measured 1) before and after a VL intraoperatively in open-chest conditions, and 2) under closed-chest conditions within 1 hour after arrival in the intensive care unit. Central venous pressure and global end diastolic volume were assessed as static preload indicators. In addition, PPV and SVV (both

TABLE 5.—Receiver Operating Characteristic and Pearson's Correlation Analysis for Several Preload Indicators as Predictors of Increase in Stroke Volume Index by more than 12% After Volume Loading in Open and Closed Chest Conditions

	Receiver Operating Characteristic Curves Predicting Increase in Stroke Volume Index ≥12%				Pearsons' Correlation with Increase in Stroke Volume Index	
Baseline Hemodynamic Indices	Area Under the Curve	Standard Error	*p* Value	95% Confidence Interval	R^2	*p* Value
Open chest						
Central venous pressure	0.578	0.168	0.678	0.248–0.907	0.0742	0.274
Global end diastolic volume index	0.756	0.130	0.173	0.500–1.011	0.4949	0.001[a]
Intrathoracic blood volume index	0.756	0.130	0.173	0.500–1.011	0.4944	0.001[a]
Pulse pressure variation	0.556	0.126	0.767	0.308–0.803	0.1046	0.190
Stroke volume variation	0.489	0.134	0.953	0.225–0.752	0.0419	0.4156
Closed chest						
Central venous pressure	0.636	0.124	0.279	0.393–0.880	0.0043	0.087
Global end diastolic volume index	0.700	0.123	0.121	0.460–0.940	0.0977	0.168
Intrathoracic blood volume index	0.682	0.123	0.159	0.441–0.923	0.0986	0.166
Pulse pressure variation	0.884	0.075	0.004[a]	0.736–1.032	0.5620	0.000[a]
Stroke volume variation	0.911	0.069	0.003[a]	0.776–1.046	0.5554	0.000[a]

[a]$p < 0.05$.

obtained with PiCCO system) were recorded. Fluid-responders were defined by an increase in stroke volume index ≥12% subsequent to the VL. Receiver operating characteristic analysis showed that all preload indicators failed to predict fluid responsiveness in open-chest conditions. Under closed-chest conditions, the areas under the receiver operating characteristic curve for PPV and SVV were 0.884 ($p = 0.004$) and 0.911 ($p = 0.003$), respectively, whereas the static and volumetric preload parameters failed to predict fluid responsiveness. A PPV of ≥10% identified fluid-responders with a sensitivity of 64% and a specificity of 100%, while a SVV of >8% identified fluid-responders with a sensitivity of 100% and a specificity of 78%.

Conclusions.—Our results suggest that the dynamic preload indicators PPV and SVV are able to predict fluid responsiveness under closed-chest conditions, whereas all static and dynamic preload indicators fail to predict fluid responsiveness under open-chest conditions (Table 5).

▶ Functional hemodynamic indices such as pulse pressure variation (PVV) and stroke volume variation (SVV) are used to determine fluid responsiveness in critically ill patients. The calculation of SVV and PVV are based on the cyclic alterations in intrathoracic pressures induced by mechanical ventilation and are critically dependent on the undisturbed transmission of airway pressure changes to cardiovascular structures within the closed thorax. Therefore, during open-chest conditions such as cardiac surgery, these changes in pleural pressure during positive pressure ventilation will be less pronounced and PPV and SVV can no longer accurately predict fluid responsiveness. This study examined the ability of PPV and SVV to predict fluid responsiveness under open chest conditions. The authors' results confirm their hypothesis that both PVV and SVV were not sensitive enough to predict fluid responsiveness under open chest conditions. The data derived from this study are in contrast to data from Reuter et al,[1] who found SVV and PVV to predict fluid responsiveness under open-chest conditions. However, their findings were solely based on significant correlations between SVV and PVV before a volume challenge and the changes in the cardiac index to that challenge. Furthermore, Reuter et al performed their measurements in the absence of pericardium, which contributes significantly to ventricular compliance.

M. Mathru, MD, FCCP

Reference

1. Reuter DA, Goepfert MS, Goresch T, Schmoeckel M, Kilger E, Goetz AE. Assessing fluid responsiveness during open chest conditions. *Br J Anaesth*. 2005;94: 318-323.

A multicenter, randomized, double-blind, placebo-controlled, dose-escalation trial assessing safety and efficacy of active site inactivated recombinant factor VIIa in subjects with acute lung injury or acute respiratory distress syndrome

Vincent J-L, Artigas A, Petersen LC, et al (Université libre de Bruxelles, Belgium; CIBER Enfermedades Respiratorias Autonomous Univ of Barcelona, Spain; Novo Nordisk, Bagsvaerd, Denmark)

Crit Care Med 37:1874-1880, 2009

Objective.—To evaluate the safety and efficacy of active site inactivated recombinant factor VIIa (FFR-rFVIIa) in patients with acute respiratory distress syndrome.

Design.—Phase II, randomized, double-blind, placebo-controlled, dose-escalation trial.

Setting.—Forty-six intensive care units (ICU) in ten countries.

Patients.—All adult (≥18 years), mechanically ventilated patients with acute onset (within 48 hour) of acute lung injury/acute respiratory distress syndrome were included.

Interventions.—Four sequential (in ascending order) treatment groups (cohorts) in single and multiple dosing strategies. Subjects were randomized in a 2:1 ratio to either FFR-rFVIIa or placebo within each cohort.

Measurements and Results.—Data were collected daily for 7 days and on days 14 and 28 for efficacy variables including hematology and coagulation parameters, plasma D-dimer levels, plasma interleukin-6 levels, vital signs, ventilator parameters, lung injury score, and Sequential Organ Failure Assessment score. The study was discontinued prematurely by the Safety Committee based on statistical analysis of the mortality in cohort 3 (4 × 400 μg/kg), which suggested that, after adjusting for prognostic covariates, 28-day mortality was significantly higher in this cohort than in the placebo group and time to death was significantly shorter. A total of 214 patients (147 male) were included in the trial, mean age 59 years (range, 24–85 years). Overall, there were no significant differences in mortality rates in treated and placebo patients (36/144 deaths FFR-rFVIIa, 15/70 placebo). There was no treatment effect of FFR-rFVIIa on vital signs, blood chemistry parameters, hematology parameters, or amount of transfusion products required. There was a trend to increased bleeding with increasing FFR-rFVIIa dose.

Conclusion.—In this randomized double-blind, placebo-controlled, dose-escalation trial, FFR-rFVIIa had no beneficial effects on morbidity or outcome overall. The cohort of patients receiving 4 × 400 μg/kg of FFR-rFVIIa had increased mortality rates compared with placebo-treated patients, and there was a trend to increased risk of serious bleeding with increasing doses (Fig 4).

▶ Tissue factor (TF) is an integral membrane glycoprotein expressed on the media and adventitia of blood vessels and acts as the cellular receptor for the coagulation factor VIIa. The formation of TF-VIIa complexes on cell surfaces triggers the coagulation cascade and, in addition, induces intracellular

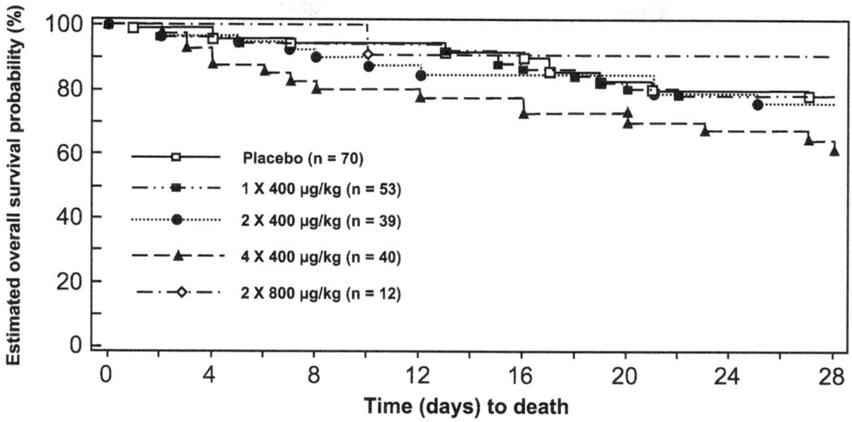

FIGURE 4.—Kaplan-Meier survival curves for the five cohorts. (Reprinted from Vincent J-L, Artigas A, Petersen LC, et al. A multicenter, randomized, double-blind, placebo-controlled, dose-escalation trial assessing safety and efficacy of active site inactivated recombinant factor VIIa in subjects with acute lung injury or acute respiratory distress syndrome. *Crit Care Med.* 2009;37:1874-1880.)

responses and specific gene regulation of inflammatory mediators. Several lines of experimental evidence suggest that inflammation is linked to coagulation via activation of the protease-activated receptors, which are activated either directly by the TF-VIIa complex or more indirectly by the coagulation factors. Therefore the TF pathway is an attractive therapeutic target in acute respiratory distress syndrome (ARDS). In this randomized, placebo-controlled trial the investigators examined the safety and efficacy of inactivated recombinant factor VIIa (FFR-rFVIIa) in patients with life threatening ARDS. Unfortunately the investigators were unable to demonstrate improved survival or efficacy outcomes in acute lung injury (ALI)/ARDS subjects treated with FFR-rFVIIa. Indeed the trial was stopped when a significant increased risk of death was observed in patients receiving higher dosage of the experimental drug. However, unlike the present clinical study in humans, treatment with FFR-rFVIIa was associated with marked attenuation of coagulopathy, inflammation, and organ injury. The reasons for the observed negative effect in this study are not clear. Possibilities for the failure include species difference, dosage of the drug, and timing of administration of the drug.

M. Mathru, MD, FCCP

A simple clinical predictive index for objective estimates of mortality in acute lung injury

Cooke CR, Shah CV, Gallop R, et al (Univ of Washington, Seattle; Univ of Pennsylvania, Philadelphia; West Chester Univ, PA; et al)

Crit Care Med 37:1913-1920, 2009

Objective.—We sought to develop a simple point score that would accurately capture the risk of hospital death for patients with acute lung injury (ALI).

Design.—This is a secondary analysis of data from two randomized trials. Baseline clinical variables collected within 24 hours of enrollment were modeled as predictors of hospital mortality using logistic regression and bootstrap resampling to arrive at a parsimonious model. We constructed a point score based on regression coefficients.

Setting.—Medical centers participating in the Acute Respiratory Distress Syndrome Clinical Trials Network (ARDSnet).

Patients.—Model development: 414 patients with nontraumatic ALI participating in the low tidal volume arm of the ARDSnet Acute Respiratory Management in ARDS study. Model validation: 459 patients participating in the ARDSnet Assessment of Low tidal Volume and elevated End-expiratory volume to Obviate Lung Injury study. Model Validation: 459 patients participating in the ARDSnet Assessment of Low tidal Volume and elevated End-expiratory volume to Obviate Lung Injury trial.

Interventions.—None.

Measurements and Main Results.—Variables comprising the prognostic model were hematocrit <26% (1 point), bilirubin ≥2 mg/dL (1 point), fluid balance >2.5 L positive (1 point), and age (1 point for age 40–64 years, 2 points for age ≥65 years). Predicted mortality (95% confidence interval) for 0, 1, 2, 3, and 4+ point totals was 8% (5% to 14%), 17% (12% to 23%), 31% (26% to 37%), 51% (43% to 58%), and 70% (58% to 80%), respectively. There was an excellent agreement between predicted and observed mortality in the validation cohort. Observed mortality for 0, 1, 2, 3, and 4+ point totals in the validation cohort was 12%, 16%, 28%, 47%, and 67%, respectively. Compared with the Acute Physiology Assessment and Chronic Health Evaluation III score, areas under the receiver operating characteristic curve for the point score were greater in the development cohort (0.72 vs. 0.67, $p = 0.09$) and lower in the validation cohort (0.68 vs. 0.75, $p = 0.03$).

Conclusions.—Mortality in patients with ALI can be predicted using an index of four readily available clinical variables with good calibration. This index may help inform prognostic discussions, but validation in nonclinical trial populations is necessary before widespread use (Figs 1 and 2).

▶ Despite progress in the treatment of the acute lung injury, the ability to predict outcome largely has eluded clinicians. The use of the acute physiology assessment and chronic health evaluation (APACHE) and other scoring tools

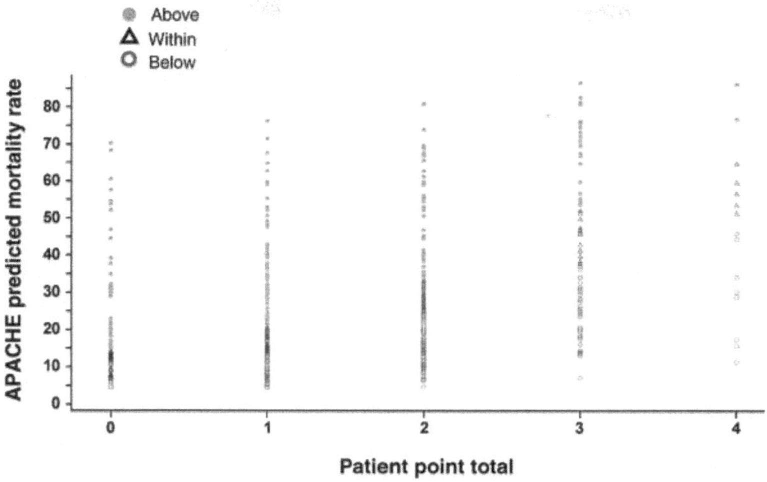

FIGURE 1.—Calibration plot. For each patient in the validation dataset, the predicted mortality estimated from the Acute Physiology Assessment and Chronic Health Evaluation (*APACHE*) III score is plotted against the point total from the custom model developed from the Acute Respiratory Distress Syndrome Network low tidal volume study. Patients with an APACHE III predicted mortality overlapping with the custom model predicted mortality in the validation cohort are shown using triangles (within). Closed circles (above) indicate patients where APACHE III predicts a greater rate of death than predicted by the simple model. Open circles (below) indicate patients where APACHE III predicts a lower rate of death than predicted by the simple model. (Reprinted from Cooke CR, Shah CV, Gallop R, et al. A simple clinical predictive index for objective estimates of mortality in acute lung injury. *Crit Care Med.* 2009;37:1913-1920.)

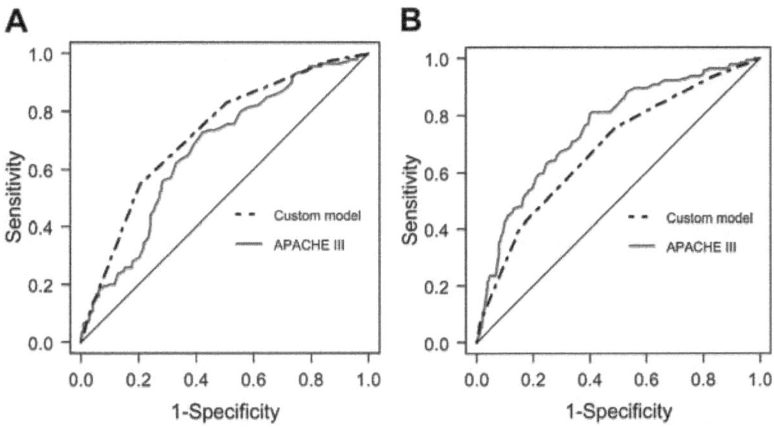

FIGURE 2.—Receiver operating characteristic (ROC) curves for the custom model. *A*, comparison of the ROC curves for the custom model and Acute Physiology Assessment and Chronic Health Evaluation (*APACHE*) III score (area 0.72 vs. 0.67, $p = 0.09$) in the development cohort. *B*, comparison between custom model and APACHE III (area 0.68 vs. 0.75, $p = 0.03$) in the validation cohort. (Reprinted from Cooke CR, Shah CV, Gallop R, et al. A simple clinical predictive index for objective estimates of mortality in acute lung injury. *Crit Care Med.* 2009;37:1913-1920.)

have been used to predict the probability of death of a patient in the ICU, but these modalities have limitations. As secondary analysis of the Acute Respiratory Distress Syndrome Clinical Trials Network (ARDSnet) low volume ventilation trial, the authors were able to identify 4 significant predictors of poor outcome (age, hematocrit, fluid status, and bilirubin) and assign these predictors a point value. The total score was compared with the APACHE score and had somewhat better receiver operator validation than the corresponding APACHE score. The authors have provided a simple and well-validated scoring system that can assist the clinician in treatment decisions in the management of patients with acute lung injury. Further validations in other populations (acute lung injury due to trauma) should be undertaken before being used as a general screening tool.

M. Mathru, MD, FCCP

Red blood cell transfusion practices in acute lung injury: What do patient factors contribute?

Murphy DJ, Howard D, Muriithi A, et al (Johns Hopkins Univ, Baltimore, MD; John H Stroger Hosp of Cook County, Chicago, IL; et al)

Crit Care Med 37:1935-1940, 2009

Objective.—To describe red blood cell (RBC) transfusion practices and evaluate the association between patient-related factors and pretransfusion hemoglobin concentration in acute lung injury (ALI).

Design.—Secondary analysis of prospectively collected data.

Setting.—Nine intensive care units (ICUs) in three teaching hospitals in Baltimore, MD.

Patients.—Two hundred forty-nine consecutive patients with ALI requiring mechanical ventilation.

Interventions.—None.

Measurements and Main Results.—Simple and multiple linear regression analyses were used to evaluate the association between the nadir hemoglobin concentration on the day of initial RBC transfusion and 20 patient-level demographic, clinical and ICU treatment factors as well as ICU type. Of 249 patients with ALI, 47% received an RBC transfusion in the ICU without evidence of active hemorrhage or acute cardiac ischemia. The mean (SD) nadir hemoglobin on the day of first transfusion was 7.7 (1.1) g/dL with 67%, 36%, 15%, and 5% of patients transfused at >7, >8, >9, and >10 g/dL, respectively. Transfused patients received a mean (SD) of 5 (6) RBC units from ALI diagnosis to ICU discharge. Prehospital use of iron or erythropoietin and platelet transfusion in the ICU were independently associated with lower pretransfusion hemoglobin concentrations. No patient factors were associated with higher hemoglobin concentrations. Admission to a surgical (vs. medical) ICU was independently associated with a 0.6 g/dL (95% confidence interval 0.1–1.1 g/dL) higher pretransfusion hemoglobin.

Conclusions.—Patients with ALI commonly receive RBC transfusions in the ICU. The pretransfusion hemoglobin observed in our study was lower than earlier studies, but a restrictive strategy was not universally adopted. Patient factors do not explain the gap between clinical trial evidence and routine transfusion practices. Future studies should further explore

TABLE 3.—Adjusted Association of Individual Patient Characteristics and ICU Type with Pretransfusion Hemoglobin Concentration

Exposure Variable[a]	Mean Change (95% CI) in Nadir Hemoglobin[b] (g/dL)	p
Patient demographic characteristic		
Age	0.002 (−0.01 to 0.02)	0.74
White	−0.06 (−0.4 to 0.3)	0.76
Patient clinical characteristics		
Charlson comorbidity index	−0.05 (−0.1 to 0.0)	0.20
Routine iron use before hospitalization	−0.5 (−1.0 to 0.1)	0.03
Routine erythropoietin use before hospitalization	−0.8 (−1.4 to −0.3)	0.005
Primary ICU admitting diagnosis Gastrointestinal	0.5 (−0.3 to 1.3)	0.20
Lung Injury Score at ALI onset	−0.1 (−0.4 to 0.2)	0.38
Patient ICU course characteristics		
Platelet transfusion[c]	−0.5 (−0.9 to −0.005)	0.048
ICU type		
Surgical (vs. Medical) ICU	0.6 (0.1 to 1.1)	0.02

ICU, intensive care unit; CI, confidence interval; ALI, acute lung injury.

[a]Exposure variables presented are those from Table 2 which were associated with a change in mean nadir hemoglobin on the day of first transfusion at $p \leq 0.15$;

[b]mean change in nadir hemoglobin concentration on day of first red blood cell transfusion associated with each 1 unit increase in continuous exposure variables (e.g., age) or each categorical exposure variable (e.g., routine iron use before hospitalization) as calculated using multiple linear regression with a fixed effect to account for clustering of the data within the 3 participating hospitals;

[c]proportion of patients receiving the ICU intervention at any time from the day of ALI onset through the day of first red blood cell transfusion.

ICU- and physician-related factors as a source of variability in transfusion practice (Table 3).

▶ Shortage of blood supply is anticipated because of the growing elderly population with increased demand for blood transfusion and the decreasing donation rate. Therefore, increased emphasis is being placed on planning for acute or sustained blood shortages. Most blood banks are establishing emergency blood emergency management plans that would be activated to deal with such eventualities. Such strategies include canceling elective surgical cases where large volumes of red blood cells are used. Recent evidence suggests that increasing proportions of the RBCC's are administered in medical patients, and the use of perioperative transfusions are decreasing in surgical patients. The goal of this study was to examine in detail the fate of RBC's issued from a single hospital blood bank to nonoperating areas of a major teaching hospital in United Kingdom and how reduced demand could be achieved safely. The study demonstrates that 89% of the RBC units are transfused outside of the operating rooms, of which 74% were to medical patients and only 22% to surgical patients. In 31% of the medical patients who had been transfused there was no evidence of surgical bleeding. Moreover, 50% of these transfusions were at least 2 RBC units and more than 50% of posttransfusion Hb concentrations were more than 9 gm/d/L. Their data confirm that an increasing proportion of the blood is transfused to medical patients rather than those undergoing surgery. The study also confirms that maintaining blood supply during acute or sustained shortage would be difficult based on interventions in surgical group alone. Furthermore, in the settings where perioperative blood conservation strategies are well established, surgical cancellations are unlikely to maintain blood supply unless shortages are approximately 10% or less. Most emergency blood plans anticipate a 30% to 50% decrease in blood supply (ie, major natural/terrorist disasters). Therefore, severe and sustained reduction in blood supply could only be addressed by controlling nonoperating room requests, especially for patients with medical diagnosis.

M. Mathru, MD, FCCP

Continuous hypertonic saline therapy and the occurrence of complications in neurocritically ill patients

Froelich M, Ni Q, Wess C, et al (Karolinska Inst, Stockholm, Sweden; New York Presbyterian Hosp)

Crit Care Med 37:1433-1441, 2009

Objective.—To evaluate potential side effects of continuous hypertonic 3% saline (CHS) as maintenance fluid in patients with brain injury.

Methods.—Retrospective chart analysis of prospectively collected data.

Patients.—Patients admitted to the neurosurgical intensive care unit for >4 days with traumatic brain injury, stroke, or subarachnoid hemorrhage with a Glasgow Coma Scale <9 and elevated intracranial pressure (ICP) or at risk of developing elevated ICP were included. Based on physician preference, one group was treated with 3% CHS at a rate of 1.5 mL/kg/bw as maintenance fluid. The other group received 0.9% normal saline (NS). Two percent saline was used in the CHS group to wean patients off 3% CHS or when sodium was above 155. Data on serum sodium, blood urea nitrogen, creatinine, ICP, infection rate, length of stay, rates of deep vein thrombosis, and pulmonary emboli and dural thrombosis were collected prospectively.

Results.—One hundred seven patients in the CHS group and 80 in the NS group met the inclusion criteria. The incidence of moderate hypernatremia (Na > 155 mmol/L) and severe hypernatremia (Na > 160 mmol/L) was significantly higher in the CHS therapy group than in the NS group. No significant relationship between CHS infusion and renal dysfunction was found. Moderate and severe hypernatremia was associated with a higher risk of elevated blood urea nitrogen and creatinine levels. Acute renal failure was not seen in these patients. A total of 53.3% in the CHS group and in 16.3% in the NS group ($p < 0.0001$) had raised ICP (>25 mm Hg), consistent with the physicians decision to use CHS in patients with elevated ICP.

Conclusions.—CHS therapy was not associated with an increased rate of infection, deep vein thrombosis, or renal failure. However, there was a significant risk of developing hypernatremia. We conclude that CHS

TABLE 4.—Complications in the Hypernatremia Group (Na > 155) and the Normal Sodium Group (Na ≤ 155)

Complications	Na > 155, n (%)	Na ≤ 155, n (%)	*p*	Adjusted Odds Ratio[a]	95% Confidence Interval	*p*
DVT, yes	16 (23.2)	12 (10.2)	0.02	2.30	(0.90–5.94)	0.08
DVT, no	53 (76.8)	106 (89.8)				
Infection, yes	57 (82.6)	99 (83.9)	0.82	1.09	(0.41–2.91)	0.87
Infection, no	12 (17.4)	19 (16.1)				
BUN >8.9	32 (47.8)	50 (41.7)	0.42	2.34	(1.13–4.88)	0.02
BUN ≤8.9	35 (52.2)	70 (58.3)				
Creatinine >132.6	21 (31.3)	25 (20.8)	0.11	2.82	(1.29–6.17)	0.01
Creatinine ≤132.6	46 (68.7)	95 (79.2)				

DVT, deep vein thrombosis; BUN, blood urea nitrogen.
[a]All four logistic regression models predict each complication for moderate hypernatremia (sodium >155) (sodium <155 used as reference), adjusting for age, gender, disease type, and log transformation of length of stay.

TABLE 5.—Complications in the Severe Hypernatremia Group (Na > 160) and the Normal Sodium Group (Na ≤ 160)

Complications	Na > 160, n (%)	Na < 160, n (%)	Chi-square *p*	Adjusted Odds Ratio[a]	95% Confidence Interval	Adjusted *p*
DVT, yes	9 (22.5)	19 (12.9)	0.13	1.66	(0.58–4.74)	0.34
DVT, no	31 (77.5)	128 (87.1)				
Infection, yes	34 (85.0)	122 (83.0)	0.76	1.95	(0.58–6.57)	0.28
Infection, no	6 (15.0)	25 (17.0)				
BUN >8.9	21 (52.5)	61 (41.5)	0.21	3.46	(1.48–8.06)	0.004
BUN ≤8.9	19 (47.5)	86 (58.5)				
Creatinine >132.6	12 (30.0)	34 (23.1)	0.37	2.23	(0.94–5.31)	0.07
Creatinine ≤132.6	28 (70.0)	113 (76.9)				

DVT, deep vein thrombosis; BUN, blood urea nitrogen.
[a]All four logistic regression models predict each complication for severe hypernatremia (sodium >160) (sodium <160 used as reference), adjusting for age, gender, disease type, and log transformation of length of stay.

administration in patients with severe injuries is safe as long as sodium levels are carefully monitored (Tables 4 and 5).

▶ Hypertonic saline remains one of the most controversial treatment modalities in the critical care arena. Hypertonic saline has been used in the neurocritical care setting for many intracranial pathologic conditions, including subarachnoid hemorrhage, stroke, and traumatic brain injury. The authors retrospectively compared 3% saline to 0.9% normal saline with a well-defined protocol in a single neurosurgical ICU. Compared with normal saline as a control, patients in the 3% saline group were more likely to experience clinically significant hypernatremia than those receiving normal saline. As opposed to earlier studies that suggested an increased incidence, the authors found no increase in infection, deep venous thrombosis, or renal failure compared with the control normal saline group. While extreme hypernatremia (>160) is detrimental for certain patient subgroups (subarachnoid hemorrhage), the benefits of hypertonic saline may outweigh the risks when frequent and diligent monitoring of sodium levels are undertaken. While somewhat difficult to perform, further multicenter prospective trials should be undertaken regarding the safety of hypertonic saline in the neurosurgical patient.

M. Mathru, MD, FCCP

Females have fewer complications and lower mortality following trauma than similarly injured males: A risk adjusted analysis of adults in the National Trauma Data Bank

Haider AH, Crompton JG, Oyetunji T, et al (Johns Hopkins Univ School of Medicine, Baltimore, MD; Howard Univ College of Medicine, WA)

Surgery 146:308-315, 2009

Background.—Studies of sexual dimorphism in trauma outcomes suggest that women have a survival advantage compared to equivalently injured men. It is unknown if this gender disparity is mediated by potentially life-threatening complications.

Objective.—To determine (1) if there is a sex-based differences in the odds of developing inpatient complications after trauma, and (2) if are these complications associated with death among trauma patients.

Methods.—Review of adult trauma patients admitted to hospitals in the National Trauma Data Bank that report complications. Patient and injury severity covariates were adjusted using multiple logistic regression and the independent effect of sex on developing complications and associated mortality was determined.

Results.—A total of 681,730 adult patients met the inclusion criteria of hospital admission ≥3 days. Women demonstrated a 21% lower adjusted risk of death compared to males (OR 0.79, 95% CI 0.76–0.83). Females had decreased adjusted odds of developing life-threatening complications including pneumonia, acute respiratory distress syndrome, acute renal failure and pulmonary embolism. However, when compared to males with life-threatening complications, females with complications were found to be at greater risk of dying.

Conclusion.—This study demonstrates that women are less likely than men to develop inpatient complications, suggesting that the survival advantage among women after traumatic injury may involve a reduced susceptibility to developing life-threatening complications (Fig 2, Table 3).

▶ Experimental research has convincingly demonstrated that gender is a determinant of mortality and morbidity after traumatic injury. Most investigators attribute this gender difference to female hormones and their immune enhancing effect. Estradiol has been shown to enhance the function of both cell- and humoral-mediated immunity. Proestrus female mice have been shown to have

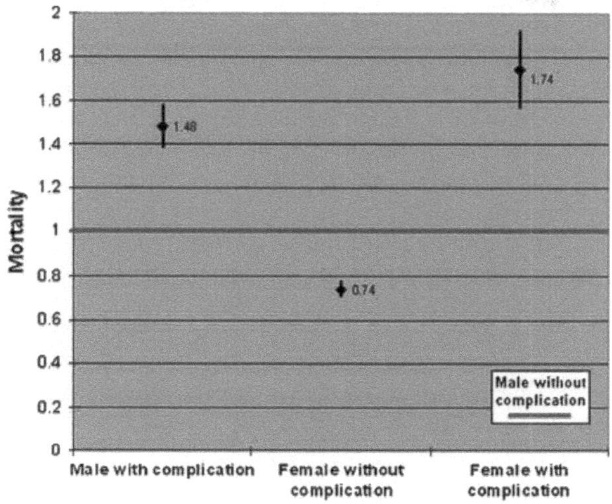

FIGURE 2.—Result of interaction analysis depicting the adjusted odds of death with the development of any complication by gender. Reference group is male patients without any complications. $n = 427,933$ patients. (Reprinted from Haider AH, Crompton JG, Oyetunji T, et al. Females have fewer complications and lower mortality following trauma than similarly injured males: a risk adjusted analysis of adults in the National Trauma Data Bank. *Surgery.* 2009;146:308-315.)

TABLE 3.—Mortality (Percent) Among Female and Male Patients for Each Life-threatening Complication

Life-threatening Complication (Number of Males with Complication; Number of Females with Complication)	Male Mortality (%)	Female Mortality (%)
Pneumonia* (males $n = 16,569$; females $n = 5,345$)	9.51	10.85
Acute respiratory distress syndrome (males $n = 4,685$; females $n = 1,609$)	17.12	18.21
Acute renal failure (males $n = 2,727$; females $n = 898$)	25.93	26.95
Pulmonary embolism (males $n = 1,890$; females $n = 729$)	10.00	7.13
Intra-abdominal abscess (males $n = 605$; females $n = 113$)	6.61	9.73

*Comparison between males and females statistically significant at the $P < .05$ level.

improved macrophage and lymphocyte responses after trauma and hemorrhagic shock. In contrast, male hormones have immunomodulating effect that suppresses the immune system, and castration of male mice has been shown to improve survival after the induction of trauma and hemorrhagic shock. However, clinical studies investigating this sexual dimorphism have produced mixed results. The authors of this study used the largest available trauma database to determine if there are sex-based differences among trauma patients in the odds of developing... common complications such as urinary tract infections and potentially life threatening complications such as acute respiratory distress syndrome (ARDS) pneumonia and renal failure. The study demonstrates 3 salient findings: (1) Adult women with equivalent injury compared with males who have a survival advantage. (2) Women have exhibited a lower odd of developing life-threatening complications when compared with men of similar age and equivalent injury following trauma. (3) Severe complications of traumatic injury such as ARDS, pneumonia, acute renal failure, pulmonary embolism, and intra-abdominal abscess are associated with greater risk of mortality in women compared with men. The exact mechanisms by which sex-based outcome disparities are promulgated in humans are still not well understood. Therefore, carefully planned, prospective outcome studies, taking into account patient characteristics, injury severity, preinjury hormone levels, and the sequelae of injury including complications are needed to accurately elucidate the pathways that lead to the improved outcomes for females after trauma.

M. Mathru, MD, FCCP

Biomarkers of sepsis

Marshall JC, for the International Sepsis Forum (Li Ka Shing Knowledge Inst, Toronto, Ontario, Canada; et al)

Crit Care Med 37:2290-2298, 2009

Background.—A complex network of biological mediators underlies the clinical syndrome of sepsis. The nonspecific physiologic criteria of sepsis syndrome or the systemic inflammatory response syndrome do not adequately identify patients who might benefit from either conventional anti-infective therapies or from novel therapies that target specific mediators of sepsis. Validated biomarkers of sepsis may improve diagnosis and therapeutic decision making for these high-risk patients.

Objectives.—To develop a methodologic framework for the identification and validation of biomarkers of sepsis.

Methods.—A small group meeting of experts in clinical epidemiology, biomarker development, and sepsis clinical trials; selective narrative review of the biomarker literature.

Results.—The utility of a biomarker is a function of the degree to which it adds value to the available clinical information in the domains of screening, diagnosis, risk stratification, and monitoring of the response to therapy. We identified needs for greater standardization of biomarker methodologies, greater methodologic rigor in biomarker studies, wider integration of biomarkers into clinical studies (in particular, early phase studies), and increased collaboration among investigators, pharmaceutical industry, biomarker industry, and regulatory agencies.

Conclusions.—Biomarkers promise to transform sepsis from a physiologic syndrome to a group of distinct biochemical disorders. This transformation could aid therapeutic decision making, and hence improve the

TABLE 3.—Summary Recommendations

We recommend that steps be taken to standardize assays for the measurement of biomarkers of sepsis, and to identify and understand the sources of differences among techniques, for example, bioassays vs. immunoassays, cell-bound vs. free protein, target biomarkers vs. levels of circulating inhibitors, and the confounding effects of inhibitors and carrier proteins. Similarly, the performance of microarray analyses must be standardized with respect to platforms, composition of arrays, and methods of data analysis
We recommend that studies of biomarkers of sepsis be performed using rigorous methodologic approaches to characterize the added value provided by the maker. Such approaches can include inception cohort studies, case–control studies, or randomized clinical trials, analyzed using multivariable techniques to define the independent diagnostic or prognostic value of the marker
We recommend wider use of validated biomarkers to assist in the decision-making process in guiding the transition from early phase clinical research to definitive trials with clinically important end points
We urge that clinical trials be used as platforms to identify and validate potentially useful biomarkers of sepsis—both to evaluate drug efficacy and to generate knowledge on variability in populations and changes with the evolution of disease
Notwithstanding the insights that can be gained from intensive evaluation within clinical trials and pooling of data across studies, we perceive a clear need for one or more large, intensive, comprehensive international study to define the biochemical natural history of sepsis, and to determine the association of biomarkers with disease progression, prognosis, and response to treatment
We urge increased collaboration between companies involved in diagnostics, and those involved in therapeutics, as well as greater collaboration among industry, clinical investigators, and regulatory agencies to advance our understanding of biomarkers in sepsis

prognosis for patients with sepsis, but will require an unprecedented degree of systematic investigation and collaboration (Table 3).

▶ Sepsis currently remains ill defined, and the current criteria is ill equipped to identify patients who might benefit from antimicrobial therapy. Furthermore, a definite microbiological diagnosis cannot be made in one-third of the patients with clinical manifestations of sepsis. Therefore, validated biomarkers may help to identify patients who may benefit from antimicrobial therapy in high-risk patients. This report is based on expert colloquium on biomarkers of sepsis convened by the international sepsis forum. A biomarker may serve 1 or more of 5 overlapping roles: (1) It may help to identify patients with increased probability of having disease. (2) It may serve as a screening test. (3) It may help to detect risk before the development of clinical disease, or it may help to identify a patient who might warrant evaluation by a more definitive, but expensive, invasive diagnostic test. Although there is widespread enthusiasm for a future role for the widespread use of biomarkers to facilitate the optimal management of sepsis the field at present is in its infancy, and this underdevelopment provides the basis for the recommendations of this colloquium.

M. Mathru, MD, FCCP

Acute systemic erythropoietin therapy to reduce delayed ischemic deficits following aneurysmal subarachnoid hemorrhage: a Phase II randomized, double-blind, placebo-controlled trial

Tseng M-Y, Hutchinson PJ, Richards HK, et al (Univ of Cambridge, UK)

J Neurosurg 111:171-180, 2009

Object.—Delayed ischemic deficits (DIDs), a major source of disability following aneurysmal subarachnoid hemorrhage (aSAH), are usually associated with severe cerebral vasospasm and impaired autoregulation. Systemic erythropoietin (EPO) therapy has been demonstrated to have neuroprotective properties acting via EPO receptors on cerebrovascular endothelia and ischemic neurons. In this trial, the authors explored the potential neuroprotective effects of acute EPO therapy following aSAH.

Methods.—Within 72 hours of aSAH, 80 patients (age range 24–82 years) were randomized to receive intravenous EPO (30,000 U) or placebo every 48 hours for a total of 90,000 U. Primary end points were the incidence, duration, and severity of vasospasm and impaired autoregulation on transcranial Doppler ultrasonography. Secondary end points were incidence of DIDs and outcome at discharge and at 6 months.

TABLE 2.—Results of Primary End Points

Primary End Points	Total (%)	Placebo (%)	EPO (%)	p Value
vasospasm*				
yes	27 (33.8)	16 (40.0)	11 (27.5)	0.24
no	53 (66.2)	24 (60.0)	29 (72.5)	
ipsilat side				
yes	24 (30.0)	14 (35.0)	10 (25.0)	0.33
no	56 (70.0)	26 (65.0)	30 (75.0)	
contralat side				
yes	17 (21.32)	11 (27.5)	6 (15.0)	0.17
no	63 (78.8)	29 (72.5)	34 (85.0)	
severe vasospasm†				
yes	14 (17.5)	11 (27.5)	3 (7.5)	0.037
no	66 (82.5)	29 (72.5)	37 (92.5)	
ipsilat side				
yes	11 (13.8)	9 (22.5)	2 (5.0)	0.014
no	69 (86.2)	31 (77.5)	38 (95.0)	
contralat side				
yes	6 (7.5)	4 (10.0)	2 (5.0)	0.43
no	74 (92.5)	36 (90.0)	38 (95.0)	

Days of Impaired Autoregulation‡	Total	Placebo	EPO	Difference	p Value
ipsilat side	5.0 ± 4.1 (4.1–5.9)	6.6 ± 4.3 (5.2–8.0)	3.5 ± 3.1 (2.5–4.4)	3.2 (1.5–4.9)	<0.001
contralat side	3.7 ± 3.6 (2.9–4.5)	4.3 ± 3.9 (3.1–5.6)	3.0 ± 3.1 (2.0–4.0)	1.3 (−0.2–2.9)	0.10

*Flow velocity (FV) > 1.2 m/second, ΔFV > 0.5 m/sec/24 hrs, Lindegaard ratio > 3.
†Flow velocity > 2.0 m/second, ΔFV > 0.5 m/sec/24 hrs, Lindegaard ratio > 3.
‡Values reflect the mean ± SD with 95% CIs in parentheses.

TABLE 3.—Results of Secondary End Points and Adverse Clinical Events

Events	Total (%)	Placebo (%)	EPO (%)	p Value
DID w/ cerebral infarcts				
ipsilat	14 (17.5)	13 (32.5)	1 (2.5)	<0.001
contralat	5 (6.3)	3 (7.5)	2 (5.0)	
no	61 (76.2)	24 (60.0)	37 (92.5)	
TCD vasospasm-related DID w/ infarcts				
ipsilat	10 (12.5)	9 (22.5)	1 (2.5)	0.014
contralat	3 (3.7)	1 (2.5)	2 (5.0)	
no	67 (83.8)	30 (75.0)	37 (92.5)	
Outcome at Discharge				
overall mRS score*				
0	0 (0)	0 (0)	0 (0)	0.18
1	23 (28.8)	7 (17.5)	16 (40.0)	
2	20 (25.0)	9 (22.5)	11 (27.5)	
3	8 (10.0)	6 (15.0)	2 (5.0)	
4	5 (6.2)	3 (7.5)	2 (5.0)	
5	15 (18.8)	10 (25.0)	5 (12.5)	
6	9 (11.2)	5 (12.5)	4 (10.0)	
favorable mRS				
0–3	51 (63.8)	22 (55.0)	29 (72.5)	0.10
unfavorable mRS				
4–6	29 (36.2)	18 (45.0)	11 (27.5)	
overall GOS score				
good recovery	38 (47.5)	14 (35.0)	24 (60.0)	0.22
mod disability	11 (13.8)	6 (15.0)	5 (12.5)	
severe disability	18 (22.5)	12 (30.0)	6 (15.0)	
vegetative	4 (5.0)	3 (7.5)	1 (2.5)	
death	9 (11.2)	5 (12.5)	4 (10.0)	
favorable GOS				
good recovery/mod disability	49 (61.2)	20 (50.0)	29 (72.5)	0.039
unfavorable GOS				
severe disability/vegetative/death	31 (38.8)	20 (50.0)	11 (27.5)	
NIHSS score in 71 survivors†				
mild (0–5)	43 (60.6)	16 (45.7)	27 (75.0)	0.014
mod (6–20)	16 (22.5)	9 (25.7)	7 (19.4)	
severe (>20)	12 (16.9)	10 (28.6)	2 (5.6)	
Outcome at 6 Mos				
mRS score				
0	12 (15.0)	8 (20.0)	4 (10.0)	0.78
1	23 (28.8)	10 (25.0)	13 (32.5)	
2	16 (20.0)	6 (15.0)	10 (25.0)	
3	9 (11.2)	5 (12.5)	4 (10.0)	
4	4 (5.0)	2 (5.0)	2 (5.0)	
5	3 (3.8)	2 (5.0)	1 (2.5)	
6	13 (16.2)	7 (17.5)	6 (15.0)	
favorable mRS				
0–3	60 (75.0)	29 (72.5)	31 (77.5)	0.61
GOS score at 6 mos				
good recovery	28 (35.0)	14 (35.0)	14 (35.0)	0.88
mod disability	27 (33.8)	12 (30.0)	15 (37.5)	
severe disability	12 (15.0)	7 (17.5)	5 (12.5)	
vegetative	0 (0)	0 (0)	0 (0)	
death	13 (16.2)	7 (17.5)	6 (15.0)	
favorable GOS				
good recovery/mod disability	55 (68.8)	26 (65.0)	29 (72.5)	0.47
unfavorable GOS				
severe disability/vegetative/death	25 (31.2)	14 (35.0)	11 (27.5)	
Adverse Clinical Events				
in-hospital death				
yes	9 (11.2)	5 (12.5)	4 (10.0)	1.0

(*Continued*)

TABLE 3. *(continued)*

Events	Total (%)	Placebo (%)	EPO (%)	p Value
no	71 (88.8)	35 (87.5)	36 (90.0)	
6-mo death				
yes	13 (16.2)	7 (17.5)	6 (15.0)	0.76
no	67 (83.8)	33 (82.5)	34 (85.0)	
ventriculitis				
yes	8 (10.0)	5 (12.5)	3 (7.5)	0.71
no	72 (90.0)	35 (87.5)	37 (92.5)	
immediate postop deficits				
yes	18 (22.5)	8 (20.0)	10 (25.0)	0.59
no	62 (77.5)	32 (80.0)	30 (75.0)	
sepsis				
yes	30 (35.7)	12 (30.0)	18 (45.0)	0.17
no	50 (62.5)	28 (70.0)	22 (55.0)	
transfusion w/ erythrocytes				
yes	16 (20.0)	12 (30.0)	4 (10.0)	0.048
no	64 (80.0)	28 (70.0)	36 (90.0)	

*On the mRS = 1 no disability, 2 = slight disability, 3 = moderately disability, 4 = moderately severe disability, unable to walk without assistance, 5 = severe disability, bedridden, and 6 = death.

†On the NIHSS there are a total of 42 points, where lower scores indicate less disability.

Results.—Randomization characteristics were balanced except for age, with the EPO group being older (mean age 59.6 vs 53.3 years, $p = 0.034$). No differences were demonstrated in the incidence of vasospasm and adverse events; however, patients receiving EPO had a decreased incidence of severe vasospasm from 27.5 to 7.5% ($p = 0.037$), reduced DIDs with new cerebral infarcts from 40.0 to 7.5% ($p = 0.001$), a shortened duration of impaired autoregulation (ipsilateral side, $p < 0.001$), and more favorable outcome at discharge (favorable Glasgow Outcome Scale score, $p = 0.039$). Among the 71 survivors, the EPO group had fewer deficits measured with National Institutes of Health Stroke Scale (median Score 2 vs 6, $p = 0.008$).

Conclusions.—This preliminary study showed that EPO seemed to reduce delayed cerebral ischemia following aSAH via decreasing severity of vasospasm and shortening impaired autoregulation (Tables 2 and 3).

▶ Subarachnoid hemorrhage (SAH) leads to severe cerebral vasospasm and impaired autoregulation. Both of these factors can contribute to delayed neurological deficits. Several lines of experimental evidence suggest that erythropoietin (EPO) therapy has neuroprotective properties acting via EPO receptors on cerebrovascular endothelia and ischemic neurons. Previous studies have recommended EPO therapy in stroke and mechanisms involve ischemic preconditioning, antiapoptosis, neurogenesis, and angiogenesis in ischemic penumbra. EPO is also known to activate the phosphorylation of endothelium-derived nitric oxide synthase (eNOS), and increase NO production and cyclic 3′,5′-guanosine monophosphate (GMP) in cerebral arteries. In experimental models of SAH, systemic administration of EPO reverses cerebral vasospasm and impaired autoregulation. In this study, the investigators have examined the neuroprotective effects of EPO in patients who sustained SAH within 72 hours. The effects of EPO on cerebral vasospasm and autoregulation was evaluated using transcranial Doppler (TCD). EPO in this series of patients did not have any effect on cerebral vasospasm. However, a multivariate analysis revealed a trend toward a sustained neuroprotective effect in these patients. The higher reticulocyte count documented after EPO therapy was not accompanied by higher hematocrit levels, suggesting that enhanced oxygen delivery by elevating the hematocrit level may not be the mechanism for the clinical benefit of EPO. The limitations of this study include small sample size and issues relating to optimal dosage and frequency were not addressed in this study. Nevertheless, the neuroprotective effects of EPO demonstrated in this study are impressive.

M. Mathru, MD, FCCP

A comparison of stroke volume variation measured by the LiDCOplus and FloTrac-Vigileo system

de Wilde RBP, Geerts BF, van den Berg PCM, et al (Leiden Univ Med Centre, The Netherlands)

Anaesthesia 64:1004-1009, 2009

The aim of this study was to compare the accuracy of stroke volume variation (SVV) as measured by the LiDCOplus system (SVVli) and by the FloTrac-Vigileo system (SVVed). We measured SVVli and SVVed in 15 postoperative cardiac surgical patients following five study interventions; a 50% increase in tidal volume, an increase of PEEP by 10 cm H_2O, passive leg raising, a head-up tilt procedure and fluid loading. Between each intervention, baseline measurements were performed. 136 data pairs were obtained. SVVli ranged from 1.4% to 26.8% (mean (SD) 8.7 (4.6)%); SVVed from 2.0% to 26.0% (10.2 (4.7)%). The bias was found to be significantly different from zero at 1.5 (2.5)%, $p < 0.001$, (95% confidence interval 1.1–1.9). The upper and lower limits of agreement were found to be 6.4 and −3.5% respectively. The coefficient of variation for the differences between SVVli and SVVed was 26%. This results in a relative large range for the percentage limits of agreement of 52%. Analysis in repeated measures showed coefficients of variation of 21% for SVVli and 22% for SVVed. The LiDCOplus and FloTrac-Vigileo system are not interchangeable. Furthermore, the determination of SVVli and SVVed are too ambiguous, as can be concluded from the high values of the coefficient of variation for repeated measures. These findings underline Pinsky's warning of caution in the clinical use of SVV by pulse contour techniques.

► Pulse contour analysis to determine stroke volume and other hemodynamic parameters is not a new subject. Remington and colleagues, and later Langewouters, developed equations to determine stroke volume based upon arterial pressure curve. Largely, until more sophisticated software was developed in the late 1990s, pulmonary artery catheterization remained largely the gold standard in hemodynamic monitoring. With the development of a lithium dilution calibration technique, accurate measurement of cardiac output could be obtained from a peripheral arterial catheter and sensor (LiDCO). A method for noncalibrated noninvasive hemodynamic monitoring system (FloTrac-Vigileo) was developed. De Wilde and colleagues present a well-designed clinical trial comparing the stoke volume variation, a clinically useful tool in ventilated patients between the 2 systems. They found a large variation between the agreements on stroke volume variation (SVV) between the 2 systems (52%) based on Bland-Altman analysis, raising concerns about the clinical use of SVV obtained by the 2 systems. They rightly concluded that the 2 systems were not equivalent and raise questions about the use of SVV in some patients. Perhaps the use of the pulmonary artery catheter may be more beneficial in selected patients.

M. Mathru, MD, FCCP

Adenosine for wide-complex tachycardia: Efficacy and safety

Marill KA, Wolfram S, deSouza IS, et al (Massachusetts General Hosp, Boston; SUNY Downstate Med. Ctr, Brooklyn, NY; et al)

Crit Care Med 37:2512-2518, 2009

Objectives.—To determine whether adenosine is useful and safe as a diagnostic and therapeutic agent for patients with undifferentiated wide QRS complex tachycardia. The etiology of sustained monomorphic wide QRS complex tachycardia is often uncertain acutely.

Design.—A retrospective observational study.

Setting.—Treatment associated with emergency visits at nine urban hospitals.

Patients.—Consecutive patients treated with adenosine for regular wide QRS complex tachycardia between 1991 and 2006.

Interventions.—Treatment with adenosine infusion.

Measurements and Main Results.—Measured outcomes included rhythm response to adenosine, if any, and all adverse effects. A positive response was defined as an observed change in rhythm including temporary atrioventricular conduction block or tachycardia termination. A primary adverse event was defined as emergent electrical or medical therapy instituted in response to an adverse adenosine effect. A rhythm diagnosis was made in each case. The characteristics of adenosine administration as a test for a supraventricular as opposed to ventricular tachycardia were determined, and the adverse event rates were calculated. A total of 197 patients were included: 104 (90%) of 116 (95% confidence interval, 83%–95%) and two (2%) of 81 (95% confidence interval, 0.3%–9%) supraventricular tachycardia and ventricular tachycardia patients demonstrated a response to adenosine, respectively. The odds of supraventricular

TABLE 5.—Rhythm and Response to Adenosine

Rhythm	Tachycardia Termination Post Adenosine	Any Response to Adenosine Yes	No
Supraventricular			
Sinus tachycardia	0	5	2
Atrial fibrillation[a]	0	4	0
Atrial flutter	1	54	4
Atrial tachycardia	2	6	1
Atrioventricular tachycardia	1	1	0
AVNRT	6	6	1
Nodo-fascicular tachycardia	1	1	0
SVT, unspecified	17	27	4
Ventricular			
VT with RV dysplasia	0	0	1
RVOT VT	0	0	3
Fascicular VT	0	0	2
Persistent recurrent VT	0	0	1
VT, unspecified	1	2	72
Totals			
All SVT		104	12
All VT		2	79

AVNRT, atrioventricular nodal tachycardia; SVT, supraventricular tachycardia; VT, ventricular tachycardia; RV, right ventricular; RVOT, right ventricular outflow tract.

[a]Atrial fibrillation with maximal R to R interval variability <5%.

TABLE 6.—Adverse Effects Associated with Adenosine Administration

Adverse Effect	Rhythm SVT	VT
Vertigo and diaphoresis	1	
Nausea and dry mouth	1	
Flushed sensation		1
Flushed sensation with headache and nausea		1
Transient increased chest pain		1
Transient increased chest pain with 6 mg adenosine and transient PVCs with 12 mg	1	
Asymptomatic PVCs	1	
Asymptomatic NSVT	1	
Decreased blood pressure and shortness of breath associated with simultaneous nitropaste administration		1
Decreased blood pressure not requiring therapy		1
None	111	76

SVT, supraventricular tachycardia; VT, ventricular tachycardia; PVCs, premature ventricular contrations; NSVT, nonsustained ventricular tachycardia.

tachycardia increased by a factor of 36 (95% confidence interval, 9–143) after a positive response to adenosine. The odds of ventricular tachycardia increased by a factor of 9 (95% confidence interval, 6–16) when there was no response to adenosine. The rate of primary adverse events for patients with supraventricular tachycardia and ventricular tachycardia was 0 (0%) of 116 (95% confidence interval, 0%–3%) and 0 (0%) of 81 (95% confidence interval, 0%–4%), respectively.

Conclusions.—Adenosine is useful and safe as a diagnostic and therapeutic agent for patients with regular wide QRS complex tachycardia (Tables 5 and 6).

▶ Adenosine, an endogenous nucleotide, causes rapid atrioventricular (AV) blockade when administered intravenously with an ultrashort half-life. Adenosine terminates most supraventricular tachycardias (SVTs) that rely on the AV node to form a re-entrant circuit. Adenosine also causes an ultrashort AV block to permit accurate diagnosis of atrial flutter, and it is unlikely to be effective in terminating ventricular tachycardia. Many clinicians are reluctant to use adenosine because of safety concerns, including paradoxic enhancement of the accessory tract conduction and acceleration of the ventricular response in the setting of atrial flutter or fibrillation with a bypass tract, persistent bradycardia or asystole, change in rhythm to atrial fibrillation, degeneration to ventricular fibrillation, myocardial ischemia due to coronary vasodilation, secondary steal syndrome or bronchospasm. The authors examined whether adenosine is safe and useful in the presence of undifferentiated wide complex tachycardia. The study demonstrates that adenosine use was safe in the presence of undifferentiated wide complex tachycardia. However, the study is limited because of the retrospective nature of this study and there were multiple potential limitations, including the risk of bias in enrollment and assessment of adenosine response by the primary physicians and the investigators, incomplete or inaccurate data collection, and nonstandardized treatment regimen. Therefore, the use and safety of adenosine administration could differ when applied to a different sample of SVT and VT patients with wide complex tachycardia.

M. Mathru, MD, FCCP

Assessing fluid responsiveness in critically ill patients: False-positive pulse pressure variation is detected by Doppler echocardiographic evaluation of the right ventricle

Mahjoub Y, Pila C, Friggeri A, et al (Amiens Univ Hosp, France)

Crit Care Med 37:2570-2575, 2009

Objectives.—To determine whether peak systolic velocity of tricuspid annular motion assessed by tissue Doppler echocardiography (Sta), a right ventricular function parameter, can discriminate patients with true- and false-positive pulse pressure variation. Pulse pressure variation is used to predict fluid responsiveness in mechanically ventilated patients. However, this parameter has been reported to be falsely positive, especially in patients with right ventricular dysfunction.

Design.—A prospective study.

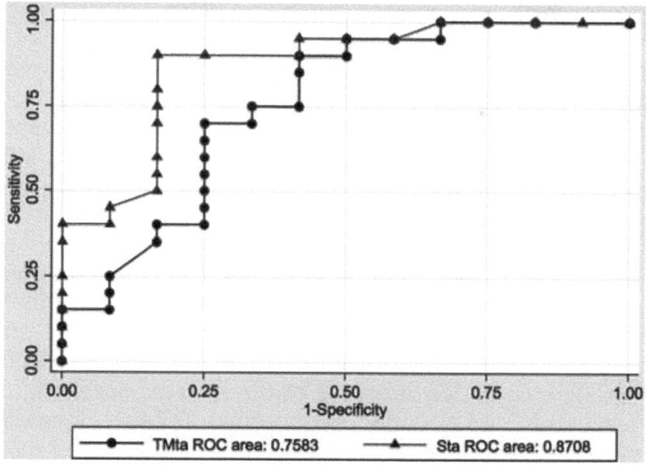

FIGURE 3.—Receiver operating characteristic (*ROC*) curves comparing the ability of tissue Doppler tricuspid annular systolic velocity (*Sta*) and tricuspid annular motion evaluated by M-mode (*TMta*) to discriminate responders (SV increase >15%) and nonresponders to volume expansion. The area under the ROC curve was better for Sta than for TMta (0.870 ± 0.0694 vs. 0.75930 ± .0973). The cutoff value for Sta was 0.15 m/s. (Reprinted from Mahjoub Y, Pila C, Friggeri A, et al. Assessing fluid responsiveness in critically ill patients: false-positive pulse pressure variation is detected by Doppler echocardiographic evaluation of the right ventricle. *Crit Care Med.* 2009;37:2570-2575.)

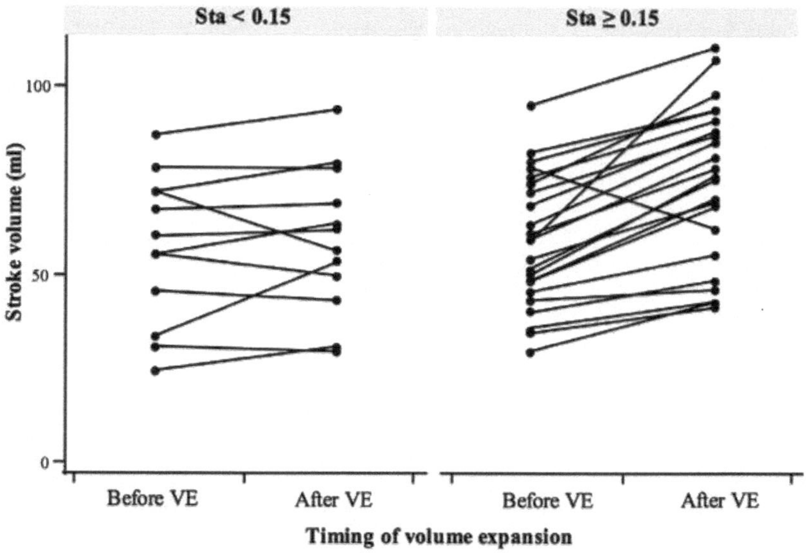

FIGURE 4.—Individual changes in stroke volume (SV) induced by volume expansion (*VE*). Patients were divided into two groups according to the prediction of fluid responsiveness by tissue Doppler tricuspid annular systolic velocity (*Sta*). Sta value <0.15 m/s (*right*) is predictive of a negative response to VE despite PPV of <12. (Reprinted from Mahjoub Y, Pila C, Friggeri A, et al. Assessing fluid responsiveness in critically ill patients: false-positive pulse pressure variation is detected by Doppler echocardiographic evaluation of the right ventricle. *Crit Care Med.* 2009;37:2570-2575.)

Setting.—Medical and surgical intensive care unit of a university hospital.

Patients.—Thirty- five mechanically ventilated patients hospitalized for >24 hrs with a pulse pressure variation of >12%.

Interventions.—Doppler echocardiography (including measurement of Sta and stroke volume) was performed before and after infusion of 500 mL of colloid solution. Patients were classified into two groups according to their response to fluid infusion: responders (at least 15% increase in stroke volume) and nonresponders.

Measurements and Main Results.—Twenty-three patients (66%) were responders (true-positive group) and 12 (34%) were nonresponders (false-positive group). Before volume expansion, Sta was statistically lower in the nonresponder group (0.13 [0.04] vs. 0.20 [0.05], $p = .0004$). The area under the curve of the receiver operating characteristic curve was 0.87 (95% confidence interval, 0.74–1). In patients with pulse pressure variation of >12%, a Sta cutoff value of 0.15 m/s discriminated between responders and nonresponders with a sensitivity of 91% (80–100) and a specificity of 83% (62–100).

Conclusions.—A Sta value of <0.15 m/s seems to be an accurate parameter to detect false-positive pulse pressure variation. Echocardiography should therefore be performed before fluid infusion in patients with pulse pressure variation of >12% (Figs 3 and 4).

▶ Respiratory variation of pulse pressure as a surrogate for stroke volume or aortic blood flow velocity variation has been demonstrated to predict accurately preload responsiveness in mechanically ventilated patients. Despite a pulse pressure variation (PPV) of >12%, some patients do not respond to volume expansion. This false-positive PPV is attributed to right ventricular (RV) dysfunction and the consequent decrease in RV ejection due to inspiratory increases in RV afterload. This study examined whether tissue Doppler derived tricuspid annular systolic velocity (Sta) can be used to recognize false-positive PPV. In this study, a PPV of >12% was associated with a 34% false-positive rate in a population of patients hospitalized for >24 hrs in whom intensivists decided to augment preload by fluid challenge. Their results also suggest that an Sta < 0.15 m/s on tissue Doppler helps to identify these false-positive results. The authors hypothesize that in the context of RV dysfunction, RV afterload increases with the increases in alveolar pressure and the failing right ventricle becomes more sensitive to increases in RV afterload and is less affected by preload variation. In the nonresponder group, PPV was not affected by volume challenge, whereas in the responder group PPV significantly decreased after volume challenge. This can be explained by the fact that, in the nonresponder group, PPV is due to RV afterload variation, whereas in the responder group PPV is due to RV preload variation. RV dysfunction is not uncommon in critically ill patients with sepsis, acute respiratory distress syndrome (ARDS), and chronic obstructive pulmonary disease (COPD).

Therefore, echocardiographic Sta should be determined before volume challenge in patients with PPV > 12%.

M. Mathru, MD, FCCP

Allogeneic human mesenchymal stem cells for treatment of *E. coli* endotoxin-induced acute lung injury in the ex vivo perfused human lung

Lee JW, Fang X, Gupta N, et al (Univ of California, San Francisco; et al)

Proc Natl Acad Sci U S A 106:16357-16362, 2009

Recent studies have suggested that bone marrow-derived multipotent mesenchymal stem cells (MSCs) may have therapeutic applications in multiple clinical disorders including myocardial infarction, diabetes, sepsis, and hepatic and acute renal failure. Here, we tested the therapeutic capacity of human MSCs to restore alveolar epithelial fluid transport and lung fluid balance from acute lung injury (ALI) in an ex vivo perfused human lung preparation injured by *E. coli* endotoxin. Intra-bronchial instillation of endotoxin into the distal airspaces resulted in pulmonary edema with the loss of alveolar epithelial fluid transport measured as alveolar fluid clearance. Treatment with allogeneic human MSCs or its conditioned medium given 1 h following endotoxin-induced lung injury reduced extravascular lung water, improved lung endothelial barrier permeability and restored alveolar fluid clearance. Using siRNA knockdown of potential paracrine soluble factors, secretion of keratinocyte growth factor was essential for the beneficial effect of MSCs on alveolar epithelial fluid transport, in part by restoring amiloride-dependent sodium transport. In summary, treatment with allogeneic human MSCs or the conditioned medium restores normal fluid balance in an ex vivo perfused human lung injured by *E. coli* endotoxin (Figs 3-5).

▶ Sepsis-induced lung injuries carry a high morbidity and mortality. Current treatment, which includes protective ventilation and fluid restriction strategy, is primarily supportive. Pharmacological strategies continue to be ineffective in the clinical arena. Several lines of experimental evidence suggest that bone marrow-derived multipotent mesenchymal stem cells (MSCs) may have therapeutic application in a variety of clinical disorders, including myocardial infarction, diabetes, sepsis, and acute hepatic and renal injury.

One experimental study in mice suggest that treatment with MSC 4 hours after endotoxin delivery to the lung improved survival and reduced pulmonary edema formation. In this study the authors examined the therapeutic role of human allogeneic MSCs in an ex vivo perfused human lung preparation injured by *Escherichia coli* endotoxin. In this human lung model, endotoxin induced lung injury, MSC reduced pulmonary edema, improved lung endothelial barrier integrity, and normalized alveolar epithelial fluid transport. The effect was mediated in part by restoring sodium dependent alveolar fluid transport. The results of their study is limited since it was studied only short-term (4 hours) and does not include the influence of perfusion of other organs such as the

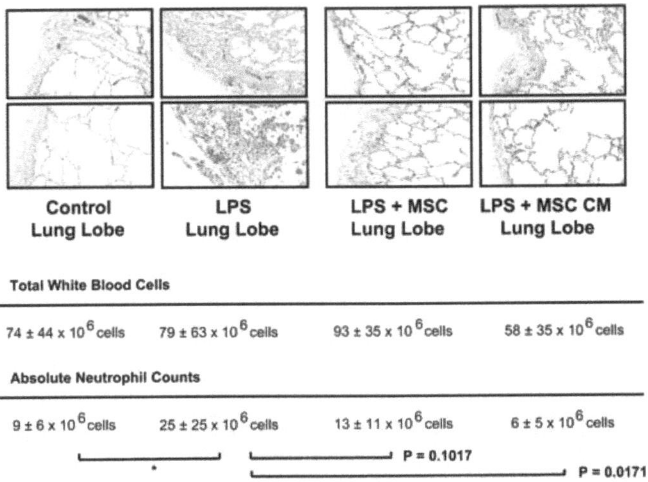

FIGURE 3.—Histology sections and neutrophil counts. Human lungs exposed to endotoxin with and without MSC or its CM were fixed in 10% formalin at 4 h. Sections were stained with hematoxylin and eosin (magnification 10×). The instillation of MSC or its CM 1 h after endotoxin injury reduced the degree of edema and cellularity in the endotoxin-injured lung lobe. Total white blood cell and neutrophil counts in the alveolar fluid of each lung lobe are shown as mean ± SD, $n = 3$–6. *, $P < 0.004$ vs. control by ANOVA (Bonferroni). Measurement of WBC in MSC-treated lung lobes was confounded by the presence of the MSC themselves. Although not quite statistically significant by ANOVA (Bonferroni), P values are shown for the comparisons between LPS vs. LPS + MSCs and LPS vs. LPS + MSC-CM. (Reprinted from Lee JW, Fang X, Gupta N, et al. Allogeneic human mesenchymal stem cells for treatment of *E. coli* endotoxin-induced acute lung injury in the ex vivo perfused human lung. *Proc Natl Acad Sci U S A.* 2009;106:16357-16362.)

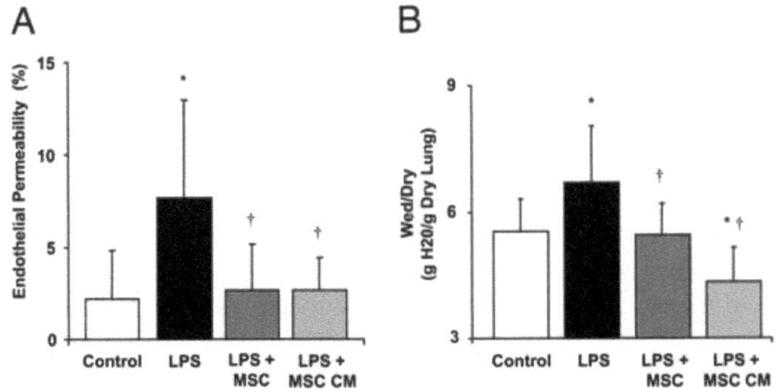

FIGURE 4.—Effect of human MSCs or its CM on lung endothelial permeability to protein and Wet/Dry Ratio. Instillation of MSCs or its CM into the endotoxin injured RML or LLL 1 h later restored lung endothelial permeability to protein (*A*) and wet/dry (W/D) ratio (*B*) to control values. Data are expressed as mean % endothelial permeability or W/D ratio ± SD, $n = 4$–5 lungs; *, $P < 0.0001$ vs. control lobe, †, $P < 0.0011$ vs. LPS (0.1 mg/kg) injured lobe for lung endothelial permeability and *, $P < 0.0014$ vs. control lobe, †, $P < 0.005$ vs. LPS (0.1 mg/kg) injured lobe for the W/D ratio by ANOVA (Bonferroni). (Reprinted from Lee JW, Fang X, Gupta N, et al. Allogeneic human mesenchymal stem cells for treatment of *E. coli* endotoxin-induced acute lung injury in the ex vivo perfused human lung. *Proc Natl Acad Sci U S A.* 2009;106:16357-16362.)

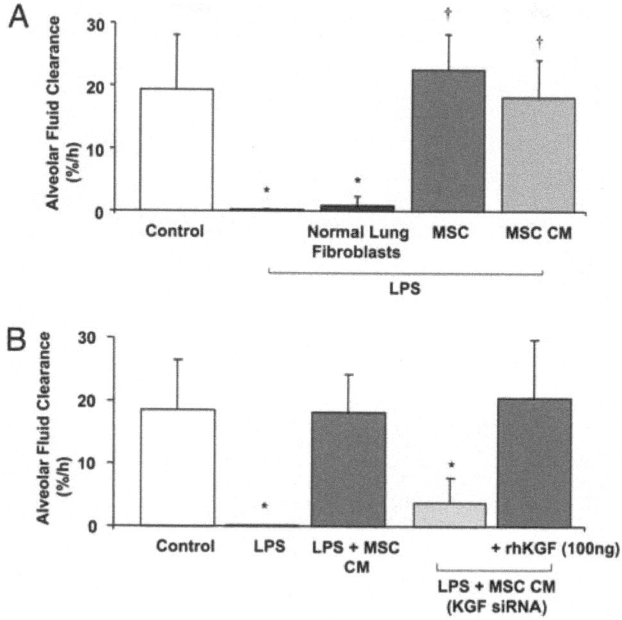

FIGURE 5.—Effect of human MSCs or its CM on alveolar fluid clearance (*A*). MSCs or its CM restored the decrease in alveolar fluid clearance in the lung lobe injured by endotoxin to control values at 4 h. $n = 3$–4; *, $P < 0.0006$ vs. control AFC; †, $P < 0.0001$ vs. LPS (0.1 mg/kg) AFC by ANOVA (Bonferroni). Effect of the CM of human MSCs pretreated with a KGF siRNA on alveolar fluid clearance (*B*). Administration of the CM of MSCs grown for 24 h pretreated with the KGF siRNA (#10818, Ambion) into the endotoxin injured lung lobe after 1 h prevented the restoration of AFC with the CM alone. The addition of recombinant KGF (100 ng) to the CM pretreated with KGF siRNA restored the decrease in AFC to control values. Data are expressed as mean AFC ± SD, $n = 4$–5 lungs; *, $P < 0.0012$ vs. control lobe by ANOVA (Bonferroni). (Reprinted from Lee JW, Fang X, Gupta N, et al. Allogeneic human mesenchymal stem cells for treatment of *E. coli* endotoxin-induced acute lung injury in the ex vivo perfused human lung. *Proc Natl Acad Sci U S A*. 2009;106:16357-16362.)

liver or spleen, which may mount significant inflammatory response. Further studies are needed to determine MSCs potential value in the treatment of human acute lung injury (ALI).

M. Mathru, MD, FCCP

Clinical Relevance of Echocardiography in Acute Severe Dyspnea

Feissel M, Maizel J, Robles G, et al (Centre Hospitalier de Belfort-Montbéliard, Belfort, France; Service de Néphrologie, Amiens, France; et al)
J Am Soc Echocardiogr 22:1159-1164, 2009

Background.—The aim of this study was to assess the most relevant echocardiographic parameter for the clinical diagnosis of acute dyspnea due to left-heart dysfunction.

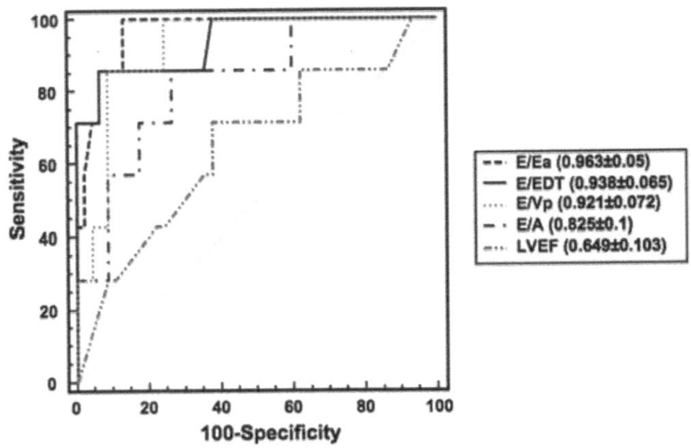

FIGURE 2.—LVEF, E/EDT, E/Ea, E/Vp, and E/A receiver operating characteristic curves and AUCs to discriminate cardiogenic and noncardiogenic dyspnea in the population with LVEFs > 45% in which all parameters were recorded (n = 58). $P < .05$ for LVEF versus E/Ea, E/EDT, and E/Vp AUC. (Reprinted from Feissel M, Maizel J, Robles G, et al. Clinical relevance of echocardiography in acute severe dyspnea. *J Am Soc Echocardiogr.* 2009;22:1159-1164, with permission from the American Society of Echocardiography.)

Methods.—Transthoracic echocardiography was performed in 88 patients in sinus rhythm admitted for respiratory distress. Two experts determined the cause of dyspnea as cardiogenic (26 patients) or noncardiogenic (62 patients).

Results.—The feasibility was 100% for the E/A ratio and the E/E deceleration time (EDT) ratio but 97%, 89%, and 85% for the E/Ea ratio, left ventricular ejection fraction (LVEF), and the E/propagation velocity (Vp) ratio, respectively. The area under the receiver operating characteristic curve for E/EDT (0.947 ± 0.035) was statistically significantly greater than that for E/A (0.753 ± 0.068) ($P = .004$). The areas under the curves for all other parameters were not statistically significantly different. In the subpopulation of patients with LVEFs > 45%, the area under the curve for LVEF was significantly smaller than those for E/Ea, E/EDT, and E/Vp.

Conclusion.—E/EDT, E/Ea, and E/Vp appear equally useful to distinguish acute dyspnea due to left-heart dysfunction from that of pulmonary origin. However, E/EDT and E/Ea can be considered the best indices with regard to feasibility (Fig 2).

▶ The evaluation of a patient who presents to the intensive care unit with acute severe dyspnea can be a diagnostic challenge. Differentiation between pulmonary and cardiac etiologies may be problematic. Pulmonary artery catheterization to determine pulmonary capillary wedge pressure has been used to differentiate pulmonary versus cardiac causes of pulmonary edema. Echocardiography has also been used to estimate pulmonary pressures as a noninvasive alternative, however, windows to assess the pulmonary vasculature may be difficult to obtain. Feissel and colleagues use standard subcostal

4 chamber views to determine mitral valve Doppler indices. Peak E and A wave velocity values were calculated, and other values (E deceleration time) were determined. Good correlation was noted between E/E/E deceleration time (EDT), E/Ea, and E/Vp values in the differentiation of cardiac versus noncardiac causes of severe dyspnea. Interestingly, the same correlation held true between patients with ejection fractions of >45% and <45%. While further studies with larger patient populations need to be performed, the use of bedside echocardiography and the use of Doppler indices show promise in the evaluation of severe dyspnea.

M. Mathru, MD, FCCP

A-Lines and B-Lines: Lung Ultrasound as a Bedside Tool for Predicting Pulmonary Artery Occlusion Pressure in the Critically Ill

Lichtenstein DA, Mezière GA, Lagoueyte J-F, et al (Hôpital Ambroise-Paré, Boulogne, France; Centre Hospitalier, Saint-Cloud, France; Hôpital Bichat, Paris, France; et al)

Chest 136:1014-1020, 2009

Background.—The risk of pulmonary edema is the main limiting factor in fluid therapy in the critically ill. Interstitial edema is a subclinical step that precedes alveolar edema. This study assesses a bedside tool for detecting interstitial edema, lung ultrasound. The A-line is a horizontal artifact indicating a normal lung surface. The B-line is a kind of comet-tail artifact indicating subpleural interstitial edema. The relationship between anterior interstitial edema detected by lung ultrasound and the pulmonary artery occlusion pressure (PAOP) value was investigated.

Method.—We performed a prospective study in medicosurgical ICUs of university-affiliated teaching hospitals. We enrolled 102 consecutive mechanically ventilated patients who all underwent pulmonary artery catheterization. We defined A-predominance as a majority of anterior A-lines and B-predominance as a majority of anterior B-lines. These patterns were correlated with PAOP.

Results.—For diagnosing PAOP $\leq$ 13 mm Hg, A-predominance had 90% specificity, 67% sensitivity, 91% positive predictive value, and 65% negative predictive value. For diagnosing PAOP $\leq$ 18 mm Hg, A-predominance had 93% specificity, 50% sensitivity, 97% positive predictive value, and 24% negative predictive value, respectively.

Conclusions.—A-predominance indicates dry interlobular septa. Specific to predicting a low PAOP value, A-predominance suggests that fluid may be given without initial concern for the development of hydrostatic pulmonary edema. B-predominance indicates interstitial syndrome, which is usually related to interstitial edema. B-predominance is observed in a wide range of PAOP values, precluding conclusions about the need for fluid therapy. This bedside potential will be appreciated by those intensivists who envision fluid therapy based on low PAOP values and who consider that using the concept of a safety factor provided by lung ultrasound is logical.

▶ Aggressive fluid resuscitation is often the first line of therapy in early hours of septic shock. The monitoring devices used by the bedside to guide fluid therapy include CVP, pulmonary artery occlusion pressure (PAOP), and arterial pressure derived indices such as pulse pressure variation, svv, and CO. The recently refined lung ultrasound is being increasingly used in the ICU to diagnose pneumothorax, pneumonia, and pulmonary embolism. The B-line generated by the ultrasound is an artifact that correlates with interstitial edema and the A-line is a horizontal artifact indicating normal lung surface. This study examined the relationship between anterior interstitial edema determined by B-lines and PAOP. Their results indicate a high specificity of A-predominance for diagnosis of low PAOP. However, B-line predominance was observed in a wide range of PAOP values precluding conclusions about fluid therapy. While using this technique to monitor fluid therapy, it should be understood that A-predominance does not define a need for fluid therapy, but rather is a criterion for lung tolerance to fluid therapy. If B-predominance replaces A-predominance following a fluid challenge, this indicates intestinal edema, likely from a hydrostatic mechanism. To determine fluid responsiveness in critically ill lung ultrasound could be coupled with other conventional devices to determine the tolerance of the lung to fluid therapy.

M. Mathru, MD, FCCP

Intensity of Continuous Renal-Replacement Therapy in Critically Ill Patients

The RENAL Replacement Therapy Study Investigators (ANZICS CTG, Australia)

N Engl J Med 361:1627-1638, 2009

Background.—The optimal intensity of continuous renal-replacement therapy remains unclear. We conducted a multicenter, randomized trial to compare the effect of this therapy, delivered at two different levels of intensity, on 90-day mortality among critically ill patients with acute kidney injury.

Methods.—We randomly assigned critically ill adults with acute kidney injury to continuous renal-replacement therapy in the form of postdilution continuous venovenous hemodiafiltration with an effluent flow of either 40 ml per kilogram of body weight per hour (higher intensity) or 25 ml per kilogram per hour (lower intensity). The primary outcome measure was death within 90 days after randomization.

Results.—Of the 1508 enrolled patients, 747 were randomly assigned to higher-intensity therapy, and 761 to lower-intensity therapy with continuous venovenous hemodiafiltration. Data on primary outcomes were available for 1464 patients (97.1%): 721 in the higher-intensity group and 743 in the lower-intensity group. The two study groups had similar

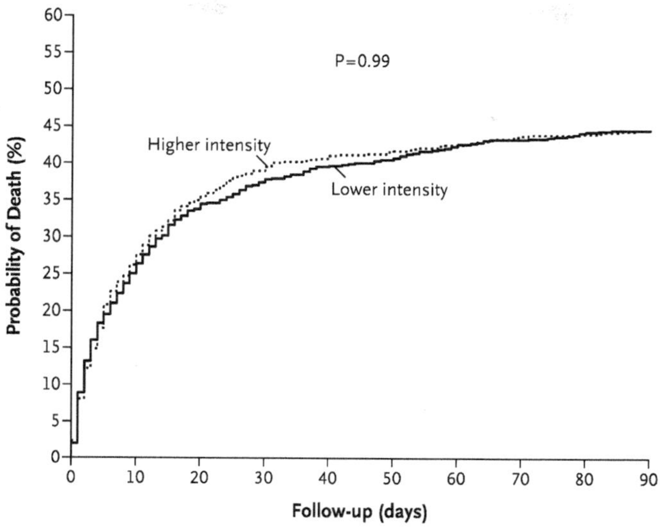

FIGURE 2.—Kaplan–Meier Estimates of the Probability of Death. Mortality at 28 days was similar in the higher-intensity and lower-intensity treatment groups (38.5% and 36.9%, respectively), and mortality at 90 days was the same (44.7%) in both groups. (Reprinted from The RENAL Replacement Therapy Study Investigators. Intensity of continuous renal-replacement therapy in critically ill patients. *N Engl J Med.* 2009;361:1627-1638, with permission from 2009 Massachusetts Medical Society. All rights reserved.)

baseline characteristics and received the study treatment for an average of 6.3 and 5.9 days, respectively (P = 0.35). At 90 days after randomization, 322 deaths had occurred in the higher-intensity group and 332 deaths in the lower-intensity group, for a mortality of 44.7% in each group (odds ratio, 1.00; 95% confidence interval [CI], 0.81 to 1.23; P = 0.99). At 90 days, 6.8% of survivors in the higher-intensity group (27 of 399), as compared with 4.4% of survivors in the lower-intensity group (18 of 411), were still receiving renal-replacement therapy (odds ratio, 1.59; 95% CI, 0.86 to 2.92; P = 0.14). Hypophosphatemia was more common in the higher-intensity group than in the lower-intensity group (65% vs. 54%, P<0.001).

Conclusions.—In critically ill patients with acute kidney injury, treatment with higher-intensity continuous renal-replacement therapy did not reduce mortality at 90 days. (ClinicalTrials. gov number, NCT00221013) (Figs 2 and 3).

▶ Once the acute kidney injury (AKI) is established, treatment is largely supportive in nature. Renal replacement therapy remains the cornerstone of management for the minority of patients who have severe AKI. The impact of renal-replacement therapy (RRT) intensity or dose on patient outcomes has been a matter of controversy. Most definitions of acute RRT dose are based on small molecule removal, as exemplified by urea, while ignoring other crucial aspects of RRT adequacy in AKI, such as volume and electrolyte control. In this

Prespecified Subgroup	Higher Intensity (N=721)	Lower Intensity (N=743)	Odds Ratio (95% CI)
	no. of deaths/no. of patients (%)		
Patients with criteria for sepsis			
Yes	168/359 (46.8)	186/363 (51.2)	0.84 (0.62–1.12)
No	154/362 (42.5)	145/379 (38.3)	1.19 (0.89–1.60)
Patients with at least one nonrenal organ failure			
Yes	299/628 (47.6)	306/649 (47.2)	1.02 (0.82–1.27)
No	23/93 (24.7)	25/93 (26.9)	0.89 (0.46–1.72)
Patients with SOFA cardiovascular score of 3 or 4			
Yes	247/510 (48.4)	254/546 (46.5)	1.08 (0.85–1.37)
No	74/210 (35.2)	75/194 (38.7)	0.86(0.58–1.29)
Patients with eGFR <60 ml/min			
Yes	114/250 (45.6)	105/222 (47.3)	0.93 (0.65–1.34)
No	81/157 (51.6)	81/185 (43.8)	1.37 (0.89–2.10)
Missing	127/314 (40.5)	146/336 (43.5)	0.88 (0.65–1.21)
Death from any cause by day 90	322/721 (44.7)	332/743 (44.7)	1.00 (0.81–1.23)

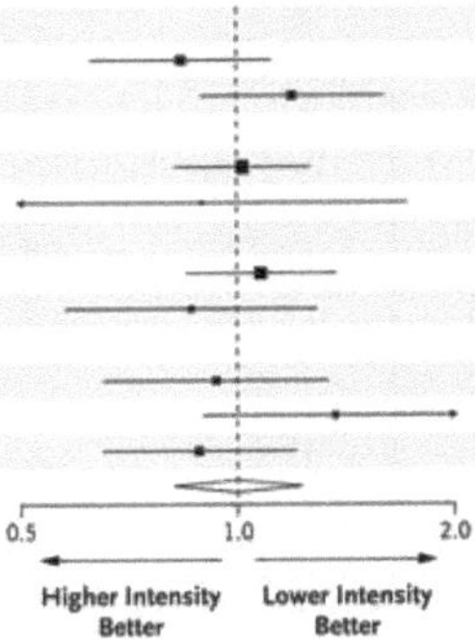

FIGURE 3.—Mortality in the Prespecified Subgroups and among All Patients. Odds ratios and 95% confidence intervals are shown for deaths in the four prespecified subgroups for both treatment pairs and for death from any cause by day 90 for all patients. CI denotes confidence interval, eGFR estimated glomerular filtration rate, and SOFA Sequential Organ Failure Assessment (range of scores, 0 to 4). Larger squares represent greater numbers of patients. (Reprinted from The RENAL Replacement Therapy Study Investigators. Intensity of continuous renal-replacement therapy in critically ill patients. *N Engl J Med.* 2009;361:1627-1638, with permission from 2009 Massachusetts Medical Society. All rights reserved.)

study, Bellomo and colleagues present the results of the randomized evaluation of normal versus augmented level replacement therapy, which was conducted in multiple centers in Australia and New Zealand. In critically ill patients with AKI, treatment with higher-intensity continuous renal replacement therapy did not reduce mortality at 90 days. The results of this study are qualitatively similar to those of the veterans affairs/National Institutes of Health (NIH) Acute Renal Failure Network Study. However, there were several differences in these 2 studies. In the Acute Renal Failure Network Study both CVVH was used in hemodynamically unstable patients, and stable patients received intermittent hemodialysis. In addition, protocol specific therapy was continued for up to 28 days, regardless of whether the patient remained in the ICU. Failure to demonstrate improved outcomes with more intensive renal replacement therapy in critically ill patients with AKI in both the Randomized Evaluation of Normal versus Augmented Level (RENAL) study and the Acute Renal Failure study imply more need to define the optimal timing. Threshold dose in RRT remains a search priority. Furthermore, more intensive therapy may be required for the treatment of severe hyperkalemia, acidemia, and severe hypercatabolism.

M. Mathru, MD, FCCP

Prevalence of Delirium with Dexmedetomidine Compared with Morphine Based Therapy after Cardiac Surgery: A Randomized Controlled Trial (DEXmedetomidine COmpared to Morphine-DEXCOM Study)

Shehabi Y, Grant P, Wolfenden H, et al (Univ of New South Wales Clinical School, Sydney, Australia; et al)

Anesthesiology 111:1075-1084, 2009

Background.—Commonly used sedatives/analgesics can increase the risk of postoperative complications, including delirium. This double-blinded study assessed the neurobehavioral, hemodynamic, and sedative characteristics of dexmedetomidine compared with morphine-based regimen after cardiac surgery at equivalent levels of sedation and analgesia.

Methods.—A total of 306 patients at least 60 yr old were randomized to receive dexmedetomidine (0.1–0.7 $\mu g \cdot kg^{-1} \cdot h^{-1}$) or morphine (10-70 $\mu g \cdot kg^{-1} \cdot h^{-1}$) with open-label propofol titrated to a target Motor Activity Assessment Scale of 2–4. Primary outcome was the prevalence of delirium measured daily *via* Confusion Assessment Method for intensive care. Secondary outcomes included ventilation time, additional sedation/analgesia, and hemodynamic and adverse effects.

Results.—Of all sedation assessments, 75.2% of dexmedetomidine and 79.6% ($P = 0.516$) of morphine treatment were in the target range. Delirium incidence was comparable between dexmedetomidine 13 (8.6%) and morphine 22 (15.0%) (relative risk 0.571, 95% confidence interval [CI] 0.256–1.099, $P = 0.088$), however, dexmedetomidine-managed patients spent 3 fewer days (2 [1–7] *versus* 5 [2–12]) in delirium (95% CI 1.09–6.67, $P = 0.0317$). The incidence of delirium was significantly less in a small subgroup requiring intraaortic balloon pump and treated with dexmedetomidine (3 of 20 [15%] *versus* 9 of 25 [36%]) (relative risk 0.416, 95% CI 0.152–0.637, $P = 0.001$). Dexmedetomidine-treated patients were more likely to be extubated earlier (relative risk 1.27, 95% CI 1.01–1.60, $P = 0.040$, log-rank $P = 0.036$), experienced less systolic hypotension (23% *versus* 38.1%, $P = 0.006$), required less norepinephrine ($P < 0.001$), but had more bradycardia (16.45% *versus* 6.12%, $P = 0.006$) than morphine treatment.

Conclusion.—Dexmedetomidine reduced the duration but not the incidence of delirium after cardiac surgery with effective analgesia/sedation, less hypotension, less vasopressor requirement, and more bradycardia *versus* morphine regimen (Table 2).

▶ Delirium in elderly patients carries a high morbidity and mortality. Given its high incidence, the consequences of delirium place a substantial burden on both patients and the health care system. Strong association has been demonstrated between inadequate pain control and the risk of postoperative delirium. Furthermore, drugs used to alleviate pain, particularly some opioids, are known to promote both delirium and postoperative cognitive loss. This paradox highlights the importance of creating a fine balance between adequate pain control,

TABLE 2.—Clinical Outcomes and Variables

Outcome Variables*	Dexmedetomidine (n = 152)	Morphine (n = 147)	*P* Value
Delirium outcomes			
Patients with delirium, n (%)	13 (8.6)	22 (15.0)	0.088
Delirium days, median (IQR)	2 [1-7]	5 [2-12]	0.031†
Patients with IABP and delirium, n (%)	3/20 (15)	9/25 (36)	0.001
Patients with valve/combined, n (%)	6/48 (12.5)	6/51 (11.8)	0.923
Study drug dose, $\mu g \cdot kg^{-1} \cdot h^{-1}$	0.48 (0.23–0.76)	49 (20–81)	NA
Time on study drug, h	18 (15–20)	17 (15–20)	0.225
MAAS within target range, n (%)			
Including all assessments ‡	1134/1507 (75.2)	1247/1567 (79.6)	0.516
6 hours after surgery	1315 (87.3)	1418 (90.5)	
Time to extubation, h	14 (10–18.5)	15 (10–22)	0.036§
ICU length of stay, h	45 (24–71)	45 (24–75)	0.148‖
Intraaortic balloon pump, h	40 (26.5–49.5)	48 (26–72)	0.648
Hospital LOS, d	8 (7–11)	8 (7–11)	0.501#
Hospital mortality, n (%)	2/152 (1.32)	4/147 (2.72)	0.442

IABP = Intraaortic aortic balloon pump; ICU = intensive care unit; IQR = interquartile range; LOS = length of stay; MAAS = motor assessment agitation scale.
*Data presented as median (interquartile range) unless otherwise stated;
†*P* value from log-rank test;
‡Including immediate post anesthesia time;
§‖#*P* value from log-rank test.

choice of analgesics, and delirium reduction. This prospective study examined the effect of an α_2 agonist based therapy dexmedetomidine, compared with a morphine based regimen at equivalent levels of analgesia and sedation, on the prevalence of delirium, ventilation time, hemodynamic profile, and the adequacy of analgesia and sedation in patients older than 60 yr after cardiac surgery. Their results demonstrate that both dexmedetomidine and morphine achieved analgesia and sedation. This trial demonstrated, specific differences even after a short period of dexmedetomidine treatment. Although the difference in the incidence of delirium failed to reach a statistical significance, the observed 42% reduction of delirium with dexmedetomidine may be clinically important, in concert with significant reduction in the duration of delirium. Furthermore, patients receiving dexmedetomidine were more likely to be extubated earlier, and they experienced less systolic hypotension, lower vasopressor requirement, but more bradycardia compared with morphine-based therapy. Their results concur with experience in general ICU population and confirm that dexmedetomidine has an antidelirium effect in cardiac surgery patients.

M. Mathru, MD, FCCP

Pulmonary Capillary Blood Flow and Cardiac Output Measurement by Partial Carbon Dioxide Rebreathing in Patients with Acute Respiratory Distress Syndrome Receiving Lung Protective Ventilation

Allardet-Servent J, Forel J-M, Roch A, et al (Service de Réanimation Médicale, France; et al)

Anesthesiology 111:1085-1092, 2009

Background.—Partial carbon dioxide rebreathing noninvasively measures the pulmonary capillary blood flow and estimates the cardiac output with the use of a predicted shunt value. It has been reported that the accuracy of the method is decreased in patients with high pulmonary shunt. The aim of this study was to investigate the agreement between partial rebreathing and thermodilution for the determination of pulmonary capillary blood flow and cardiac output in the setting of acute respiratory distress syndrome.

Methods.—Twenty consecutive patients with the acute respiratory distress syndrome were enrolled. Ventilator settings include low tidal volume ($6\ ml \cdot kg^{-1}$) and positive end-expiratory pressure + $2\ cm\ H_2O$ higher than the lower inflection point if present or $10\ cm\ H_2O$ if not. Seven pairs of cardiac output and pulmonary capillary blood flows were recorded every 20 min over a 2-h period. The authors determined bias, SD, limit of agreement (95% confidence interval) and percentage error.

Results.—Bias and agreement for cardiac output measurement were $0.8 \pm 1.2 l \cdot min^{-1}$ (-2.1 to $3.7 l \cdot min^{-1}$), and percentage error was 36%. Bias and agreement for pulmonary capillary blood flow measurement were $-0.1 \pm 0.8 l \cdot min^{-1}$ (-2.1 to $1.9 l \cdot min^{-1}$), and percentage error was 35%. Dead space, arteriovenous oxygen content difference, mean pulmonary arterial pressure, and baseline cardiac output were independently associated with differences between methods.

Conclusions.—In patients with the acute respiratory distress syndrome, partial rebreathing cannot yet replace thermodilution for measuring pulmonary capillary blood flow or cardiac output. However, accuracy of the method is close to the boundary of clinical relevance.

► In critically ill patients, the associated sepsis, hypovolemia, and mechanical ventilation with positive end expiratory pressure (PEEP) can have significant impact on cardiac output (CO). The standard for determining CO is the thermodilution principle performed in a clinical setting with an indwelling pulmonary artery catheter. In addition, PA catheter allows calculation of shunt fraction and, therefore, it indirectly gives pulmonary blood flow. However, the insertion of pulmonary catheter is invasive and its use in critically ill patients is being increasingly debated. Partial carbon dioxide rebreathing method is being increasingly used to determine CO using Fick principle to carbon dioxide. As a result, principle flow is proportional to the elimination rate by the lung (vCO_2) and to the difference between mixed venous ($Cvco_2$) and arterial ($Caco_2$) content. Pulmonary capillary blood flow can be calculated as the change in Vco_2 between the nonbreathing and rebreathing periods divided by change in $Cvco_2$ and minus $Caco_2$.The accuracy of the partial rebreathing method to estimate CO has been validated in the operating room environment. This study examined the agreement between partial rebreathing and thermodilution for the determination of pulmonary capillary blood flow and CO in patients with acute respiratory distress syndrome (ARDS) requiring mechanical ventilation and PEEP. The principle finding of this study was that in patients with ARDS receiving mechanical ventilation, partial rebreathing method cannot replace thermodilution for the measurement of CO or pulmonary capillary blood flow because it slightly overpasses the boundary of clinical relevance. In this population percentage error was 36% for CO and 35% for pulmonary capillary blood flow. The main factors that could have contributed to this difference between the methods were the mean pulmonary artery pressure, the dead space fraction, arteriovenous oxygen difference, and the baseline CO. Future research should address the issue of improving the algorithm of partial carbon dioxide rebreathing for ARDS patients.

M. Mathru, MD, FCCP

Haemoglobin A1c as a predictor of postoperative hyperglycaemia and complications after major colorectal surgery

Gustafsson UO, Thorell A, Soop M, et al (Ersta Hosp, Stockholm, Sweden; Univ of Auckland, New Zealand; et al)

Br J Surg 96:1358-1364, 2009

Background.—Hyperglycaemia following major surgery increases morbidity, but may be improved by use of enhanced-recovery protocols. It is not known whether preoperative haemoglobin (Hb) A1c could predict hyperglycaemia and/or adverse outcome after colorectal surgery.

Methods.—Some 120 patients without known diabetes underwent major colorectal surgery within an enhanced-recovery protocol. HbA1c was measured at admission and 4 weeks after surgery. All patients received an oral diet beginning 4 h after operation. Plasma glucose was monitored five times daily. Patients were stratified according to preoperative levels of HbA1c (within normal range of 4·5–6·0 per cent, or higher).

Results.—Thirty-one patients (25·8 per cent) had a preoperative HbA1c level over 6·0 per cent. These had higher mean(s.d.) postoperative glucose (9·3(1·5) *versus* 8·0(1·5) mmol/l; $P < 0{\cdot}001$) and C-reactive protein (137(65) *versus* 101(52) mg/l; $P = 0{\cdot}008$) levels than patients with a normal HbA1c level. Postoperative complications were more common in patients with a high HbA1c level (odds ratio 2·9 (95 per cent confidence interval 1·1 to 7·9)).

Conclusion.—Postoperative hyperglycaemia is common among patients with no history of diabetes, even within an enhanced-recovery protocol. Preoperative measurement of HbA1c may identify patients at higher risk

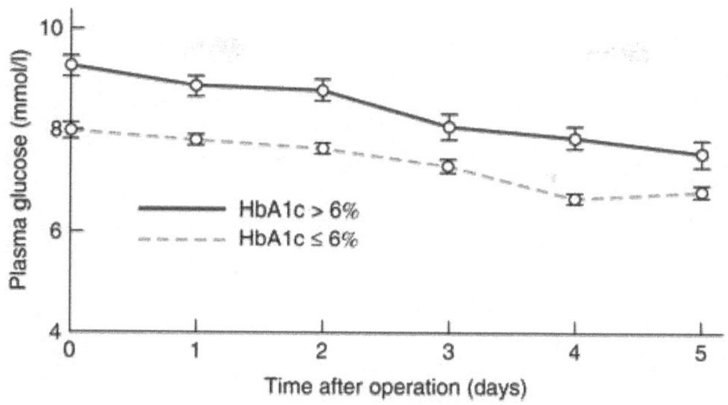

FIGURE 1.—Mean (s.e.m.) of five daily capillary plasma glucose concentrations following colorectal resection in patients stratified according to preoperative haemoglobin (Hb) A1c level. Glucose concentrations were raised throughout the 5 days among patients with a HbA1c level over 6 per cent and the difference between groups remained constant over time ($P < 0{\cdot}001$, repeated-measures ANOVA). (Reprinted from Gustafsson UO, Thorell A, Soop M, et al. Haemoglobin A1c as a predictor of postoperative hyperglycaemia and complications after major colorectal surgery. *Br J Surg*. 2009;96:1358-1364, with permission from 2009 British Journal of Surgery Society Ltd.)

TABLE 3.—Inflammatory Response and Recovery After Colorectal Surgery

	HbA1c >6·0%	HbA1c ≤6·0%	Crude *P**	Adjusted *P*†
C-reactive protein, postop. days 1–3 (mg/l)	137(65)	101(52)	0·003	0·008
Time to oral food only, no drip (days)	5·9(4·3)	3·3(6·2)	0·012	0·013
Time to first bowel movement (days)	3·4(3·1)	2·9(1·9)	0·261	0·995
Time to EDA removal (days)	4·1(1·9)	3·9(2·4)	0·606	0·770
Time to fulfil discharge criteria	6·6(4·8)	5·3(4·3)	0·206	0·244
Length of hospital stay (days)	8·5(5·4)	7·3(5·6)	0·337	0·482

Values are mean(s.d.). EDA, epidural anaesthesia.
*Two-tailed *t* test.
†Adjusted for age, sex, body mass index, American Society of Anesthesiologists physical status grade, preoperative bleeding and duration of surgery (multiple linear regression).

of poor glycaemic control and postoperative complications (Fig 1, Tables 3 and 4).

▶ Tight glucose control in the perioperative period is known to reduce morbidity and mortality in patients undergoing surgery. Furthermore, the use of minimally invasive surgery, epidural anesthesia, and preoperative oral carbohydrate treatment (enhanced recovery protocols) results in better perioperative glucose control. Currently it is not known whether preoperative blood sugar control is a determinant of postoperative outcome. Assuming that is the case, early identification of patients at risk for hyperglycemia may allow the institution of specific protocols to control blood sugar in the perioperative period and may improve the postoperative recovery phase. Plasma HbA1c is formed by the nonenzymatic glycation of valine and lysine residues in the Hb molecule, and reflects mean ambient fasting and postprandial hyperglycemia over a 2- to

TABLE 4.—Complications After Colorectal Surgery

	HbA1c >6·0% ($n = 31$)	HbA1c ≤6·0% ($n = 89$)
Respiratory failure	0	1
Plural fluid	1	0
Cardiac failure	0	1
Cardiac arrhythmia	1	2
Postop. bleed	1	4
Postop. ileus	3	1
Anastomotic leak	0	2
Stoma necrosis	1	0
Wound infection	2	7
Pneumonia	3	3
Sepsis	0	1
Urinary infection	3	3
Other infection	1	1
Total no.	16	26
No. of patients with complications	14 (45)	22 (25)
No. of patients with infection	9 (29)	15 (17)

Values in parentheses are percentages. Six patients had more than one complication, two with a haemoglobin (Hb) A1c level above 6·0 per cent and four with a level of 6·0 per cent or less.

3-month period. Raised Hb1Ac reflects chronic hyperglycemia and has therefore been suggested as an alternative to the oral glucose tolerance test. In this study the authors examined whether HbA1c can be used in nondiabetic patients undergoing surgery to correlate, with postoperative glucose control, the magnitude of the inflammatory response, postoperative recovery, and 30-day morbidity after colorectal surgery. In this study, high preoperative Hb1Ac levels in nondiabetic patients were associated with significantly raised glucose levels after surgery. Furthermore, these patients with high Hb1Ac levels had almost 3-fold increased risk of overall complications than patients with normal levels. Main differences were found with regard to the rates of pneumonia, urinary tract infections, pleural effusion, and postoperative ileus. In addition, the complication rates were higher in patients with high Hb1Ac levels despite the use of enhanced recovery protocol, which is supposed to reduce surgical metabolic stress and insulin resistance. This study convincingly demonstrates that preoperative Hb1Ac may be used to identify patients at a higher risk of poor postoperative glycemic control and postoperative complications after major abdominal surgery.

M. Mathru, MD, FCCP

The Effect of Intravenous Alanyl-Glutamine Supplementation on Plasma Glutathione Levels in Intensive Care Unit Trauma Patients Receiving Enteral Nutrition: The Results of a Randomized Controlled Trial

Eroglu A (Karadeniz Technical Univ, Trabzon, Turkey)

Anesth Analg 109:502-505, 2009

Background.—We sought to investigate the effect of IV alanyl-glutamine supplementation on plasma glutathione levels in severely traumatized patients receiving enteral nutrition.

Methods.—Forty adult patients with severe trauma according to the Injury Severity Score >20 were enrolled in this randomized, controlled study. The patients were assigned to two groups: Group G received $0.5\ g \cdot kg^{-1} \cdot d^{-1}$ of alanyl-glutamine dipeptide supplementation IV, and Group C received a control solution without alanyl-glutamine for 7 days. Blood samples were taken for analysis of glutathione before the initiation of supplementation and on the 3rd, 7th, and 10th days of feeding.

Results.—Total plasma glutathione levels significantly increased in Group G when compared with Group C on Days 7 and 10 ($1.34 \pm 0.20\ \mu M$ vs $1.13 \pm 0.14\ \mu M$, and $1.38 \pm 0.19\ \mu M$ vs $1.12 \pm 0.16\ \mu M$) ($P < 0.001$).

Conclusions.—This study demonstrates that IV alanyl-glutamine supplementation for 7 days increases total plasma glutathione levels in critically ill trauma patients receiving standard enteral nutrition.

▶ Glutathione is a critical antioxidant in human tissues. In addition to its antioxidant effect it has cytoprotective effects and is also involved in detoxification and metabolism of a number of substances in the liver. Tissue glutathione levels are depleted in critically ill patients and in trauma patients. Plasma glutathione levels are maintained primarily by a balance secretion from the liver and by the degradation by kidney and other tissues. The regulation of glutathione concentration involves the release of glutathione precursors from peripheral tissues, *de novo* synthesis within the cells, and transportation into plasma. Previous studies have shown that glutamine-enriched parenteral nutrition enhanced plasma stores glutathione and the glutamine was rate limiting for glutathione biosynthesis during parenteral nutrition. In addition, studies have also shown that enteral and intravenous supplementation of IV glutamine replenishes tissue levels of glutathione. This study examined the effect of IV alanyl-glutamine dipeptide supplementation on plasma glutathione levels in severely traumatized patients. The study demonstrates that IV supplementation of glutamine for 7 days increases total plasma glutathione levels in critically ill trauma patients receiving standard enteral nutrition. Despite the impressive results, this study is limited by its sample size and limited follow-up of patients to determine the outcome.

M. Mathru, MD, FCCP

Hydrogen Sulfide Improves Survival After Cardiac Arrest and Cardiopulmonary Resuscitation via a Nitric Oxide Synthase 3–Dependent Mechanism in Mice

Minamishima S, Bougaki M, Sips PY, et al (Massachusetts General Hosp, Boston, MA; et al)

Circulation 120:888-896, 2009

Background.—Sudden cardiac arrest (CA) is one of the leading causes of death worldwide. We sought to evaluate the impact of hydrogen sulfide (H_2S) on the outcome after CA and cardiopulmonary resuscitation (CPR) in mouse.

Methods and Results.—Mice were subjected to 8 minutes of normothermic CA and resuscitated with chest compression and mechanical ventilation. Seven minutes after the onset of CA (1 minute before CPR), mice received sodium sulfide (Na_2S) (0.55 mg/kg IV) or vehicle 1 minute before CPR. There was no difference in the rate of return of spontaneous circulation, CPR time to return of spontaneous circulation, and left ventricular function at return of spontaneous circulation between groups. Administration of Na_2S 1 minute before CPR markedly improved survival rate at 24 hours after CPR (15/15) compared with vehicle (10/26; $P = 0.0001$ versus Na_2S). Administration of Na_2S prevented CA/CPR-induced oxidative stress and ameliorated left ventricular and neurological dysfunction 24 hours after CPR. Delayed administration of Na_2S at 10 minutes after CPR did not improve outcomes after CA/CPR. Cardioprotective effects of Na_2S were confirmed in isolated-perfused mouse hearts subjected to global ischemia and reperfusion. Cardiomyocyte-specific overexpression of cystathionine γ-lyase (an enzyme that produces H_2S) markedly improved outcomes of CA/CPR. Na_2S increased phosphorylation of nitric oxide synthase 3 in left ventricle and brain cortex, increased serum nitrite/nitrate levels, and attenuated CA-induced mitochondrial injury and cell death. Nitric oxide synthase 3 deficiency abrogated the protective effects of Na_2S on the outcome of CA/CPR.

Conclusions.—These results suggest that administration of Na_2S at the time of CPR improves outcome after CA possibly via a nitric oxide synthase 3–dependent signaling pathway.

► Hydrogen sulfide (H_2S) exerts a variety of biological effects that range from cytotoxic to cytoprotective effects. Low concentrations of H_2S reduces metabolism and improves survival in experimental hemorrhagic shock. H_2S also has antiapoptotic and anti-inflammatory effects following an ischemia-reperfusion event in heart, liver, and kidney. The impact of H_2S on global ischemia-reperfusion (cardiac arrest/cardiopulmonary resuscitation [CA/CPR]) has not been investigated. In this elegant experimental study, the authors examined the impact of H_2S on the outcome of CA/CPR in mouse. This study demonstrated that administration of H_2S at the time of CPR improves myocardial and neurological function and survival after CA/CPR in mice. This protective effect is attributed to activation of antiapoptotic pathway and also prevention of systemic oxidative stress and acceleration of mitochondrial permeability transition in the heart. The study also suggests that H_2S administration improves outcome by nitric oxide (NO)-dependent pathway. Their observation if extrapolated to clinical scenario in human beings may be highly clinically relevant because their results suggest that sodium sulfide administration can improve outcome of sudden CA at the time of CPR when intravenous access is obtained. Future studies are needed to elucidate the impact of exogenous and endogenous H_2S on the long-term outcome of CA and CPR complicated by post-CA syndrome.

M. Mathru, MD, FCCP

Development and Validation of a Prediction Score for Postoperative Acute Renal Failure Following Liver Resection

Slankamenac K, Breitenstein S, Held U, et al (Univ Hosp of Zurich, Switzerland)

Ann Surg 250:720-728, 2009

Objective.—To develop and validate a score to predict postoperative acute renal failure (ARF) after liver resection.

Background.—Postoperative ARF after major surgery is associated with morbidity and mortality. Early identification of patients at risk of ARF is important in order to provide protective kidney treatment.

Methods.—Postoperative ARF was prospectively assessed in consecutive patients undergoing liver resection. In randomly selected two-third of the total number of patients, multivariate logistic regression analysis was used to develop a new prediction score (including a full and a reduced model), based on the preoperative parameters of age, gender, preexisting chronic renal dysfunction, cardiovascular disease, diabetes, bilirubin, and alanine aminotransferase (ALT) levels. In the remaining last third of the patients, the new score was validated by calibrating the accuracy of the score (ClinicalTrials.gov NCT 00743132).

Results.—Postoperative ARF occurred in 15.1% (86 of 569 consecutive patients) from 2002 to 2007 and was highly associated with mortality (22.5% vs. 0.8% without ARF, $P < 0.001$). In the 380 (two-third of the population) patients selected for the development of the prediction score, preoperatively elevated ALT, preexisting cardiovascular disease, chronic renal failure, and diabetes were the strongest predictors of ARF. Validating the full prediction model (0–22 points) to the remaining 189 patients (one-third of the population), the risk could be predicted accurately (mean predicted risk of 11.5% vs. an observed risk of 14.8%) without significant differences between predicted and observed risks across different risk categories ($P = 0.98$). Prediction with the reduced model including the 4 strongest predictors (0–7 points) was almost as accurate as with the full model (11.4% predicted vs. 14.8% observed) and also without significant differences across different risk categories ($P = 0.75$).

TABLE 4.—Postoperative Outcome

	All Patients n = 569	Postoperative Non-ARF* n = 483	Postoperative ARF* n = 86
Overall morbidity	295 (51.8%)	220 (45.5%)	75 (87.2%)
No postoperative complications	274 (48.2%)	263 (54.5%)	11 (12.8%)
Overall mortality	24 (4.2%)	4 (0.8%)	20 (23.2%)
Mortality based on			
Acute renal failure	12 (2.1%)	0%	12 (13.9%)
Intraabdominal infection	4 (0.7%)	0%	4 (4.7%)
Liver insufficiency	3 (0.5%)	3 (0.6%)	0%
Cardiac insufficiency	3 (0.5%)	1 (0.2%)	2 (2.3%)
Sepsis, unknown focus	2 (0.4%)	0%	2 (2.3%)

*ARF indicates acute renal failure.

TABLE 6.—Development of Predictor Score Based on Multivariate Logistic Regression Model

Predictor	Categories	Regression Coefficient β*	Odds Ratio (β)	P	Shrinked Coefficient βs†	Shrinked Odds Ratio (βs)	Risk Score‡
Cardiovascular disease	No	1.19	3.29	0.004	1.02	2.78	0
	Yes						5
Chronic renal failure	No	1.13	3.08	0.003	0.98	2.63	0
	Yes						4
Diabetes	No	0.85	2.34	0.045	0.73	2.07	0
	Yes						3
ALT	≤35/50 U/L§	1.21	3.34	0.001	1.03	2.82	0
	>35/50 U/L§						5
Age	<60 yr	0.29	1.34	0.456	0.25	1.29	0
	60–69 yr	0.62	1.86	0.146	0.53	1.70	1
	≥ 70 yr						3
Bilirubin	<17 μmol/L	0.23	1.26	0.521	0.20	1.22	0
	≥17 μmol/L						1
Female	No	0.27	1.31	0.412	0.23	1.26	0
	Yes						1

*Compared with reference category, which is no cardiovascular disease, no chronic renal failure, no diabetes, ALT ≤35/50 U/L for women/men, age <60 yr, bilirubin <17 μmol/L, and male gender, respectively. Constant = −3.297.
†Shrinkage coefficient: 0.86
‡One point is assigned per 10 yr increase of age = coefficient of 0.25 (reference category). Points rounded to the next integer.
§Cut-offs for women/men.

Conclusions.—The new prediction score (the full as well as the reduced model) accurately predicted postoperative ARF after liver resection. The use of these scores allows early identification of patients at high risk of ARF, and may support decision making for protective kidney interventions perioperatively (Tables 4 and 6).

▶ Acute renal failure (ARF) in the presence of liver disease carries a high morbidity and mortality. Currently there is very little information available in the literature regarding the incidence and outcome of ARF in patients following liver resection. Identifying patients preoperatively who are at high risk for developing ARF postoperatively will help to formulate preventive strategies in the perioperative period. The authors developed and validated an easily applicable score to predict the risk for ARF in patients undergoing liver resection. The score based on 7 parameters showed good discrimination and calibration. The 4 strongest predictors for ARF include pre-existing cardiovascular disease, chronic renal failure, diabetes, and high levels of alanine aminotransferase (ALT). This short list predicted the risk of ARF nearly as accurately as the full score. This current scoring system may support decision making for the kidney-protective interventions during the entire perioperative period, which could potentially improve outcome. A number of preoperative predictors identified in this study such as cardiac dysfunction, renal dysfunction, diabetes, and cholestasis are treatable and could be modified. This scoring system needs to be validated in a larger population, and future studies should compare the predictive performance of the full and reduced scores to evaluate whether the reduced score can be used safely without much loss on information. Further studies are needed to evaluate the impact of possible pre-, intra-, and postoperative targets for optimizing, treating, and influencing the postoperative renal function following liver resection and the occurrence of ARF following surgery.

M. Mathru, MD, FCCP

Initiation of Inappropriate Antimicrobial Therapy Results in a Fivefold Reduction of Survival in Human Septic Shock

Kumar A, Ellis P, Arabi Y, et al (Univ of Manitoba, Winnipeg, Canada; Univ of Toronto, Canada; King Saud Bin Abdulaziz Univ for Health Sciences, Riyadh, Saudi Arabia; et al)

Chest 136:1237-1248, 2009

Objective.—Our goal was to determine the impact of the initiation of inappropriate antimicrobial therapy on survival to hospital discharge of patients with septic shock.

Methods.—The appropriateness of initial antimicrobial therapy, the clinical infection site, and relevant pathogens were retrospectively determined for 5,715 patients with septic shock in three countries.

Results.—Therapy with appropriate antimicrobial agents was initiated in 80.1% of cases. Overall, the survival rate was 43.7%. There were marked differences in the distribution of comorbidities, clinical infections, and pathogens in patients who received appropriate and inappropriate initial antimicrobial therapy ($p < 0.0001$ for each). The survival rates after appropriate and inappropriate initial therapy were 52.0% and 10.3%, respectively (odds ratio [OR], 9.45; 95% CI, 7.74 to 11.54; $p < 0.0001$). Similar differences in survival were seen in all major epidemiologic, clinical, and organism subgroups. The decrease in survival with inappropriate initial therapy ranged from 2.3-fold for pneumococcal infection to 17.6-fold with primary bacteremia. After adjustment for acute physiology and chronic health evaluation II score, comorbidities, hospital site, and other potential risk factors, the inappropriateness of initial antimicrobial therapy remained most highly associated with risk of death (OR, 8.99; 95% CI, 6.60 to 12.23).

Conclusions.—Inappropriate initial antimicrobial therapy for septic shock occurs in about 20% of patients and is associated with a fivefold reduction in survival. Efforts to increase the frequency of the appropriateness of initial antimicrobial therapy must be central to efforts to reduce the mortality of patients with septic shock.

▶ Mortality remains high despite the use of potent antibiotics and aggressive supportive management. Several clinical studies suggest that effective use of antimicrobial agents is central to the ultimate outcome in life-threatening infections in critically ill patients. The same group of investigators in a previous large retrospective study demonstrated that delay in the initiation of effective antimicrobial therapy following the onset of hypotension is the critical determinant of outcome in septic shock. The authors hypothesized that the initiation of treatment with inappropriate antimicrobial agents (in relation to the subsequently demonstrated sensitivity of the pathogens) as the initial empiric therapy may be the single most common cause of prolonged delay in the introduction of effective therapy, and this inappropriate choice of antibiotics may have a negative outcome. In this retrospective multicenter study the investigators examined the relationship between the appropriateness of initial empiric antimicrobial therapy and survival in patients with septic shock. Their results suggest that provision of inappropriate initial antimicrobial therapy has a substantial negative effect on outcome in patients with septic shock. The study also confirms that the incidence of the initiation of organism inappropriate empiric therapy is surprisingly common. Overall, the survival dropped 5-fold from 52.0% to 10.3%. The primary weakness of this study is that it was observational in nature. Future prospective studies should address the issue of selection of initial antimicrobial regimen with coverage against the inciting isolated or presumed pathogens is required for the best possible survival in septic shock.

M. Mathru, MD, FCCP

Utility of Thoracic Computed Tomography after Blunt Trauma: When is Chest Radiograph Enough?

Barrios C, Malinoski D, Dolich M, et al (Univ of California, Orange)
Am Surg 75:966-969, 2009

The purpose of this study was to identify the utility of thoracic computed tomography (TCT) in blunt trauma patients with a normal admission chest radiograph (CXR). A retrospective study was performed of 200 consecutive blunt trauma patients who received both CXR and TCT. One hundred and forty-three patients had a normal screening CXR; 36 of these patients (25%) had an abnormal TCT. TCT changed the management in only nine of these patients (6%): two required serial

CXR for occult pneumothorax, four received additional imaging of the spine, and three were admitted to a monitored bed. Fifty-seven patients had an abnormal initial CXR. Of these, 41 (81%) had an abnormal TCT. TCT changed management in 21 (37%) of these patients: two aortic injuries identified, 12 aortic injuries excluded, two chest tubes placed, one patient taken to the Operating Room, and four patients required further diagnostic evaluation. TCT was significantly more likely to alter management in patients with an abnormal admission CXR (6% *vs* 37%, $P < 0.001$). TCT is of limited utility in patients with a normal admission CXR. A diagnostic strategy of obtaining TCT only in patients with abnormal CXR or high-risk mechanism of injury can result in significant cost savings without adversely affecting patient outcomes.

▶ Plain chest X-ray was commonly used to diagnose blunt chest trauma injuries, including pneumothorax, hemothorax, and rib fractures. However, with the recent advent of thoracic computed tomography (TCT) and with its increased sensitivity and specificity, TCT is being increasingly used to diagnose blunt chest trauma. Despite its widespread use, the clinical significance of occult findings on TCT has not been proven. This study examined the utility of TCT in blunt trauma patients with a normal admission chest X-ray. This study, similar to previous studies, demonstrates low likelihood that patients with a normal chest X-ray will have a life-threatening occult injury such as aortic dissection, which is usually only identified on TCT. Due to its increased sensitivity and specificity, TCT will result in increased diagnoses of blunt chest trauma. This study clearly suggests that in patients with a normal screening chest X-ray, TCT is not useful. Occult injuries identified are unlikely to be life threatening. However, TCT resulted in a change of management in a significant number of patients with an abnormal initial chest X-ray. The cost and radiation risks associated should be taken into consideration by clinicians while ordering TCT in patients with blunt trauma and normal chest X-ray (Table 2 in the original article).

M. Mathru, MD, FCCP

Extracorporeal Membrane Oxygenation for 2009 Influenza A(H1N1) Acute Respiratory Distress Syndrome

The Australia and New Zealand Extracorporeal Membrane Oxygenation (ANZ ECMO) Influenza Investigators (Alfred Hosp, Melbourne, Victoria, Australia)

JAMA 302:1888-1895, 2009

Context.—The novel influenza A(H1N1) pandemic affected Australia and New Zealand during the 2009 southern hemisphere winter. It caused an epidemic of critical illness and some patients developed severe acute respiratory distress syndrome (ARDS) and were treated with extracorporeal membrane oxygenation (ECMO).

Objectives.—To describe the characteristics of all patients with 2009 influenza A(H1N1)–associated ARDS treated with ECMO and to report incidence, resource utilization, and patient outcomes.

Design, Setting, and Patients.—An observational study of all patients (n = 68) with 2009 influenza A(H1N1)–associated ARDS treated with ECMO in 15 intensive care units (ICUs) in Australia and New Zealand between June 1 and August 31, 2009.

Main Outcome Measures.—Incidence, clinical features, degree of pulmonary dysfunction, technical characteristics, duration of ECMO, complications, and survival.

Results.—Sixty-eight patients with severe influenza-associated ARDS were treated with ECMO, of whom 61 had either confirmed 2009 influenza A(H1N1) (n = 53) or influenza A not subtyped (n = 8), representing an incidence rate of 2.6 ECMO cases per million population. An additional 133 patients with influenza A received mechanical ventilation but no ECMO in the same ICUs. The 68 patients who received ECMO had a median (interquartile range [IQR]) age of 34.4 (26.6-43.1) years and 34 patients (50%) were men. Before ECMO, patients had severe respiratory failure despite advanced mechanical ventilatory support with a median (IQR) $Pa{O_2}$/fraction of inspired oxygen ($F{IO_2}$) ratio of 56 (48-63), positive end-expiratory pressure of 18 (15-20) cm H_2O, and an acute lung injury score of 3.8 (3.5-4.0). The median (IQR) duration of

TABLE 1.—Comparison of Patients With Influenza A Who Received ECMO and Those Who Received Mechanical Ventilation But Without ECMO at ECMO Centers[a]

Parameter	ECMO (n = 61)	Mechanical Ventilation But Without ECMO (n = 133)	*P* Value
Age, median (IQR), y	36 (27-45)	44 (31-54)	.02
Male sex	29 (48)	63 (47)	.54
BMI, median (IQR)	29 (23-36)	29 (24-37)	.92
Chronic lung disease	18 (30)	35 (26)	.64
APACHE III comorbidity[b]	5 (8)	30 (23)	.02
Pregnancy or postpartum	10 (16)	12 (9)	.21
Diabetes mellitus	9 (15)	23 (17)	.64
H1N1 positive	56 (92)	107 (80)	.05
At ICU admission			
Mechanical ventilation	53 (87)	117 (88)	.80
Vasopressor	35 (57)	46 (34)	.02
Renal replacement therapy	5 (8)	9 (7)	.95
Duration or length of stay, median (IQR), d			
Mechanical ventilation	18 (9-27)	8 (4-14)	.001
ICU	22 (13-32)	12 (7-18)	.001
Hospital	28 (15-43)	20 (13-31)	.07
Mortality			
in ICU	14 (23)	12 (9)	.01
in hospital	14 (23)	17 (13)	.06

Abbreviations: APACHE, Acute Physiology and Chronic Health Evaluation; BMI, body mass index (calculated as weight in kilograms divided by height in meters squared); ECMO, extracorporeal membrane oxygenation; ICU, intensive care unit; IQR, interquartile range.

[a]Data are presented as No. (%) unless otherwise specified.

[b]The presence or not of at least 1 comorbidity.

TABLE 3.—Patient Outcomes[a]

Outcome Measure	2009 Influenza A(H1N1) Confirmed Infection (n = 53)	2009 Influenza A(H1N1) Suspected Infection (n = 15)	All Infections (N = 68)
Length of stay, median (IQR), d			
ICU	26 (16-35)	31 (15-38)	27 (16-37)
Hospital	35 (24-45)	40 (27-54)	39 (23-47)
Duration, median (IQR), d			
Mechanical ventilation	24 (13-31)	28 (13-34)	25 (13-34)
ECMO support	10 (7-14)	11 (10-16)	10 (7-15)
Survival at ICU discharge	38 (72)	10 (67)	48 (71)
Still in ICU	4 (8)	2 (13)	6 (9)
Survival at hospital discharge	22 (42)	10 (67)	32 (47)
Still in hospital[b]	14 (26)	2 (13)	16 (24)
Ambulant at hospital discharge[c]	21 (95)	10 (100)	31 (97)
SaO_2 on room air at hospital discharge, median (IQR), %[c]	97 (95-98)	97 (95-98)	97 (95-98)
Discharge destination			
Died	11 (21)	3 (20)	14 (21)
Home	18 (34)	4 (27)	22 (32)
Other hospital	0	1 (7)	1 (1)
Rehabilitation facility	4 (8)	5 (33)	9 (13)
Cause of death[d]			
Hemorrhage	3 (27)	1 (33)	4 (29)
Intracranial hemorrhage	4 (36)	2 (66)	6 (43)
Infection	1 (9)	0	1 (7)
Intractable respiratory failure	3 (27)	1 (33)	4 (29)

Abbreviations: ECMO, extracorporeal membrane oxygenation; ICU, intensive care unit; IQR, interquartile range; SaO_2, arterial oxygen saturation.

[a]Data are presented as No. (%) unless otherwise specified.

[b]Not including patients still in the ICU.

[c]For survivors only.

[d]Data are shown as No. (% of deaths) and patients could have more than 1 cause contributing to death.

ECMO support was 10 (7-15) days. At the time of reporting, 48 of the 68 patients (71%; 95% confidence interval [CI], 60%-82%) had survived to ICU discharge, of whom 32 had survived to hospital discharge and 16 remained as hospital inpatients. Fourteen patients (21%; 95% CI, 11%-30%) had died and 6 remained in the ICU, 2 of whom were still receiving ECMO.

Conclusions.—During June to August 2009 in Australia and New Zealand, the ICUs at regional referral centers provided mechanical ventilation for many patients with 2009 influenza A(H1N1)–associated respiratory failure, one-third of whom received ECMO. These ECMO-treated patients were often young adults with severe hypoxemia and had a 21% mortality rate at the end of the study period (Tables 1 and 3).

► The novel influenza A (H1N1) pandemic affected the entire hemisphere. A proportion of these patients developed severe respiratory distress syndrome. In some cases when conventional measures such as mechanical ventilation and lung recruitment maneuvers fail, extracorporeal membrane oxygenation (ECMO) was recommended for the treatment of refractory hypoxemia. In this case series the authors report clinical features, severity of respiratory failure, technical characteristics, duration of extracorporeal support, and survival in patients with severe influenza-related acute respiratory distress syndrome (ARDS). This is the first multicenter study on the use of ECMO in influenza-associated ARDS. In previous studies where ECMO was used in ARDS of heterogeneous etiology the mortality rates were betwen 30% and 48%, whereas in this series of patients ECMO use was associated with 21% mortality. The reduced mortality associated with ECMO use was attributed to the younger age group and better ECMO technology (ie, heparin coated cannulae, rotary pumps, and small efficient long lasting oxygenators). Will ECMO use reduce mortality in influenza-associated refractory ARDS? Of course casual inference should not be drawn from an uncontrolled case series. Recent data suggest that patients who might be considered for ECMO often may survive without it. Nonetheless, based on the data presented here, it seems likely that the mortality rate would have been higher than 21% without the use of the ECMO. The study is limited because allocation to receive ECMO was not conducted in a randomized control trial. Since the expense associated with the use of ECMO in these patients will be prohibitive, institutions must develop explicit policies to equitably determine who will and who will not receive life support systems such as ECMO should absolute scarcity occur.

M. Mathru, MD, FCCP

Bedside Sublingual Video Imaging of Microcirculation in Assessing Bacterial Infection in Cirrhosis

Sheikh MY, Javed U, Singh J, et al (Univ of California San Francisco-Fresno Med Education Program)

Dig Dis Sci 54:2706-2711, 2009

Bacterial infections are common in cirrhosis and can lead to life-threatening complications. Sidestream dark-field (SDF) imaging has recently emerged as a noninvasive tool for capturing real-time video images of sublingual microcirculation in critically ill patients with sepsis. The objective of this study was to assess the utility of SDF in determining underlying infection in patients with cirrhosis. Sublingual microcirculation was compared among patients with compensated cirrhosis (Group A, $n = 13$), cirrhosis without sepsis (Group B, $n = 18$), cirrhosis with sepsis (Group C, $n = 14$), and sepsis only (Group D, $n = 10$). The blood flow was semi-quantitatively evaluated in four equal quadrants in small (10–25 mm); medium (26–50 mm); and large (51–100 mm) sublingual capillaries. The blood flow was described as no flow (0), intermittent flow (1), sluggish flow (2), and continuous flow (3). The overall flow score or microvascular flow index (MFI) was measured for quantitative assessment of microcirculation and predicting power for concurrent infection in cirrhosis. Marked impairment was observed at all levels of microvasculature in Groups B and C when compared with Group A. This effect was restricted to small vessels only when Group B was compared with

TABLE 2.—Microvascular Flow Index (MFI) in the Four Study Groups in Relation to Vessel Size

Vessel	Group	MFI (mean ± SD)	95% CI
Small	A	2.40 ± 0.46	2.07–2.73
	B	1.40 ± 0.52	1.03–1.77
	C	0.80 ± 0.48	0.45–1.15
	D	1.15 ± 0.34	0.45–1.39
Medium	A	2.35 ± 0.42	2.05–2.64
	B	1.40 ± 0.32	1.17–0.62
	C	1.25 ± 0.48	0.90–0.59
	D	1.55 ± 0.28	1.34–0.75
Large	A	2.75 ± 0.35	2.50–3.00
	B	1.90 ± 0.77	1.35–0.45
	C	1.65 ± 0.47	1.31–1.99
	D	2.10 ± .52	1.73–0.47
Mean[a]	A	2.50 ± 0.21	2.35–2.64
	B	1.56 ± 0.35	1.31–1.81
	C	1.23 ± 0.24	1.06–1.40
	D	1.60 ± 0.32	1.37–1.82

Group A, compensated cirrhosis; Group B, decompensated cirrhosis without infection/sepsis; Group C, decompensated cirrhosis with infection/sepsis; Group D, sepsis without cirrhosis.

[a]Mean of all vessel types in an individual study group.

Group C. MFI < 1.5 was found to have highest sensitivity (100%) and specificity (100%) for infection in decompensated cirrhosis. SDF imaging of sublingual microcirculation can be a useful bedside diagnostic tool to assess bacterial infection in cirrhosis (Table 2).

▶ Preserved integrity of the microcirculation is critical for adequate tissue oxygenation during infection and sepsis. As microvascular bed is the site of exchange for nutrient and oxygen, the persistence of microcirculatory abnormalities can lead to tissue hypoxia, organ failure, and death. Previous experimental and clinical studies have demonstrated perturbations in microcirculation in sepsis. Recently refined sidestream dark field (SDF) imaging has emerged as a noninvasive bedside tool that provides high-contrast, real-time video images of microcirculation in critically ill patients with sepsis. This study was designed to assess sublingual changes in microcirculation with SDF video imaging in decompensated cirrhosis with and without infection. This study demonstrates that sublingual microcirculation in decompensated cirrhosis shows perturbations in microcirculation similar to septic patients, but with less intensity. Marked microcirculatory abnormalities were observed in patients with sepsis. The precise mechanisms responsible for these changes are not elucidated by this study. Possible mechanisms include alterations in gut flora and bacterial translocation, deficient phagocytic activity, lower complement levels, and poor opsonization. Increased plasma levels, proinflammatory cytokines, and endothelin could also play a role in the disturbed microcirculation. Early noninvasive monitoring of microcirculation in infections such as spontaneous bacterial peritonitis can help physicians to decide the timing of the initiation of antibiotic therapy, thus preventing life-threatening complications of cirrhosis. Their results need to be validated in a larger series of patients.

M. Mathru, MD, FCCP

A genetic variant of hypoxia-inducible factor-1α is associated with adverse outcomes in acute kidney injury

Kolyada AY, Tighiouart H, Perianayagam MC, et al (Caritas St Elizabeth's Med Ctr, Boston, MA; Tufts Med Ctr, Boston, MA)

Kidney Int 75:1322-1329, 2009

Hypoxia-inducible factor-1α (HIF-1α) is a transcription factor that mediates many cellular responses to tissue hypoxia, a common feature of acute kidney injury (AKI). Here we studied 241 patients with AKI and determined the relationship to adverse outcome of a non-synonymous polymorphism in the coding region of the HIF-1α gene where a C to T substitution occurs at position +85 in exon 12, a change known to enhance transactivation. The baseline characteristics of the patients were not different among genotype groups except for a significantly higher prevalence of shock and number of failed organs in T-allele carriers. A significant genotype-phenotype association was found for plasma levels of vascular endothelial growth factor-A but not angiopoietin-2, two downstream targets of HIF-1α. Compared to the CC genotype, T-allele carriers had significantly higher adjusted odds for dialysis requirement or in-hospital death; assisted mechanical ventilation or dialysis requirement; and the composite of assisted mechanical ventilation, dialysis requirement or in-hospital death. The trend for higher plasma angiopoietin-2 levels was associated with significantly higher adjusted odds for in-hospital death; dialysis requirement or in-hospital death; and the composite outcome of assisted mechanical ventilation, dialysis, or in-hospital death. Despite

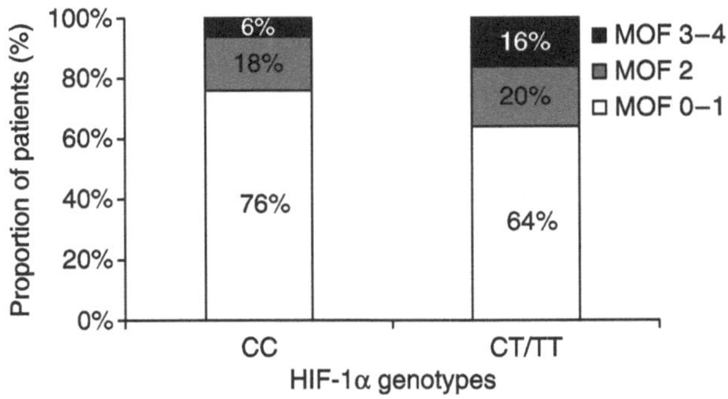

FIGURE 1.—Multiple organ failure (MOF) score stratified by HIF-1α genotypes. $P = 0.04$ by χ^2-test. (Reprinted from Kolyada AY, Tighiouart H, Perianayagam MC, et al. A genetic variant of hypoxia-inducible factor-1α is associated with adverse outcomes in acute kidney injury. *Kidney Int*. 2009;75:1322-1329, with permission from Macmillan Publishers Ltd.)

TABLE 3.—Association of HIF-1α Exon 12 (+85) Genotypes with Adverse Clinical Outcomes in Patients with AKI

HIF-1α CT/TT Genotypes (vs CC Genotype)	OR	95% CI	*P*-Value
In-hospital death			
Unadjusted	1.64	0.86, 3.13	0.14
Adjusted for race, sex, and APACHE II score	1.53	0.72, 3.29	0.27
Adjusted for race, sex, APACHE II score, and shock	1.49	0.69, 3.24	0.31
Dialysis requirement or in-hospital death			
Unadjusted	2.89	1.56, 5.36	<0.001
Adjusted for race, sex, and APACHE II score	3.61	1.77, 7.39	<0.001
Adjusted for race, sex, APACHE II score, and shock	3.87	1.87, 8.01	<0.001
Assisted mechanical ventilation or dialysis requirement			
Unadjusted	2.58	1.39, 4.78	0.003
Adjusted for race, gender, and APACHE II score	3.39	1.60, 7.19	0.001
Adjusted for race, sex, APACHE II score, and shock	3.67	1.70, 7.89	0.001
Assisted mechanical ventilation, dialysis requirement, or in-hospital death			
Unadjusted	3.28	1.71, 6.29	0.0004
Adjusted for race, gender, and APACHE II score	4.74	2.16, 10.43	0.0001
Adjusted for race, sex, APACHE II score, and shock	4.73	2.14, 10.47	0.0001

AKI, acute kidney injury; 95% CI, 95% confidence interval for the odds ratio (OR); HIF-1α, hypoxia-inducible factor-1α.

the limited cohort size, our study found this particular HIF-1α genetic variant to be associated with disease severity and adverse outcomes in AKI. Larger studies are needed to confirm these relationships (Fig 1, Table 3).

▶ Several lines of experimental evidence suggest that polymorphism of host-response candidate genes have emerged as potentially important determinants of disease severity and adverse outcome in acute kidney injury (AKI). A nonsynonymous polymorphism in the coding region of the hypoxia-inducible factor-1α (HIF-1α) gene resulting in proline to serine substitution has recently been shown and described to increase the transactivation potential of the transcription factor. In this study, the investigators examined the association of this HIF-1α genetic variant with measures of disease severity and adverse outcomes in a cohort of hospitalized patients with established AKI, focusing mainly on dialysis requirement, assisted mechanical ventilation, and in-hospital mortality. Their results demonstrate that the genetic variance of this gene has associated higher prevalence of in-hospital mortality, more organ failure, increased dialysis requirement, and assisted mechanical ventilation. Given the importance of this gene in mediating cellular responses to hypoxia, this data seems to contradict experimental observation that hypoxic preconditioning and subsequent HIF-1α activation protects against ischemic and nephrotoxic injury. The precise mechanisms underlying the association of the HIF-1α T-allele with higher requirement for organ support are unknown. The poor outcome associated with this gene polymorphism may be due, in part, to the slower degradation of the mutated HIF-1α after reversal of tissue hypoxia, that is, when oxygen supply is restored, thereby creating an effective state of "hypoxia extension." This maladptation might be conducive to aberrant cytokine activation pattern that has been described previously in sepsis and linked to HIF-1α activation.

M. Mathru, MD, FCCP

Acid–base disorders evaluation in critically ill patients: we can improve our diagnostic ability

Boniatti MM, Cardoso PRC, Castilho RK, et al (Hosp de Clínicas de Porto Alegre, Brazil)

Intensive Care Med 35:1377-1382, 2009

Purpose.—To determine whether Stewart's approach can improve our ability to diagnose acid–base disorders compared to the traditional model.

Methods.—This prospective cohort study took place in a university-affiliated hospital during the period of February–May 2007. We recorded clinical data and acid–base variables from one hundred seventy-five patients at intensive care unit admission.

Results.—Of the 68 patients with normal standard base excess (SBE) (SBE between −4.9 and +4.9), most ($n = 59$; 86.8%) had a lower effective strong ion difference (SIDe), and of these, 15 (25.4%) had SIDe < 30 mEq/L.

TABLE 3.—Examples of acid–base disorders

	Patient 1	Patient 2
Measured variables		
Sodium (mmol/L)	151	146
Potassium (mmol/L)	3.4	3.8
Calcium (mg/dl)	7.0	7.2
Magnesium (mmol/L)	2.0	1.8
Phosphate (mmol/L)	1.0	2.0
Albumin (g/L)	27.0	27.0
Chloride (mmol/L)	121	124
pH	7.48	7.43
$PaCO_2$ (mmHg)	29.0	30.2
Lactate (mmol/L)	2.0	1.3
Derived variables		
HCO_3 (mmol/L)	21.5	20.0
SBE (mmol/L)	−0.7	−3.8
AG (mmol/L)	12.4	6.3
SIDa (mmol/L)	34.4	27.4
SIDe (mmol/L)	29.9	28.8
SIG (mmol/L)	4.5	−1.4

HCO_3 serum bicarbonate, *SBE* standard base excess, *AG* anion gap, *SID_a* apparent strong ion difference, *SID_e* effective strong ion difference, *SIG* strong ion gap

Thus, the evaluation according to Stewart's method would allow an additional diagnosis of metabolic disorder in 33.7% patients.

Conclusions.—The Stewart approach, compared to the traditional evaluation, results in identification of more patients with major acid–base disturbances (Table 3).

▶ Stewart's physiochemical approach is attaining popularity among intensivists for the assessment of acid-base derangement. This approach is used instead of the conventional measures, which include anion gap (AG), standard base excess (SBE), and bicarbonate (HCO_3). The physiochemical approach is mechanistic and helps to identify hidden metabolic disorders in the critically ill; the approach is also of prognostic value. In this study the investigators examined whether the diagnostic evaluation of acid-base disorders in a population of critically ill patients can be improved using Stewart's method compared with the traditional model. The salient finding of this study is that it demonstrates the greater sensitivity of physiochemical evaluation in identifying acid-base disorders in critically ill patients. In this study the physiochemical method compared with the traditional method based on SBE, allowed an additional diagnosis of metabolic disorders in one third of the patients. In the 2 examples cited, SBE failed to identify important metabolic disorders due to the alkalinizing effect of hypoalbuminemia and hypophosphatemia. In both cases there was hyperchloremic acidosis, which could have been prevented by the use of more balanced solution such as ringers lactate. This study was limited by the small sample size and failure to evaluate possible changes in treatment based on a change in diagnostic evaluation.

M. Mathru, MD, FCCP

A potential role for inducible nitric oxide synthase in the cerebral response to acute hemodilution

McLaren AT, Mazer CD, Zhang H, et al (Univ of Toronto, Canada)

Can J Anesth 56:502-509, 2009

Purpose.—Acute anemia increases the cerebral expression of hypoxic molecules including neuronal nitric oxide synthase (nNOS) and hypoxia inducible factor-1α (HIF-1α). This study assessed the effects of acute hemodilution on inducible NOS (iNOS) and systemic inflammatory cytokines.

Methods.—Anesthetized rats ($n = 5–7$ per group) underwent 50% hemodilution with pentastarch, whole blood exchange or no fluid exchange. Cerebral cortical nNOS and iNOS protein levels were characterized using Western blot analysis and immunostaining (1 and 18 h). Plasma cytokine levels were assessed by enzyme-linked immunosorbent assay (1, 4, and 18 h). Data were analyzed by two-way analysis of variance to determine significance ($P < 0.05$, mean ± SD).

Results.—No differences in mean arterial blood pressure or arterial blood gases were observed between groups after hemodilution. A comparable hemoglobin target (~70 g · L^{-1}) was achieved in all groups following hemodilution. Cerebral cortical iNOS protein levels were increased in anemic rats, relative to controls. The nNOS protein levels increased to a greater degree ($P < 0.05$ for both). Immunostaining demonstrated that iNOS localized to endothelium, glial fibrillary acidic protein (GFAP) positive (astrocytes) and GFAP negative cells within the brain. Plasma cytokine levels (tumour necrosis factor α, interleukin (IL)-1β and IL-6) increased transiently, to the same levels, in both control and hemodiluted rats.

Conclusions.—Cerebral cortical iNOS and nNOS protein levels were both increased in anemic rats. The nNOS response was predominant. This suggests that NOS-derived NO may be an important signalling pathway which is activated in the brain during anemia. These cellular responses could maintain cerebral homeostasis, or contribute to neuronal injury, during acute hemodilutional anemia.

▶ Whole body responses to anemia include increases in CO, redistribution of perfusion, increases in oxygen extraction, and vasodilation. Moreover, anemia tolerance varies between organs. This is attributed to organ specific adaptive and maladaptive mechanisms within the organs. The authors in previous experimental studies have demonstrated that hypoxia inducible factor-1α (HIF-α) and neuronal nitric oxide synthase (nNOS) protein levels are increased in the brain during acute anemia in rats. However, experimental studies have not yet demonstrated whether inducible NOS (iNOS) protein levels are also increased in the brain during acute anemia. iNOS has been shown to contribute to both adaptive (ischemic preconditioning) and maladaptive inflammatory mechanisms within the brain. In this study the investigators examined the effects of acute isovolemic anemia on inducible NOS (iNOS) and inflammatory cytokines. This experimental study demonstrated that both iNOS and nNOS protein levels increased in the cerebral cortex of anemic rats following acute hemodilution. However, plasma cytokine did not appear to contribute to the observed increase in cerebral iNOS expression. Potential NOS signaling pathways within the perivascular cerebral tissue include tissue hypoxia in remote organs (ie, the kidney), which could send afferent signals to the central nervous system activating appropriate afferent responses, including an increase nNOS derived NO from perivascular neurons or vascular smooth muscle. Alternatively, hemodilutional anemia may activate receptors within the vascular lumen, which results in the upregulation of perivascular NOS derived NO. iNOS derived NO may be maladaptive and may contribute to anemia-induced cerebral injury. A clearer understanding of the cellular responses during acute anemia is required to determine the potential mechanisms of injury.

M. Mathru, MD, FCCP

Predictors of Prolonged Postoperative Endotracheal Intubation in Patients Undergoing Thoracotomy for Lung Resection

Cywinski JB, Xu M, Sessler DI, et al (Cleveland Clinic, OH)

J Cardiothorac Vasc Anesth 23:766-769, 2009

Objective.—The aim of this study was to identify predictors of delayed endotracheal extubation defined as the need for postoperative ventilatory support after open thoracotomy for lung resection.

Design.—An observational cohort investigation.

Setting.—A tertiary referral center.

Participants.—The study population consisted of 2,068 patients who had open thoracotomy for pneumonectomy, lobectomy, or segmental lung resection between January 1996 and December 2005.

Interventions.—Not applicable.

Measurements and Main Results.—Preoperative and intraoperative variables were collected concurrently with the patient's care. Risk factors were identified using logistic regression with stepwise variable selection procedure on 1,000 bootstrap resamples, and a bagging algorithm was used to summarize the results. Intraoperative red blood cell transfusion, higher preoperative serum creatinine level, absence of a thoracic epidural catheter, more extensive surgical resection, and lower preoperative FEV_1 were associated with an increased risk of delayed extubation after lung resection.

Conclusion.—Most predictors of delayed postoperative extubation (ie, red blood cell transfusion, higher preoperative serum creatinine, lower preoperative FEV_1, and more extensive lung resection) are difficult to modify in the perioperative period and probably represent greater severity of underlying lung disease and more advanced comorbid conditions. However, thoracic epidural anesthesia and analgesia is a modifiable factor that was associated with reduced odds for postoperative ventilatory support. Thus, the use of epidural analgesia may reduce the need for post-thoracotomy mechanical ventilation.

▶ Mechanical ventilation and prolonged intubation in patients undergoing lung resection, increases the cost and could potentially increase morbidity such as nosocomial pneumonia. Furthermore, after lung resection, mechanical ventilation can increase the stress on the remaining lung and potentially increase postoperative air leak. The goal of this study was to identify preoperative variables associated with delayed postoperative extubation after thoracotomy for lung resection. The authors identified several factors, which were predictive of delayed extubation, including intraoperative transfusion, preoperative renal dysfunction, lower preoperative forced expiratory volume in 1 second (FEV1), and extent of the lung resection. Intraoperative activation of the epidural catheter reduces the postoperative opioid requirement, which can presumably improve respiratory function. Consistent with this theory, the authors found that the use of thoracic epidural anesthesia (TEA) improved the odds of operating room (OR) extubation in their series of patients.

Recognizing the predictive importance of these factors may help to identify patients at risk for extended postoperative mechanical ventilation and help to allocate postoperative resources. TEA is one intervention that may reduce the odds of prolonged postoperative ventilation.

M. Mathru, MD, FCCP

Surviving blood loss without blood transfusion in a swine poly-trauma model

Alam HB, Shuja F, Butt MU, et al (Massachusetts General Hosp/Harvard Med School, Boston)

Surgery 146:325-333, 2009

Background.—We have demonstrated previously that valproic acid (VPA), a histone deacetylase inhibitor, can improve survival in lethal models of hemorrhagic shock. This study investigated whether VPA treatment would improve survival in a clinically relevant large animal model of poly-trauma/hemorrhagic shock, and whether the protective effects are executed through the Akt survival pathway.

Methods.—Yorkshire swine were subjected to a poly-trauma protocol including: (1) Pre-hospital phase- Femur fracture, 60% hemorrhage, 30 min of shock (mean arterial pressure [MAP]: 25–30 mmHg), and infusion of 154mM NaCl (3 × shed blood); (2) Early hospital phase A Grade V liver injury (simulating rupture of a previously contained hematoma) followed by liver packing; (3) Treatment/monitoring phase randomization to 3 treatment groups ($n = 6$–8/group): no treatment (control), fresh whole blood (FWB), and intravenous VPA (400 mg/kg, given during the pre-hospital phase). Animals were monitored for 4 h, with survival being the primary endpoint. Liver tissue was subjected to Western blot analysis.

Results.—FWB ($n = 6$) and VPA treatments ($n = 7$) significantly increased survival (100% and 86%, respectively) compared to control group ($n = 8$) (25%). The protocol produced significant anemia (Hb<6 g/dL) and lactic acidosis (lactate 3–5 mmol/L). Acidosis improved after blood transfusion and worsened in the other two groups. VPA treatment increased phospho-Akt (activated), phospho-GSK-3β (Glycogen synthase kinase 3β), β-catenin and Bcl-2 (B-cell leukemia/lymphoma 2) protein levels compared to control group ($P = .01$, .01, .03, and .02, respectively). There was no significant difference in the level of these proteins between the control and FWB groups.

Conclusion.—Treatment with VPA without blood transfusion improves early survival in a highly lethal poly-trauma and hemorrhagic shock model. The survival advantage is due not to improvement in resuscitation but to better tolerance of shock by the cells, in part due to the preservation of the Akt survival pathway (Figs 1, 3 and 7).

▶ Prompt resuscitation with colloids or crystalloids and restoring perfusion remains as the critical element in the management of hemorrhagic shock.

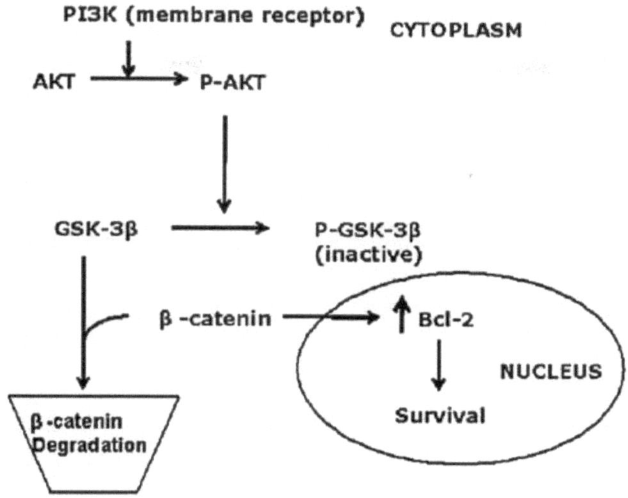

FIGURE 1.—PI3K/Akt survival pathway. *P-AKT,* Phospho-Akt; *P-GSK-3β,* phospho-GSK-3β. (Reprinted from Alam HB, Shuja F, Butt MU, et al. Surviving blood loss without blood transfusion in a swine poly-trauma model. *Surgery.* 2009;146:325-333, with permission from Mosby, Inc.)

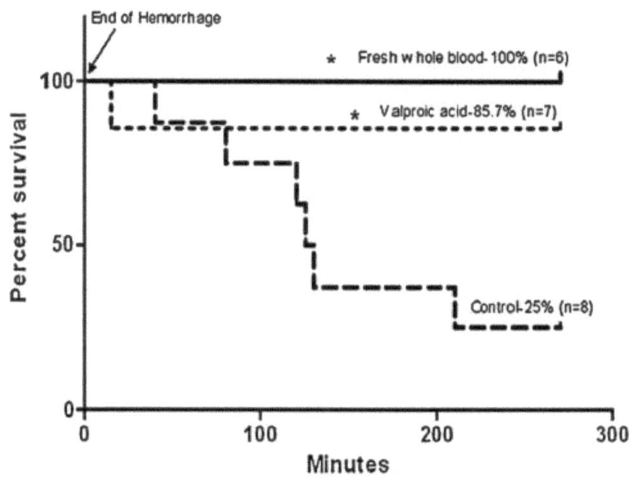

FIGURE 3.—Kaplan-Meier survival curves. $^{*}P < .05$ compared to control. (Reprinted from Alam HB, Shuja F, Butt MU, et al. Surviving blood loss without blood transfusion in a swine poly-trauma model. *Surgery.* 2009;146:325-333, with permission from Mosby, Inc.)

However, the efficacy of current resuscitation regimens remains controversial. Several lines of experimental evidence suggest that severe shock and resuscitation may act as a model of global ischemia reperfusion with a generation of reactive oxygen species and can also prime and activate various inflammatory cells. This realization has lead to designing novel resuscitation strategies, which have been shown to decrease immune/inflammatory activation and

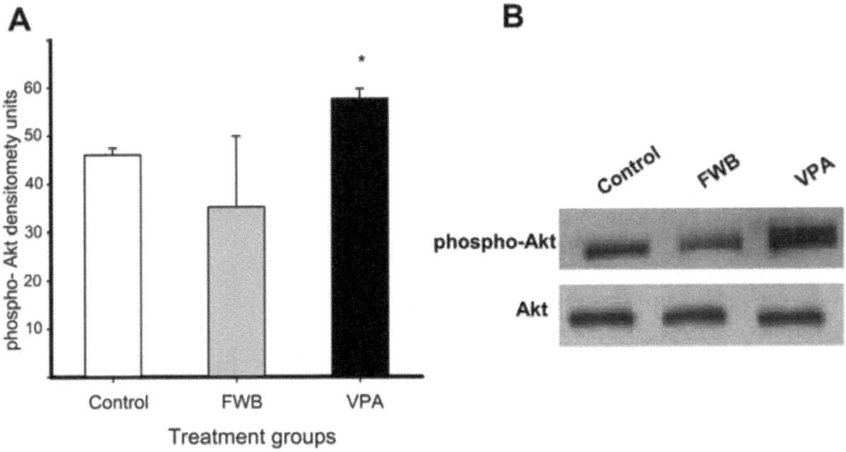

FIGURE 7.—Effect of VPA on Akt activity after polytrauma and hemorrhagic shock. (*A*) Protein bands quantified by densitometry were expressed as mean values of 3 experiments ± SEM. *FWB*, Fresh whole blood; *VPA*, valproic acid alone. (*B*) Representative protein bands from Western blots for phospho-Akt (Ser473) and total Akt. VPA preserves the levels of phospho-Akt compared to control group. $^{*}P < .05$ compared to control. (Reprinted from Alam HB, Shuja F, Butt MU, et al. Surviving blood loss without blood transfusion in a swine poly-trauma model. *Surgery.* 2009;146:325-333, with permission from Mosby, Inc.)

alter the rate of cellular survival. In previous studies the authors established the concept of pharmacological resuscitation involving drugs (ie, histone deacetylase inhibitors [HDACI]) that modulates pathways involving inflammation, immune activation, and cell survival. In this study, the investigators examined whether valproic acid, an HDACI would increase survival in a swine model of hemorrhagic shock. They also tested whether this would be through its activation of the Akt/protein kinase B (PKB) cascade, a well established cell survival signaling pathway. In this lethal model, VPA treatment provided an impressive survival advantage (86%) without any additional resuscitation. The increase in tolerable ischemia time was attributed to the activation of prosurvival molecular pathways such as the Akt signaling pathway.

M. Mathru, MD, FCCP

Non-invasive ventilation after extubation in hypercapnic patients with chronic respiratory disorders: randomised controlled trial

Ferrer M, Sellarés J, Valencia M, et al (Universitat de Barcelona, Spain; et al)
Lancet 374:1082-1088, 2009

Background.—Non-invasive ventilation can prevent respiratory failure after extubation in individuals at increased risk of this complication, and enhanced survival in patients with hypercapnia has been recorded. We aimed to assess prospectively the effectiveness of non-invasive

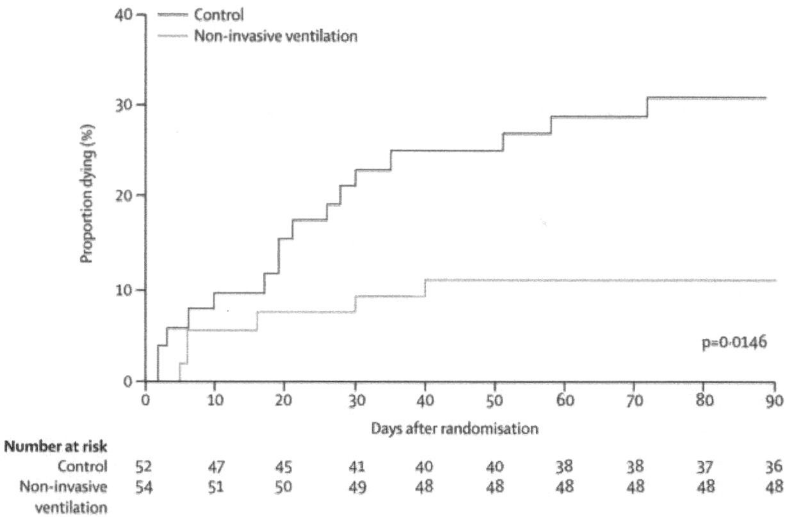

FIGURE 3.—Kaplan-Meier 90-day mortality curve. (Reprinted from Ferrer M, Sellarés J, Valencia M, et al. Non-invasive ventilation after extubation in hypercapnic patients with chronic respiratory disorders: randomised controlled trial. *Lancet*. 2009;374:1082-1088.)

ventilation after extubation in patients with hypercapnia and as rescue therapy when respiratory failure develops.

Methods.—We undertook a randomised controlled trial in three intensive-care units in Spain. We enrolled 106 mechanically ventilated patients with chronic respiratory disorders and hypercapnia after a successful spontaneous breathing trial. We randomly allocated participants by computer to receive after extubation either non-invasive ventilation for 24 h (n=54) or conventional oxygen treatment (n=52). The primary endpoint was avoidance of respiratory failure within 72 h after extubation. Analysis was by intention to treat. This trial is registered with clinicaltrials.gov, identifier NCT00539708.

Findings.—Respiratory failure after extubation was less frequent in patients assigned non-invasive ventilation than in those allocated conventional oxygen therapy (8 [15%] *vs* 25 [48%]; odds ratio 5·32 [95% CI 2·11–13·46]; p<0·0001). In patients with respiratory failure, non-invasive ventilation as rescue therapy avoided reintubation in 17 of 27 patients. Non-invasive ventilation was independently associated with a lower risk of respiratory failure after extubation (adjusted odds ratio 0·17 [95% CI 0·06–0·44]; p<0·0001). 90-day mortality was lower in patients assigned non-invasive ventilation than in those allocated conventional oxygen (p=0·0146).

Interpretation.—Early non-invasive ventilation after extubation diminished risk of respiratory failure and lowered 90-day mortality in patients with hypercapnia during a spontaneous breathing trial. Routine

TABLE 1.—Baseline Characteristics of Patients at Entry into the Study

	Non-invasive Ventilation (n = 54)	Control (n = 52)
Age (years)	67 (10)	70 (9)
Men	44 (81%)	36 (69%)
APACHE-II score on admission	20 (7)	20 (7)
APACHE-II score at entry into the study	11 (3)	11 (3)
Previous duration of mechanical ventilation (days)	5 (3)	4 (2)
Forced expiratory volume in 1 s (% predicted)	34 (13)	38 (11)
Type of chronic respiratory disease		
COPD or chronic bronchitis*	38 (70%)	36 (69%)
Sequelae of pulmonary tuberculosis	7 (13%)	6 (12%)
Bronchiectasis	2 (4%)	4 (8%)
Obesity-hypoventilation syndrome	5 (9%)	4 (8%)
Chest-wall deformity	1 (2%)	1 (2%)
Chronic persistent asthma	1 (2%)	1 (2%)
Other comorbidities		
Chronic heart disorders†	19 (35%)	27 (52%)
Immunosuppression‡	2 (4%)	2 (4%)
Diabetes mellitus	11 (20%)	13 (25%)
Liver cirrhosis	3 (6%)	1 (2%)
Neoplasm	2 (4%)	4 (8%)
Chronic renal failure	1 (2%)	1 (2%)
Previous use of non-invasive ventilation in hospital	7 (13%)	7 (13%)
Causes of mechanical ventilation		
Exacerbation of chronic respiratory disorder	28 (52%)	25 (48%)
Pneumonia	7 (13%)	7 (13%)
Congestive heart failure	5 (9%)	8 (15%)
Neurological disease	1 (2%)	2 (4%)
Sepsis	6 (11%)	5 (10%)
Postoperative respiratory failure	3 (6%)	2 (4%)
Other	4 (7%)	3 (6%)

Data are mean (SD) or number of patients (%). APACHE-II=acute physiology and chronic health evaluation-II. COPD=chronic obstructive pulmonary disease. Pulmonary function tests were available in 66 (62%) patients.

*Chronic bronchitis defined by history of dyspnoea, cough, expectoration, and smoke consumption without pulmonary function testing.

†Includes coronary-artery disease, hypertensive or valvular heart diseases, and dilated myocardial disease of any cause.

‡Includes neutropenia after chemotherapy or bone-marrow transplant, drug-induced immunosuppression in solid-organ transplant or as a result of corticosteroids or cytotoxic therapy, and HIV-related disorders.

implementation of this strategy for management of mechanically ventilated patients with chronic respiratory disorders is advisable (Fig 3, Table 1).

▶ Reintubation after failed weaning is an independent risk factor for nosocomial pneumonia, mortality, and extended hospital stay. Previous studies suggest that noninvasive ventilation should be a promising therapy for respiratory failure with potential to avoid reintubation. However, previous randomized trials failed to show any benefit in terms of reintubation in patients who developed respiratory failure after extubation. This study examined the early use of noninvasive ventilation during the initial period of extubation to assess whether it would prevent reintubation and enhance survival of patients with chronic respiratory disorders who had hypercapnia during spontaneous breathing trial before extubation. Noninvasive ventilation reduced the frequency of reintubation due to respiratory failure and lowered the 90-day mortality in patients with hypercapnia during a spontaneous breathing trial. The positive results obtained in this study in contrast to the previous studies may be related to the use of high-performance ventilators specifically designed for this procedure, which includes control of Fio2, effective compensation for leaks, real-time assessment of mask pressure, and a sensitive and rapid response by flow trigger. Furthermore, noninvasive ventilation was used continuously in this study. This study confirms the effectiveness of noninvasive ventilation in this clinical setting and provides convincing scientific evidence for routine implementation of this strategy for management of mechanically ventilated patients with chronic respiratory disorders.

M. Mathru, MD, FCCP

Effects of Ventilatory Mode During One-Lung Ventilation on Intraoperative and Postoperative Arterial Oxygenation in Thoracic Surgery

Cruz Pardos P, Garutti I, Piñeiro P, et al (Hosp General Universitario "Gregorio Marañón", Madrid, Spain)

J Cardiothorac Vasc Anesth 23:770-774, 2009

Objective.—The purpose of this study was to investigate the relationship between the ventilatory mode used during one-lung ventilation (OLV) and intraoperative and early postoperative arterial oxygenation in patients undergoing thoracic surgery.

Methods.—A prospective, randomized clinical trial.

Setting.—A tertiary care university hospital single institution.

Participants.—One hundred ten patients scheduled for thoracic surgery with at least 1 hour of OLV.

Interventions.—Patients were prospectively randomized into 2 groups depending on the ventilatory mode used during OLV: volume-controlled ventilation (VCV) or pressure-controlled ventilation (PCV). In VCV, the authors used a tidal volume (Vt) of 8 mL/kg and in the PCV group an inspiratory pressure to provide a tidal volume of 8 mL/kg.

Measurements and Main Results.—Airway pressures and arterial blood gases were obtained at 20, 30, and 40 minutes after OLV. The authors recorded the ratio of arterial oxygen tension to inspired oxygen fraction (PaO_2/F_IO_2) at 4 hours (RU1) and 24 hours (RU2) after surgery. During OLV, there were no differences in arterial oxygenation, airway plateau pressure, and mean pressure between groups, although peak pressure was higher in the VCV group ($p < 0.01$). The PaO_2/F_IO_2 ratio at RU1 was 312.6 ± 106 in the VCV group and 322.1 ± 104. In the PCV group at RU2, it was 402.4 ± 105 and 389.6 ± 114, respectively, and there were no significant differences between the groups.

TABLE 3.—Intraoperative Variables for the Different Study Groups

Variable	Group	Baseline	OLV + 20	OLV + 30	OLV + 40	End of Surgery
PaO_2 (mmHg)	VCV	362 (79)	103.7 (65)*	133.4 (74)*	131.6 (81)*	353.6 (85)
	PCV	348 (80)	103.2 (53)*	134.1 (75)*	129.2 (67)*	332.5 (95)
Compliance (mL/cmH_2O)	VCV	45.4 (14)	28.7 (8)*	33.9 (10)*	34.1 (10)*	45.5 (15)
	PCV	45.5 (12)	27.8 (6)*	34.1 (10)*	33 (9)*	46.2 (13)
Ppeak (cmH_2O)	VCV	19.1 (5)	25.7 (5)*	25.4 (5)*	25.3 (5)*	20.9 (5)†
	PCV	18.8 (4)	22.4 (4)*‡	22.3 (4)*‡	22.6 (5)*§	19.8 (4)†
Pplateau (cmH_2O)	VCV	16.9 (5)	22.2 (5)*	21.7 (5)*	21.7 (5)*	18.8 (5)†
	PCV	16.9 (4)	21.8 (4)	21.9 (4)*	22.2 (4)*	19.2 (4)*
Pmean (cmH_2O)	VCV	6.2 (3)	7.9 (2)*	9.9 (2)*	9.9 (2)*	8.5 (2)*
	PCV	6.2 (2)	8.1 (2)*	10.6 (1)*	10.6 (1)*	9.6 (2)*§
$PaCO_2$ (mmHg)	VCV	40.8 (6)	42.6 (7)†	41.9 (7)†	42.3 (6)†	42.3 (5)†
	PCV	39 (6)	43.1 (8)*	42 (8)†	42.5 (8)†	40.3 (7)
SaO_2	VCV	99.9 (0.3)	94.6 (5)*	96.6 (5)*	96.5 (5)*	99.9 (0.4)
	PCV	99.9 (0.2)	94.1 (6)*	96.7 (4)	96.7 (4)*	99.8 (0.5)

NOTE. Values expressed as mean (standard deviation).
*$p < 0.001$ (baseline *v* others periods).
†$p < 0.05$ (baseline *v* others periods).
‡$p < 0.001$ (PCV *v* VCV).
§$p < 0.01$ (PCV *v* VCV).

TABLE 4.—Postoperative Data

	VCV	PCV	
PaO_2/FIO_2 at RU1	312.6 (106)	322.1 (104)	$p = 0.66$
PaO_2/FIO_2 at RU2	402.4 (105)	389.6 (114)	$p = 0.58$
Days in recovery unit	1.2 (0.7)	1.6 (3)	$p = 0.27$
Days in hospital	7 (4)	7 (3)	
Readmission to recovery unit (n)	2	1	
ARDS (n)	0	1	
Mortality at 30 days (n)	0	0	

NOTE. Values expressed as mean (standard deviation) or number of patients (n). Days in hospital is reported as median (interquartile range).

Conclusions.—In patients undergoing thoracic surgery, the use of PCV compared with VCV during OLV with the same Vt of 8 mL/kg does not affect arterial oxygenation during OLV or early postoperative oxygenation (Tables 3 and 4).

▶ Endothelial injury occurs in the lung of patients undergoing lung resection, which is attributed to the high airway pressure used during one-lung ventilation (OLV). Some studies advocate limiting pressure peak and pressure plateau to prevent postpneumonectomy pulmonary edema and lung injury. Licker et al stated that high airway pressure during OLV was an independent risk factor for acute lung injury (ALI) in the postoperative period. Pressure controlled ventilation (PCV) unlike volume controlled ventilation (VCV) uses a decelerating flow, which minimizes peak airway pressure and keeps the set inspiratory pressure constant. However, the effects of PCV on intraoperative oxygenation during OLV have shown conflicting results. This study was designed to investigate the effects of PCV on intraoperative and postoperative oxygenation in patients undergoing thoracotomy. The authors compared PCV with VCV on intraoperative and postoperative oxygenation. This prospective study shows that ventilatory mode per se used during OLV does not affect intraoperative and postoperative arterial oxygenation. The conclusion of this study is limited by its sample size.

M. Mathru, MD, FCCP

Management of Inadvertent Arterial Catheterisation Associated with Central Venous Access Procedures

Pikwer A, Acosta S, Kölbel T, et al (Malmö Univ Hosp, Sweden)
Eur J Vasc Endovasc Surg 38:707-714, 2009

Objective.—This study aims to describe the clinical management of inadvertent arterial catheterisation after attempted central venous catheterisation.

Methods.—Patients referred for surgical or endovascular management for inadvertent arterial catheterisation during a 5-year period were identified from an endovascular database, providing prospective information on techniques and outcome. The corresponding patient records and radiographic reports were analysed retrospectively.

Results.—Eleven inadvertent arterial (four common carotid, six subclavian and one femoral) catheterisations had been carried out in 10 patients. Risk factors were obesity ($n = 2$), short neck ($n = 1$) and emergency procedure ($n = 4$). All central venous access procedures but one had been made using external landmark techniques. The techniques used were stent-graft placement ($n = 6$), percutaneous suture device ($n = 2$), external compression after angiography ($n = 1$), balloon occlusion and open repair ($n = 1$) and open repair after failure of percutaneous suture device ($n = 1$). There were no procedure-related complications within a median follow-up period of 16 months.

Conclusions.—Inadvertent arterial catheterisation during central venous cannulation is associated with obesity, emergency puncture and lack of ultrasonic guidance and should be suspected on retrograde/pulsatile catheter flow or local haematoma. If arterial catheterisation is recognised, the catheter should be left in place and the patient be referred for percutaneous/endovascular or surgical management (Figs 1 and 3).

► Central venous access procedures are often performed by intensivists. Inadvertent arterial catheterization associated with central venous cannulation occurs in 6% of patients when the vein is cannulated using anatomical landmarks. Arterial catheterization can lead to hemorrhage, pseudoaneurysm, neurological injury, and severe airway compression. The purpose of this study was to identify potential risk factors for, and clinical signs of, inadvertent arterial catheterization after attempted central venous cannulation, and to review the

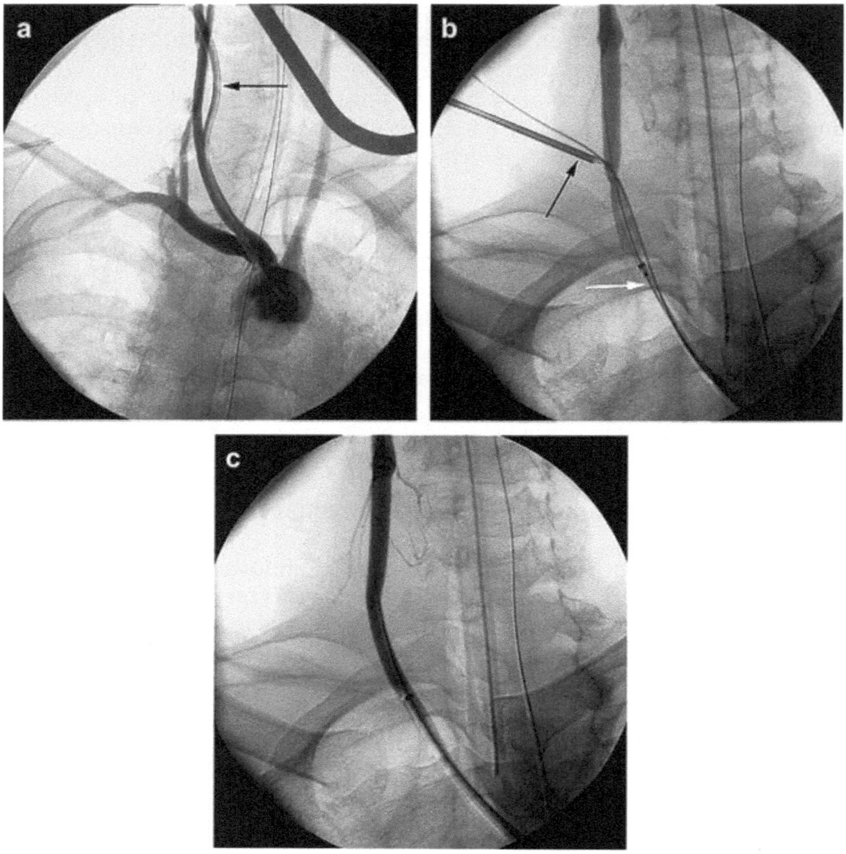

FIGURE 1.—a. Angiogram made via a 12 Fr catheter (arrow), inadvertently placed in the proximal right common carotid artery with the tip positioned in the aortic arch of a 37 year-old male patient. b. The central venous catheter, inadvertently placed in the carotid artery, replaced by a Perclose® suturing device, and arterial sutures applied to the puncture site. The sliding knot was tied with a knot pusher (black arrow). The guide wire was withdrawn after haemostasis had been confirmed. A transfemorally introduced angioplasty balloon catheter (white arrow) in its introducer sheath was kept at ready for inflation in case of haemorrhage. c. Completion angiogram showing no extravasation or stenosis. (Reprinted from Pikwer A, Acosta S, Kölbel T, et al. Management of inadvertent arterial catheterisation associated with central venous access procedures. *Eur J Vasc Endovasc Surg*. 2009;38:707-714, with permission from the European Society for Vascular Surgery.)

author's experience of minimally invasive clinical management. In agreement with previous studies, obesity, short neck, emergency catheterization, and hypovolemia were risk factors for inadvertent arterial catheterization. The study also demonstrates that the use of ultrasound reduces the risk of arterial puncture during central venous catheterization. Accidental arterial catheterization should be suspected immediately on excessive or pulsatile backflow of well-oxygenated blood through the catheter or local hematoma at the site of catheterization. Factors that are associated with an increased risk for serious complications after catheter removal are catheter diameter, time since catheter

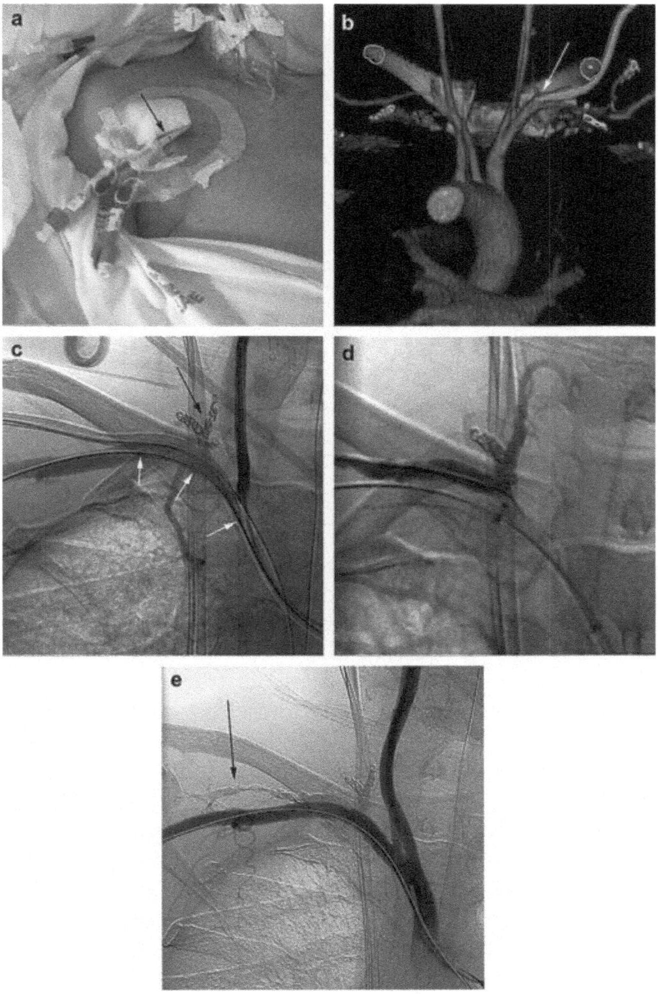

FIGURE 3.—a. In a 61 year old female a 16 Fr double-lumen catheter (arrow) was inadvertently inserted into the subclavian artery, and thereafter another 16 Fr double-lumen catheter was correctly positioned in the internal jugular vein. b. Posterior–anterior three-dimensional reconstruction of computed tomographic angiography showing the 16 Fr double-lumen catheter inadvertently passing caudally to the right clavicle into the right subclavian artery. The arrow indicates the vascular site of catheter entry at the branching of the thyreocervical trunk from the right subclavian artery. c. Angiogram made before withdrawal of the 16 Fr catheter inadvertently placed in the right subclavian artery. An 8 × 50 mm Gore Viabahn® stent graft (white arrows) was placed across the puncture site distally to the right vertebral artery, catheterised separately to secure access in case of overstenting. A 0.018-inch guide-wire passing through the inadvertently placed 16 Fr catheter proved to be most useful after withdrawal of the catheter (d and e). The thyreocervical trunk was embolized with metallic coils (black arrow) to prevent retrograde bleeding. d. Angiogram after withdrawal of a catheter inadvertently placed in the right subclavian artery showing continuous extravasation along the 0.018-inch safety guide partially withdrawn into the subcutaneous channel. e. Completion angiogram showing no further extravasation after embolization with N-butyl cyano-acrylate (Histoacryl; Braun, Melsungen, Germany) mixed with iodised oil (Lipiodol; Laboratoire Guerbet, Roissy, France). The arrow points at the glue in the subcutaneous channel of the inadvertently placed catheter. (Reprinted from Pikwer A, Acosta S, Kölbel T, et al. Management of inadvertent arterial catheterisation associated with central venous access procedures. *Eur J Vasc Endovasc Surg*. 2009;38:707-714, with permission from European Society for Vascular Surgery.)

insertion, and the puncture site. Treatment strategies for inadvertent arterial catheterization include local compression, open surgical treatment with direct arterial repair, and percutaneous/endovascular treatment. Any suspected intra-arterial catheter position should be verified radiographically and the catheter be left in place on referral for repair. Withdrawal of an arterial catheter may result in considerable hemorrhage, stroke, or as seen in one of their patients, pseudoaneurysm.

M. Mathru, MD, FCCP

Comparison of routine and on-demand prescription of chest radiographs in mechanically ventilated adults: a multicentre, cluster-randomised, two-period crossover study

Hejblum G, Chalumeau-Lemoine L, Ioos V, et al (Institut National de la Santé et de la Recherche Médicale, Paris, France; Assistance Publique-Hôpitaux de Paris, France; et al)

Lancet 374:1687-1693, 2009

Background.—Present guidelines recommend routine daily chest radiographs for mechanically ventilated patients in intensive care units. However, some units use an on-demand strategy, in which chest radiographs are done only if warranted by the patient's clinical status. By comparison between routine and on-demand strategies, we aimed to establish which strategy was more efficient and effective for optimum patient care.

Methods.—In a cluster-randomised, open-label crossover study, we randomly assigned 21 intensive care units at 18 hospitals in France to use a routine or an on-demand strategy for prescription of chest radiographs during the first of two treatment periods. Units used the alternative strategy in the second period. Each treatment period lasted for the time taken for enrolment and study of 20 consecutive patients per intensive care unit; patients were monitored until discharge from the unit or for up to 30 days' mechanical ventilation, whichever was first. Units enrolled 967 patients, but 118 were excluded because they had been receiving mechanical ventilation for less than 2 days. The primary outcome measure was the mean number of chest radiographs per patient-day of mechanical ventilation. Analysis was by intention to treat. This study is registered with ClinicalTrials.gov, number NCT00893672.

Findings.—11 intensive care units were randomly allocated to use a routine strategy to order chest radiographs in the first treatment period, and 10 units to use an on-demand strategy. Overall, 424 patients had 4607 routine chest radiographs (mean per patient-day of mechanical ventilation 1·09, 95% CI 1·05–1·14), and 425 had 3148 on-demand chest radiographs (mean 0·75, 0·67–0·83), which corresponded to a reduction of 32% (95% CI 25–38) with the on-demand strategy ($p<0·0001$).

Interpretation.—Our results strongly support adoption of an on-demand strategy in preference to a routine strategy to decrease use of chest radiographs in mechanically ventilated patients without a reduction in patients' quality of care or safety (Fig 3, Tables 2 and 3).

▶ Chest radiographs are commonly obtained on a daily basis in mechanically ventilated, critically ill patients. This practice is based on the premise that potentially life threatening complications (eg, barotrauma) that might otherwise fail to be diagnosed can be discovered and treated promptly. However, several lines of evidence suggest that on-demand strategy might reduce unnecessary radiation exposure and provide substantial cost savings. Furthermore, very few routine chest radiographs lead to therapeutic or diagnostic interventions. This study was designed to investigate the efficiency and effectiveness of routine versus on-demand chest radiographs for optimum care of mechanically ventilated patients using a prospective two-period cluster-randomized design. Their results demonstrate a substantial reduction in use of chest radiographs with the on-demand strategy, corresponding to a 32% decrease overall

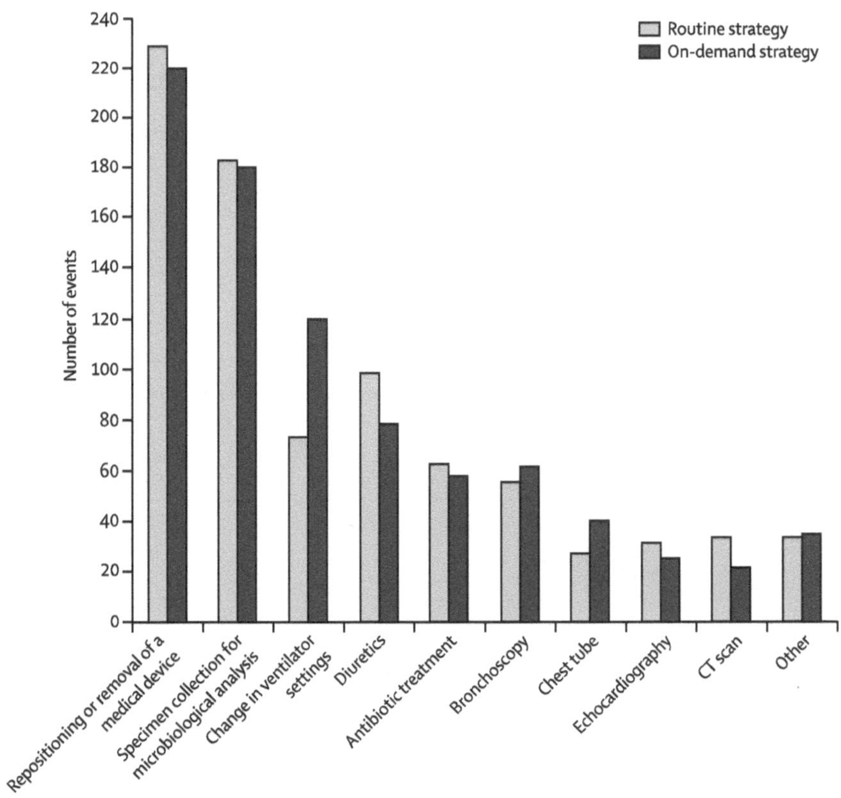

FIGURE 3.—Distribution of diagnostic procedures or therapeutic interventions done after findings from chest radiographs. (Reprinted from Hejblum G, Chalumeau-Lemoine L, Ioos V, et al. Comparison of routine and on-demand prescription of chest radiographs in mechanically ventilated adults: a multicentre, cluster-randomised, two-period crossover study. *Lancet*. 2009,374:1687-1693, with permission from Elsevier Ltd.)

TABLE 2.—Patient Characteristics at Baseline

	Routine Strategy (n = 424)	On-Demand Strategy (n = 425)
Age (years)	61 (51–74)	63 (49–74)
SAPS II score; predicted hospital mortality*	52 (40–66); 51·0%	52 (39–66); 51·6%
Men	257 (61%)	271 (64%)
Reason for starting mechanical ventilation		
Thoracic diseases	171 (40%)	153 (36%)
ARDS or ALI	55 (32%)	46 (30%)
Pneumonia (without ARDS or ALI criteria)	42 (25%)	34 (22%)
Acute respiratory failure with chronic respiratory insufficiency	29 (17%)	47 (31%)
Cardiogenic oedema	14 (8%)	11 (7%)
Acute respiratory failure with immunodeficiency	17 (10%)	6 (4%)
Acute asthma	7 (4%)	1 (1%)
Other	7 (4%)	8 (5%)
Extrathoracic diseases	209 (49%)	228 (54%)
Shock	104 (50%)	106 (46%)
Coma (excluding coma due to intoxication)	64 (31%)	80 (35%)
Coma due to intoxication	34 (16%)	35 (15%)
Other	7 (3%)	7 (3%)
Postoperative care	42 (10%)	41 (10%)
Unknown	2 (1%)	3 (1%)

Data are median (IQR), percentage, or number (%). SAPS II = simplified acute physiology score II. ARDS = acute respiratory distress syndrome. ALI = acute lung injury.

*Percentage derived from the mean of all patients' probabilities of predicted hospital mortality, therefore number of patients is not given.

TABLE 3.—Number of Chest Radiographs, Length of Stay, Duration of Mechanical Ventilation, and Mortality in Intensive Care Units

	Routine Strategy (n = 424)	On-Demand Strategy (n = 425)	p Value
Chest radiographs per patient-day of mechanical ventilation (total number; mean [95% CI])*	4607; 1·09 (1·05–1·14)	3148; 0·75 (0·67–0·83)	<0·0001
Morning rounds†	3779; 0·90 (0·86–0·93)	2224; 0·54 (0·47–0·60)	<0·0001
Unscheduled†	780; 0·18 (0·15–0·22)	893; 0·20 (0·16–0·25)	0·24
Days of mechanical ventilation (total number; mean [SD]; median [IQR])*	4172; 9·82 (8·24); 7 (4–13)	4226; 9·94 (8·75); 7 (3–14)	0·90
Length of stay (days; mean [SD]; median [IQR])	13·96 (11·61); 10 (5–19)	13·21 (11·01); 10 (5–19)	0·28
Mortality	131 (31%)	136 (32%)	0·79

Data are number (%) unless otherwise indicated.

*Data were censored to 30 days of mechanical ventilation; patients with more than 30 days of mechanical ventilation were regarded as having 30 days of mechanical ventilation in all calculations.

†For 48 chest radiographs done for patients on the routine strategy and 31 done for those on the on-demand strategy (p = 0·9), whether the chest radiograph was done during the morning round or was unscheduled was not recorded.

compared with the routine strategy. Their results are similar to 3 previous studies that favored on-demand strategy. The strength of this study is its prospective nature, and the cluster-randomized crossover design accounted for variation between the intensive care units. Although this study did not investigate whether the on-demand strategy was associated with missed findings that resulted in adverse events or delay in treatment, the authors convincingly demonstrated that the on-demand strategy did not change the number of radiographs that lead or contributed to diagnostic or therapeutic interventions, duration of mechanical ventilation, or stay in intensive care unit or mortality.

M. Mathru, MD, FCCP

Dexmedetomidine vs Midazolam for Sedation of Critically Ill Patients: A Randomized Trial

Riker RR, Shehabi Y, Bokesch PM, et al (Univ of Vermont College of Medicine and Maine Med Ctr, Portland, ME; Univ of New South Wales Clinical School, Australia; Hospira Inc, Lake Forest, IL)

JAMA 301:489-499, 2009

Context.—γ-Aminobutyric acid receptor agonist medications are the most commonly used sedatives for intensive care unit (ICU) patients, yet preliminary evidence indicates that the α_2 agonist dexmedetomidine may have distinct advantages.

Objective.—To compare the efficacy and safety of prolonged sedation with dexmedetomidine vs midazolam for mechanically ventilated patients.

Design, Setting, and Patients.—Prospective, double-blind, randomized trial conducted in 68 centers in 5 countries between March 2005 and August 2007 among 375 medical/surgical ICU patients with expected mechanical ventilation for more than 24 hours. Sedation level and delirium were assessed using the Richmond Agitation-Sedation Scale (RASS) and the Confusion Assessment Method for the ICU.

Interventions.—Dexmedetomidine (0.2-1.4 μg/kg per hour [n = 244]) or midazolam (0.02-0.1 mg/kg per hour [n = 122]) titrated to achieve light sedation (RASS scores between −2 and +1) from enrollment until extubation or 30 days.

Main Outcome Measures.—Percentage of time within target RASS range. Secondary end points included prevalence and duration of delirium, use of fentanyl and openlabel midazolam, and nursing assessments. Additional outcomes included duration of mechanical ventilation, ICU length of stay, and adverse events.

Results.—There was no difference in percentage of time within the target RASS range (77.3% for dexmedetomidine group vs 75.1% for midazolam group; difference, 2.2% [95% confidence interval {CI}, −3.2% to 7.5%]; P = .18). The prevalence of delirium during treatment was 54% (n = 132/244) in dexmedetomidinetreated patients vs 76.6% (n = 93/122) in midazolam-treated patients (difference, 22.6% [95% CI, 14% to 33%]; P < .001). Median time to extubation was 1.9 days shorter in dexmedetomidine-treated patients (3.7 days [95% CI, 3.1 to 4.0] vs 5.6 days [95% CI, 4.6 to 5.9]; $P = .01$), and ICU length of stay was similar (5.9 days [95% CI, 5.7 to 7.0] vs 7.6 days [95% CI, 6.7 to 8.6]; $P = .24$). Dexmedetomidinetreated patients were more likely to develop bradycardia (42.2% [103/244] vs 18.9% [23/122]; $P < .001$), with a nonsignificant increase in the proportion requiring treatment (4.9% [12/244] vs 0.8% [1/122]; $P = .07$), but had a lower likelihood of tachycardia (25.4% [62/244] vs 44.3% [54/122]; $P < .001$) or hypertension requiring treatment (18.9% [46/244] vs 29.5% [36/122]; $P = .02$).

Conclusions.—There was no difference between dexmedetomidine and midazolam in time at targeted sedation level in mechanically ventilated ICU patients. At comparable sedation levels, dexmedetomidine-treated patients spent less time on the ventilator, experienced less delirium, and developed less tachycardia and hypertension. The most notable adverse effect of dexmedetomidine was bradycardia.

Trial Registration.—clinicaltrials.gov Identifier: NCT00216190.

▶ I think the conclusion of this multicenter study article says it all—dexmedetomidine is a major advance in our critical care armamentarium—as patients spend less time on the ventilator, experience less delirium, and develop tachycardia and hypertension. I think I should thank Mervin Mays for persistence in bringing this drug to our society. Thanks, Mervin.

M. F. Roizen, MD

8 Other Perioperative Patient Care Issues

Effect of thigh strength on incident radiographic and symptomatic knee osteoarthritis in a longitudinal cohort

Segal NA, Torner JC, Felson D, et al (Univ of Iowa; Boston Univ, MA; et al)
Arthritis Rheum 61:1210-1217, 2009

Objective.—To assess whether knee extensor strength or hamstring:quadriceps (H:Q) ratio predicts risk for incident radiographic tibiofemoral and incident symptomatic whole knee osteoarthritis (OA) in adults ages 50-79 years.

Methods.—We followed 1,617 participants (2,519 knees) who, at the baseline visit of the Multicenter Osteoarthritis (MOST) Study, did not have radiographic tibiofemoral OA and 2,078 participants (3,392 knees) who did not have symptomatic whole knee OA (i.e., did not have the combination of radiographic OA and frequent knee symptoms). Isokinetic strength was measured at baseline, and participants were followed for development of incident radiographic tibiofemoral OA, or incident symptomatic whole knee OA at 30 months. Generalized estimating equations accounted for 2 knees per subject, and multivariable models adjusted for age, body mass index (BMI), hip bone mineral density, knee surgery or pain, and physical activity score.

Results.—In the studies of incident radiographic and incident symptomatic knee OA, mean ± SD ages were 62.4 ± 8.0 years and 62.3 ± 8.0 years, respectively, and mean ± SD BMI scores were 30.6 ± 5.8 kg/m^2 and 30.2 ± 5.5 kg/m^2, respectively. Knee extensor strength and H:Q ratio at baseline significantly differed between men and women. Neither knee extensor strength nor the H:Q ratio was predictive of incident radiographic tibiofemoral OA. Compared with the lowest tertile, the highest tertile of knee extensor strength protected against development of incident symptomatic whole knee OA in both sexes (adjusted odds ratio 0.5-0.6). H:Q ratio was not predictive of incident symptomatic whole knee OA in either sex.

Conclusion.—Thigh muscle strength does not appear to predict incident radiographic OA, but does seem to predict incident symptomatic knee OA.

► Your muscles provide shock absorbers for the knee in preventing osteoarthritis. Why they do it for symptomatic and not for radiographic osteoarthritis is beyond the scope of my knowledge. But what it does mean is that when you are sitting behind the screen not doing anything special, then do some exercises that strengthen your leg muscles, especially your upper leg muscles. Squats are great; you can do them in an OR, or leaning against the wall while you are watching the monitor intently.

M. F. Roizen, MD

Duration and magnitude of the postoperative risk of venous thromboembolism in middle aged women: prospective cohort study

Sweetland S, Green J, Liu B, et al (Univ of Oxford, UK; et al)

BMJ 339:b4583, 2009

Objective.—To examine the duration and magnitude of increased risk of venous thromboembolism after different types of surgery.

Design.—Prospective cohort study (Million Women Study).

Setting.—Questionnaire data from the Million Women Study linked with hospital admission and death records.

Participants.—947 454 middle aged women in the United Kingdom recruited in 1996-2001 and followed by record linkage to routinely collected NHS data on hospital admissions and deaths. During follow-up 239 614 admissions were for surgery; 5419 women were admitted, and a further 270 died, from venous thromboembolism.

Main Outcome Measures.—Adjusted relative risks and standardised incidence rates for hospital admission or death from venous thromboembolism (pulmonary embolism or deep vein thrombosis), by time since and type of surgery.

Results.—Compared with not having surgery, women were 70 times more likely to be admitted with venous thromboembolism in the first six weeks after an inpatient operation (relative risk 69.1, 95% confidence interval 63.1 to 75.6) and 10 times more likely after a day case operation (9.6, 8.0 to 11.5). The risks were lower but still substantially increased 7-12 weeks after surgery (19.6, 16.6 to 23.1 and 5.5, 4.3 to 7.0, respectively). This pattern of risk was similar for pulmonary embolism (n = 2487) and deep venous thrombosis (n = 3529). The postoperative risks of venous thromboembolism varied considerably by surgery type, with highest relative risks after inpatient surgery for hip or knee replacement and for cancer—1-6 weeks after surgery the relative risks were, respectively, 220.6 (187.8 to 259.2) and 91.6 (73.9 to 113.4).

Conclusion.—The risk of deep vein thrombosis and pulmonary embolism after surgery is substantially increased in the first 12 postoperative weeks, and varies considerably by type of surgery. An estimated 1 in 140 middle aged women undergoing inpatient surgery in the UK will be admitted with venous thromboembolism during the 12 weeks after surgery (1 in 45 after hip or knee replacement and 1 in 85 after surgery for cancer), compared with 1 in 815 after day case surgery and only 1 in 6200 women during a 12 week period without surgery.

▶ Increased risk of DVT is present for at least 12 postoperative weeks. An estimated 1 in 140 women undergoing inpatient surgery are admitted for venous thromboembolism in the United Kingdom, and 1 in 815 are admitted after day care surgery compared with only 1 in 6200 women who do not have surgery. What that means is that even in day care surgery we will have a major role in advising patients. We should advise them to resume their aspirin as soon as possible if they are not on other prophylaxis that contraindicates aspirin, and to get walking. Whether those recommendations actually will help the risks return to normal, we don't know.

M. F. Roizen, MD

Depression After Coronary Artery Disease Is Associated With Heart Failure

May HT, Horne BD, Carlquist JF, et al (Intermountain Med Ctr, Murray, UT; et al)

J Am Coll Cardiol 53:1440-1447, 2009

Objectives.—The purpose of this study was to evaluate the influence of post-coronary artery disease (CAD) depression diagnosis on heart failure (HF) incidence.

Background.—Depression has been shown to be a risk factor for poor outcomes among CAD patients. However, little is known about the influence of depression on HF development in CAD patients.

Methods.—Patients ($n = 13{,}708$) without a diagnosis of HF and depression (International Classification of Diseases-Ninth Revision [ICD-9] codes: 296.2 to 296.36 and 311) and who were not prescribed antidepressant medication (ADM) at the time of CAD diagnosis ($\geq$70% stenosis) were studied. For those with available medication records ($n = 7{,}719$), patients subsequently diagnosed with depression were stratified by use of ADM. Patients were followed until HF diagnosis (physician-diagnosed or ICD-9 code: 428) or death. Results were analyzed by Cox proportional hazards regression models.

Results.—A total of 1,377 patients (10.0%) had a post-CAD clinical depression diagnosis. The incidence of HF among those without a post-CAD depression diagnosis was 3.6 per 100 compared with 16.4 per 100 for those with a post-CAD depression diagnosis. Depression was associated with an increased risk for HF incidence (adjusted hazard ratio [HR]: 1.50, $p < 0.0001$). Results were similar among those with available follow-up medication information (vs. no depression: depression without ADM use [HR: 1.68, $p < 0.0001$]; depression with ADM use [HR: 2.00, $p < 0.0001$]). No difference was found between depressed patients with and without ADM treatment (HR: 0.84, $p = 0.24$).

Conclusions.—Depression diagnosis was shown to be associated with an increased incidence of HF after CAD diagnosis, regardless of ADM treatment. This finding suggests the need to further study the effect of depression on HF risk among CAD patients.

▶ There is often a high incidence of depression after coronary bypass procedures and even after vascular procedures. This study showed that there is often subclinical heart failure that accompanies depression, and that heart failure often presents in the years following depression. Postoperatively, the depressed patient is one to worry about for not only this reason, but because of the shortened lifespan and increased disability that patient will have.

M. F. Roizen, MD

Effect of the preliminary hydration on gastric emptying time for water in healthy volunteers

Umenai T, Arai N, Chihara E (Kyoto Prefectural Univ of Medicine, Japan; Meiji Univ of Integrative Medicine, Kyoto, Japan)
Acta Anaesthesiol Scand 53:223-226, 2009

Background.—International guidelines allow healthy patients to drink clear liquid up to 2 h before general anesthesia. Recently, MRI measurements have been used for tracking gastric volume in humans. Hence, we used MRI to examine the gastric emptying rate of water in healthy volunteers with or without prior water loading.

Methods.—Fifteen healthy volunteers were enrolled. The participants had MRI examinations on separate days under two different protocols: The preliminary hydration protocol (group H) and the water restriction protocol (group R). After the intake of water, MR imaging was performed every 10 min for 60 min. The gastric content was outlined as area of interest (AOI), and the AOI area of each slice was summated to calculate the volume of gastric contents.

Results.—The 50% reduction time of gastric volume in group R and group H was 18 ± 9 and 16 ± 8 min (mean ± SD), respectively. There were no significant changes between the two groups.

Conclusion.—The gastric emptying time for water evaluated with MRI was not affected by preliminary hydration, which shows the safety of repeated oral hydrations in the pre-operative period.

▶ When physicians and perioperative nurses tell patients that they may have clear fluids up to 2 hours preoperatively, the intent is not that they drink liquids continuously. In this study, subjects consumed either 4 mL/kg (more than 10 oz for an 80kg person) at 1 and 2 hours before study or nothing for at least 4 hours before study. Based on the results of this study, gastric emptying times are no slower in individuals consuming large amounts of water than those of less-hydrated individuals, and residual gastric volume is no greater in patients who had taken clear water, 4 mL/kg, the hour before the study.

Interestingly, subjects in this study were instructed to have lunch 4 hours before the initial MRI to establish baseline gastric volume. This oral intake is not consistent with the more common recommendation for perioperative consumption of food in many hospitals where patients are instructed to remain NPO for a minimum of 6 hours following a light meal. While the average gastric volume in this study decreased below baseline within 60 minutes of oral intake of water in both groups of study patients—those who were relatively dehydrated before the 4 mL/kg intake of water and those who had consumed 12 mL/kg of water in total—one wonders if it would have been greater or less had the subjects not had lunch 4 hours previously. While that study remains to be done, it seems, based on the results of this study, that ongoing oral hydration with water does not decrease the rate of gastric emptying, and that as long as oral intake of clear liquids is stopped 1 hour preoperatively, the amount consumed, as long as it is less than 8 ml/kg, will not slow gastric emptying. Because gastric volumes return to baseline within 60 minutes of ingestion of water, one wonders how early patients have to stop their P.O. intake. Healthy patients undergoing elective procedures could perhaps have water until 1 hour before their scheduled procedure. More conservative guidelines, though, remain prudent for patients with comorbidities such as gastroesophageal reflux disease, intra-abdominal pathology, opioid administration, and emergent surgery.

C. A. Lien, MD

Effect of preoperative smoking cessation interventions on postoperative complications and smoking cessation

Thomsen T, Tønnesen H, Møller AM (Herlev Univ Hosp, Denmark; Bispebjerg Univ Hosp, Copenhagen, Denmark)

Br J Surg 96:451-461, 2009

Background.—The aim of this study was to examine the effect of preoperative smoking cessation interventions on postoperative complications and smoking cessation itself.

Methods.—Relevant databases were searched for randomized controlled trials (RCTs) of preoperative smoking cessation interventions. Trial inclusion, risk of bias assessment and data extraction were performed by two authors. Risk ratios for the above outcomes were calculated and pooled effects estimated using the fixed-effect method.

Results.—Eleven RCTs were included containing 1194 patients. Smoking interventions were intensive, medium intensity and less intensive. Follow-up for postoperative complications was 30 days. For smoking cessation it was from the day of surgery to 12 months thereafter. Overall, the interventions significantly reduced the occurrence of complications (pooled risk ratio 0·56 (95 per cent confidence interval 0·41 to 0·78); $P < 0 \cdot 001$). Intensive interventions increased smoking cessation rates both before operation and up to 12 months thereafter. The effects of medium to less intensive interventions were not significant. Meta-analysis of the effect on smoking cessation was not done owing to heterogeneity of data.

Conclusion.—Surgical patients may benefit from intensive preoperative smoking cessation interventions. These include individual counselling initiated at least 4 weeks before operation and nicotine replacement therapy.

▶ Not surprisingly, this review of 11 randomized controlled trials describing results in almost 1200 patients found that preoperative interventions in smokers reduced the incidence of smoking-related complications and increased the rate of smoking cessation. Surprisingly though, it was only the patients who received intensive intervention, described as weekly individual counseling by trained specialists for a period of 4 weeks before surgery as well as nicotine replacement therapy, that experienced these benefits. Patients offered less intensive forms of intervention had no reduction in postoperative complications or increase in smoking cessation.

Based on these few trials, effective preoperative management for the patient who smokes requires more than a casual preoperative recommendation to stop smoking. That being said, it is unlikely that anesthesiologists would not, in spite of apparent lack of efficacy, take advantage of the preoperative visit to counsel patients to quit smoking.

Setting up systems to effectively manage cigarette smokers preoperatively would require a concentrated effort by departments and institutions in addition to individuals. While the cost of offering this more effective intervention may seem substantial, the cost of not doing so—in terms of managing postoperative complications and the long-term morbidities associated with ongoing nicotine use—are likely to be considerably greater.

C. A. Lien, MD

Levels of Consciousness During Regional Anesthesia and Monitored Anesthesia Care: Patient Expectations and Experiences

Esaki RK, Mashour GA (Univ of Michigan Med School)

Anesth Analg 108:1560-1563, 2009

Complaints of "intraoperative awareness" after regional anesthesia and monitored anesthesia care have been reported. We hypothesized that this may be due to either unmet expectations regarding levels of consciousness or states of consciousness resembling general anesthesia. A structured interview assessing expected and experienced levels of consciousness was given to 117 patients who underwent regional anesthesia or monitored anesthesia care. Complete unconsciousness was the state most often expected and subjectively experienced. Furthermore, only 58% of patients had expectations set by the anesthesia provider. These data indicate that, from the patient's perspective, the boundary between general and nongeneral anesthesia is obscured.

▶ This study is interesting, in that it found that less than 20% of patients studied expected to be conscious during their surgical procedure with either regional or monitored anesthesia care. This is indicative of a significant degree of patient lack of understanding of the differences between different types of anesthesia and different depths of anesthesia. Sedation, as might be provided during a monitored anesthetic or to accompany a regional anesthetic, can be minimal, moderate, or deep. None guarantees lack of consciousness or awareness during a surgical procedure. This misalignment of patient expectations and what should have been anticipated based on the anesthetic provided occurred in spite of the anesthetic being explained to patients in more than half of the cases studied by an anesthesia care provider. At least 2 factors may have contributed to this. Patients may have wanted to be unaware during the course of their anesthetic regardless of whether or not they had a perfectly functioning regional anesthetic. Additionally, the anesthesia provider explaining the procedure to the patient may not have seen the preoperative visit as an opportunity to educate the patients about the different depths of anesthesia that were likely to be provided as part of their anesthetic.

While the authors did not report patient satisfaction with the intraoperative experience, their results speak to the import of the anesthesiologist's preoperative interaction with the patient. Patient satisfaction is related to their understanding of what will happen in the perioperative period—avoiding unpleasant and unexpected surprises. The preoperative visit is the anesthesiologist's opportunity to speak with patients and educate them about what they can realistically expect during the perioperative period. It also provides an opportunity to allay patients' fears. As found in this study, increased anxiety was a factor leading to a decreased level of consciousness in the operating room. Excessive levels of sedation are more likely to be avoided with appropriate preparation of the patient in the preoperative area.

C. A. Lien, MD

Improved Function From Progressive Strengthening Interventions After Total Knee Arthroplasty: A Randomized Clinical Trial With an Imbedded Prospective Cohort

Petterson SC, Mizner RL, Stevens JE, et al (Univ of Delaware, Newark, NJ; Eastern Washington Univ, Spokane; Health Sciences Ctr and Univ of Colorado at Denver)

Arthritis Rheum 61:174-183, 2009

Objective.—To determine the effectiveness of progressive quadriceps strengthening with or without neuromuscular electrical stimulation (NMES) on quadriceps strength, activation, and functional recovery after total knee arthroplasty (TKA), and to compare progressive strengthening with conventional rehabilitation.

Methods.—A randomized controlled trial was conducted between July 2000 and November 2005 in an academic outpatient physical therapy clinic. Two hundred patients who had undergone primary, unilateral TKA for knee osteoarthritis were randomized to 1 of 2 interventions 4 weeks after surgery, and 41 patients eligible for enrollment who did not participate in the intervention were tested 12 months after surgery (standard of care group). All randomized patients received 6 weeks of outpatient physical therapy 2 or 3 times per week through 1 of 2 intervention protocols: an exercise group (volitional strength training) or an exercise-NMES group (volitional strength training and NMES). Treatment effects were evaluated by a burst superimposition test to assess quadriceps strength and volitional activation 3 and 12 months postoperatively. The Medical Outcomes Study Short Form 36 and Knee Outcome Survey were completed. Knee range of motion, Timed Up and Go, Stair-Climbing Test, and 6-Minute Walk were also measured.

Results.—Strength, activation, and function were similar between the exercise and exercise-NMES groups at 3 and 12 months. The standard of care group was weaker and exhibited worse function at 12 months compared with both treatment groups.

Conclusion.—Progressive quadriceps strengthening with or without NMES enhances clinical improvement after TKA, achieving similar short- and long-term functional recovery and approaching the functional level of healthy older adults. Conventional rehabilitation does not yield similar outcomes.

▶ It is clear from the data on lifestyle changes that involve food, physical activity, and stress management, that whether one looks at diabetics or cardiac patients, or patients with prostate cancer, strengthening after knee replacement, that one thing we as physicians should advocate for, is almost mandatory inclusion of lifestyle programs to help people never get recurrences or get better functional recovery from the surgical procedures they do get. This study is again a great tribute to the benefits of continuing lifestyle treatments after the patient leaves the hospital.

M. F. Roizen, MD

An assessment of the predictors of difficult intubation in patients with acromegaly

Ali Z, Bithal PK, Prabhakar H, et al (All India Inst of Med Sciences, New Delhi, India)

J Clin Neurosci 16:1043-1045, 2009

Various clinical signs have been used for assessing difficult intubation in patients with acromegaly. These signs include the modified Mallampati classification, measurement of thyromental distance and head and neck movements. Some authors have also tried to establish a relationship between growth hormone levels and difficult intubation. We hypothesized that duration of symptoms in patients with acromegaly may have an association with difficult airway and difficult laryngoscopy. In this prospective study we evaluated tests of airway assessment such as: (i) the Mallampati grade; (ii) the thyromental distance; and (iii) the laryngoscopic grade (Cormack-Lehane). The growth hormone levels and the duration of disease symptoms were also examined. Significant correlation was observed between the Cormack-Lehane and Mallampati gradings ($p = 0.05$; $\rho = 19.3\%$), and between the thyromental distance and the duration of the symptoms ($p = 0.03$; $\rho = 26.9\%$). The incidence of Mallampati III and IV grades was higher in patients with acromegaly. Increased thyromental distance was noted in patients with a long duration of disease. However, increased thyromental distance was not associated with difficult laryngoscopy.

► Acromegalic patients are not infrequently difficult to intubate. What is most unsettling within this group of patients is that it is often not possible to anticipate who will be difficult to intubate. This prospective trial in 66 patients confirms that of the measures tested (ie, growth hormone, thyromental distance, Mallampati grade, and duration of symptoms) none was predictive of inability to intubate a patient's trachea. Mallampati grade III or IV correlated positively with a difficult laryngoscopy as determined by Cormack-Lehane classification.

Clinicians will have to continue to assess all aspects of the airway in their acromegalic patients understanding that there is no single predictive factor for a difficult intubation in these patients. Regardless of that assessment, they should anticipate that intubation will be more difficult than expected.

C. A. Lien, MD

Extra Calories Cause Weight Gain–But How Much?

Katan MB, Ludwig DS (VU Univ, Amsterdam, the Netherlands; Children's Hosp, Boston, MA)

JAMA 303:65-66, 2010

How much weight would an individual gain by eating an extra chocolate chip cookie every day for life? One approach to answering this question, frequently used in textbooks and scientific articles, is based on the assumption that a pound (454 g) of fat tissue has about 3500 kilocalories (kcal). Thus, a daily 60-kcal cookie would be expected to produce 0.2 kg (0.5 lb) weight gain in a month, 2.7 kg (6 lb) in a year, 27 kg (60 lb) in a decade, and many hundreds of pounds in a lifetime. This of course does not happen. In this article, the physiology of weight gain and loss

is reviewed, and the amount of reduction of caloric intake necessary to avoid becoming overweight or obese is estimated.

▶ This is actually an eye-opening article by Katan and Ludwig. What it basically says is that as you plan to lose weight (for example, elimination of 3500 calories would help you lose a pound, and you could do so by eliminating roughly 105 calories a day for 30 days of a month), you need to understand what happens to your metabolic rate. After you lost that pound, you then don't have to support that pound with energy so that you plateau and lose less as you go on. In fact, at one point you start to gain weight back; as the amount of calories you drop increases your assentote at a weight that is above where you want to be, because the amount of weight you lost requires you to use less energy to support its metabolic needs. What is really truly remarkable is that this article explains a lot about calorie intake. Since 1983 Americans have eaten 2% more calories a day. Americans ate 20 more calories in 1984, 40 more calories in 1985, 60 more calories in 1986, 88 more calories in 1987, and so forth (start compounding that 2% yearly if you will). Thus, now we are eating some 600 more calories per day than we were in 1983, and in fact from 1858-1983 every year we had been eating roughly the same number of calories (around 1800) and now we are consuming around 2400 calories a day as Americans. That explains why we have gained a little over a pound a year since 1984 (ie, 60-year-olds in the year 2005 weigh about 25 pounds more than 60-year-olds did in the year 1984).

This change in energy balance means not only is it tougher to lose weight, but it is also tougher to gain weight, although you wouldn't know it. Thus, eating 10 calories more per day doesn't add 1 pound a year forever, it adds 1 pound a year until you use up the extra calories that you consume so that eating (roughly what would gain you one pound a year roughly 10 calories more per day than you expend) actually yields a gain of only about 6 pounds over a 25 year period. The take home: we Americans really do have to decrease calorie intake and increase physical activity because it is unlikely that we (Americans in general) will increase physical activity a person by 600 calories a day, which is approximately how much we have to do to get back to our close to ideal weights. I guess we shouldn't be surprised because we have been producing so much extra food that we are seeing larger patients in preoperative clinics in the year 2010 than your predecessor or I saw in the year 1975.

M. F. Roizen, MD

Association Between Dietary Nutrient Composition and the Incidence of Cirrhosis or Liver Cancer in the United States Population

Ioannou GN, Morrow OB, Connole ML, et al (Veterans Affairs Puget Sound Health Care System, Seattle, WA)

Hepatology 50:175-184, 2009

Little is known about the impact of dietary factors on the progression of liver disease. Our aim was to determine whether dietary intake was associated with the risk of cirrhosis-related or liver cancer–related death or hospitalization in the U.S. population. Participants included 9221 persons aged 25-74 years without evidence of cirrhosis at entry into the study or during the first 5 years of follow-up, who were subsequently followed for a mean of 13.3 years as part of the first National Health and Nutrition Examination Survey. Dietary intake was ascertained at baseline using a 24-hour dietary recall questionnaire. During follow-up, 123 of 9221 participants had a diagnosis of cirrhosis (n = 118) or liver cancer (n = 5) in hospitalization records or death certificates, including 36 who were diagnosed only on the basis of death certificates. Participants who reported a diet high in protein were at a higher risk of hospitalization or death due to cirrhosis or liver cancer ($P = 0.001$), whereas those who reported a diet high in carbohydrates were at a lower risk ($P = 0.003$), after adjusting for potential confounders (daily consumption of protein, carbohydrate, fat, tea or coffee, and alcohol, gender, race, age, educational attainment, U.S. geographical region, diabetes, body mass index, and subscapular-to-triceps skinfold ratio). Although total fat consumption was not significantly associated with the risk of cirrhosis or liver cancer, cholesterol consumption was associated with higher risk ($P = 0.007$), whereas serum cholesterol level was not associated with risk of cirrhosis or liver cancer.

Conclusion.—Diet may be an important and potentially modifiable determinant of liver disease.

▶ I clearly knew that extra protein was an important component of kidney disease and something you wanted to avoid if someone had an elevated blood urea nitrogen (BUN) level—and be careful about feeding them high protein concentrates in the ICU or high protein diets afterwards. But I didn't know that was true for progression of liver disease as well. As the incidence of non-alcoholic fatty liver disease is increased from 1% in 1990 to over 35% in 2005, I guess it behooves us to be aware of the nutrients that modify it. Of course the whole thing could largely be avoided if we avoided obesity in the country.

M. F. Roizen, MD

Which Regions of the Operating Gown Should be Considered Most Sterile?

Bible JE, Biswas D, Whang PG, et al (Yale Univ School of Medicine, New Haven, CT)

Clin Orthop Relat Res 467:825-830, 2009

Various guidelines have been proposed regarding which portions of a surgical gown may be considered sterile. Unfortunately, the validity of these recommendations has not been definitively established. We therefore evaluated gown sterility after major spinal surgery to assess the legitimacy of these guidelines. We used sterile culture swabs to obtain samples of gown fronts at 6-inch increments and at the elbow creases of 50 gowns at the end of 29 spinal operations. Another 50 gowns were swabbed immediately after they were applied to serve as negative controls. Bacterial growth was assessed using semiquantitative plating techniques on a nonselective, broad-spectrum media. Contamination was observed at all locations of the gown with rates ranging from 6% to 48%. Compared with the negative controls, the contamination rates were greater at levels 24 inches or less and 48 inches or more relative to the ground and at the elbow creases. The section between the chest and operative field had the lowest contamination rates. Based on these results, we consider the region between the chest and operative field to be the most sterile and any contact with the gown outside this area, including the elbow creases, should be avoided to reduce the risk of infection.

▶ Many guidelines are established with the lack of supporting data. The area of perioperative infection is receiving new attention as efforts are being made to reduce its incidence. To this end, documentation of timely administration of prophylactic antibiotics, maintenance of patient temperature, and wearing of cap, mask, and sterile gowns and gloves with the placement of central lines have become increasingly important. Significant amounts of time are spent teaching new medical students, nurses, and scrub technicians how to scrub for surgery and how to appropriately don gown and gloves. Yet, in the best of circumstances, what portion of the garment is sterile? The Association of periOperative Registered Nurses (AORN) suggests that it is the portion of the gown between the chest and the operating field.[1] Other texts suggest that the sterile area of the gown is below the neckline and axilla and the arms proximal to the elbow crease.[2-4] Bible and colleagues report in this article that more limited areas of the gown can actually be considered sterile and that all areas produce some bacterial growth when swabbed and plated. The greatest bacterial growth occurred from cultures obtained below the level of the operating room (OR) table, above the chest region and the arms from the elbow creases to the axilla. These data imply that even strict aseptic technique does not guarantee that a surgical gown will remain free of bacteria. While these results are very concerning, no study has to date correlated gown infection with perioperative infections. In 2008, these same authors documented contamination of the C-arm drape for intraoperative fluoroscopy.[5] For anyone who has ever worked in an OR with a draped C-arm for fluoroscopy or a draped microscope or a robot, the findings of this study are hardly surprising. In fact, it is more the notion that these routine adjuncts to modern-day surgery should ever be considered sterile after rotating around the operating table, having arms brushed over them or being near the face and then adjusted with sterile operating hands is surprising. The standards for draping of these additional pieces of equipment vary widely from institution to institution and from operating suite to operating suite, indicating that there is no known ideal standard for practice. In some ORs, microscopes are not draped and never touched by someone scrubbed in for surgery unless an additional pair of gloves are donned and then discarded after adjusting the microscope. In others, microscopes and C-arms are draped, and then the person who has placed the drape changes his or her gloves before rejoining the operating team. This study can easily lead one to believe that nothing in the OR is sterile. The significance of any of the contaminants found on surgical gowns and C-arms has not been established. In both studies, the authors recommend limiting exposure to potentially contaminated areas by not allowing elbows to touch the OR table and reducing the number of times the C-arm is brought into the operating field. While this recommendation makes sense based on the data provided, there are no data to indicate that either the incidence or severity of infection is increased based on either the degree of contamination of the surgical gown or the C-arm or the number of times the C-arm is brought into or elbows are near the surgical field. Certainly, use of a sterile gown and gloves are standard for any surgical procedure. However, even the rationale behind standard practices needs to be examined to determine whether improvement is possible.

C. A. Lien, MD

References

1. AORN Recommended Practices Committee. Recommended practices for maintaining a sterile field. *AORN J*. 2006;83:402-404.
2. Boess-Lott R, Stecik S. *The ophthalmic Surgical Assistant*. 1st ed. Thorofare, NJ: Slack Inc; 1999.
3. Spry C. *Essentials of Perioperative Nursing*. 2nd ed. Gaithersburg, MD: Aspen Publishers; 1997.
4. Whalan C. *Assisting at Surgical Operations: A Practical Guide*. Cambridge, UK: Cambridge University Press; 2006.
5. Biswas D, Bible JE, Whang PG, Simpson AK, Grauer JN. Sterility of C-arm fluoroscopy during spinal surgery. *Spine*. 2008;33:1913.

Hypertension is an independent predictor of survival disparity between African-American and white breast cancer patients

Braithwaite D, Tammemagi CM, Moore DH, et al (Univ of California, San Francisco; Brock Univ, Ontario, Canada; et al)

Int J Cancer 124:1213-1219, 2009

The objective of this study was to determine whether comorbidity, or pre-existing conditions, can account for some of the disparity in survival between African-American and white breast cancer patients. A historical cohort study was conducted of 416 African-American and 838 white women diagnosed with breast cancer between 1973 and 1986, and followed through 1999 in the Kaiser Permanente Northern California Medical Care Program. Information on comorbidity, tumor characteristics and breast cancer treatment was obtained from medical records, and Surveillance, Epidemiology and End Results, Northern California Cancer Center Registry. Associations between comorbidity and survival were analyzed with multiple Cox proportional hazards regression. Over a mean follow-up of 9 years, African Americans had higher overall crude mortality than whites: 165 (39.7%) *versus* 279 (33.3%), respectively. When age, race, tumor characteristics and breast cancer treatment were controlled, the presence of hypertension was associated with all cause survival [hazard ratio (HR) = 1.33, 95% confidence intervals (CI) 1.07-1.67] and it accounted for 30% of racial disparity in this outcome. Hypertension-augmented Charlson Comorbidity Index was a significant predictor of survival from all causes (HR = 1.32, 95%CI 1.18-1.49), competing causes (HR = 1.52, 95%CI 1.32-1.76) and breast cancer specific causes (HR = 1.18, 95%CI 1.03-1.35). In conclusion, hypertension has prognostic significance in relation to survival disparity between African-American and white breast cancer patients. If our findings are replicated in contemporary cohorts, it may be necessary to include hypertension in the Charlson Comorbidity Index and other comorbidity measures.

▶ We have never understood why African American women don't survive breast cancer treatment as well as Caucasian women. Maybe 30% of the difference or more is the concomitant greater presence of hypertension in African American women who have breast cancer. It does not appear that the increase in hypertension is caused by the breast cancer treatment, but was just a bystanding effect of it.

M. F. Roizen, MD

Does television viewing predict dietary intake five years later in high school students and young adults?

Barr-Anderson DJ, Larson NI, Nelson MC, et al (Univ of Minnesota, Minneapolis)

Int J Behav Nutr Phys Act 6:7, 2009

Background.—Prior research has found that television viewing is associated with poor diet quality, though little is known about its long-term impact on diet, particularly during adolescence. This study examined the associations between television viewing behavior with dietary intake five years later.

Methods.—Survey data, which included television viewing time and food frequency questionnaires, were analyzed for 564 middle school students (younger cohort) and 1366 high school students (older cohort) who had complete data available at Time 1 (1998–1999) and five years later at Time 2 (mean age at Time 2, 17.2 ± 0.6 and 20.5 ± 0.8 years, respectively). Regression models examined longitudinal associations between Time 1 television viewing behavior and Time 2 dietary intake adjusting for sociodemographic characteristics, Time 1 dietary intake, and Time 2 total daily energy intake.

Results.—Respondents were categorized as limited television users (<2 hours/daily), moderately high television viewers (2–5 hours/daily), and heavy television viewers (≥5 hours/daily). Among the younger cohort, Time 1 heavy television viewers reported lower fruit intake and higher sugar-sweetened beverage consumption than the other two groups. Among the older cohort, watching five or more hours of television per day at Time 1, predicted lower intakes of fruits, vegetables, whole grain and calcium-rich foods, and higher intakes of trans fat, fried foods, fast food menu items, snack products, and sugar-sweetened beverages (products commonly advertised on television) five years later.

Conclusion.—Television viewing in middle and high school predicted poorer dietary intake five years later. Adolescents are primary targets of advertising for fast food restaurants, snack foods, and sugar-sweetened beverages, which may influence their food choices. Television viewing, especially during high school, may have long-term effects on eating choices and contribute to poor eating habits in young adulthood.

▶ I guess this is one easy way to get an indication of how healthy your patients' diet is—just ask them what their average amount of time watching TV is. The problem then is, will they tell you the truth. But clearly, if you watch more than 2 hours of TV your dietary habits are likely to be poor whether you are a middle school student, high school student, or an adult. These 5-hour TV viewers seem to be great targets for fast food restaurants, snack foods, sugar sweetened beverages, and in fact, they predict their own obesity in young and middle age. This article speaks to one of the real reasons why children should not have a TV in their bedroom and should have strict limits on TV time. We always say 5, 4, 3, 2, 1, 0 at the Cleveland Clinic—the 2 relates to less than 2 hours of TV, the 5, of course, is the number of fruits and vegetables you have a day; you will have to log on to our Web site to find out what the other numbers relate to. I can tell you that one of the numbers corresponds with the number of compliments you should give each day.

M. F. Roizen, MD

9 Patient Safety, Complications, and Mishaps in Anesthesia

Is After-Hours Orthopaedic Surgery Associated with Adverse Outcomes? A Prospective Comparative Study

Ricci WM, Gallagher B, Brandt A, et al (Washington Univ School of Medicine, St. Louis, MO; Swedish Med Ctr, Englewood, CO; Med College of Georgia, Augusta; et al)

J Bone Joint Surg Am 91:2067-2072, 2009

Background.—Treatment of fractures is sometimes performed after normal daytime operating hours and in such instances may be performed under less than ideal conditions. The consequence of performing operations under such conditions is largely unknown and was therefore studied in the context of intramedullary nail fixation of tibial and femoral shaft fractures.

Methods.—Two hundred and three consecutive patients with either a femoral or tibial shaft fracture (Orthopaedic Trauma Association classification 32 or 42) treated with intramedullary nail fixation were included in a prospective, multicenter, nonrandomized study. Patients were divided into an after-hours group defined as an operation beginning from 4:00 P.M. to 6:00 A.M. or a daytime group defined as an operation beginning from 6:00 A.M. to 4:00 P.M. These groups were further divided on the basis of the injured bone into the following subgroups: after-hours femoral fracture (fifty-five patients), daytime femoral fracture (forty-four patients), after-hours tibial fracture (forty-eight patients), and daytime tibial fracture (fifty-six patients). The demographic and fracture characteristics were similar among the subgroups. All patients were treated with the same type of femoral antegrade, femoral retrograde, or tibial nail fixation with reaming. Data for fracture-healing, complications, operative time, and fluoroscopy time were collected prospectively.

Results.—The healing rates were similar between daytime and after-hours surgery groups for both the tibial and femoral nailing. On the basis of univariate analysis, operative times were shorter in the after-hours group compared with the daytime group for both the tibial and femoral nail fixation groups ($p < 0.02$), but regression analysis failed to identify time of surgery as an independent variable associated with operative time. Radiation exposure was similar for the after-hours group and the daytime group for both tibial and femoral nail fixation ($p > 0.05$). The after-hours group had more unplanned reoperations than the daytime group ($p < 0.02$). Removal of painful hardware was more frequent in the after-hours femoral fracture group (27%) than in the daytime femoral fracture group (3%) ($p < 0.02$), and after-hours surgery was an independent variable associated with the need for removal of painful femoral fracture hardware ($p < 0.05$).

Conclusions.—Rates of nonunion, infectious complications, and radiation exposure are similar for after-hours and daytime surgery for intramedullary nail fixation of both femoral and tibial fractures. After-hours femoral nail fixation was associated with an increased frequency for removal of painful hardware, which may be related to technical errors associated with nonideal conditions and shorter operative times. An increase in the allocated amount of daytime operative time for orthopaedic trauma surgery has the potential to reduce minor complication rates for intramedullary nail fixation.

▶ Because operating room staffing and fatigue levels differ between day and night-time hours, it was not surprising to find in this study that the incidence of complications was different in patients operated on at different times. Frequently, support staff most familiar with specialized procedures will not work late into the night hours when their particular expertise may not be required as much. Additionally, there is, as noted by the authors, increasing evidence that physicians do not perform optimally when fatigued.[1-4] There is no obvious reason that these same findings would not apply to ancillary personnel.

It would have been interesting had the authors divided the workday into more than 2 portions. Had they looked at procedures done between 12 AM and 6 AM, would the incidence of complications have been significantly higher than in those operations done between 12 noon and 6 PM? Also of interest is the shorter operating time found for those patients with surgeries beginning after 6 PM. The authors do not speculate on why this may have occurred. They state that there was always an attending surgeon present. Might there have been more of a sense of having to rush through the procedure to get it done so that staff could leave for home? The authors report on the frequency of surgery on tibial and femoral fractures during day and night-time hours. However, did the patients having after-hours surgery have greater severity of fractures than those having surgery in the daytime hours? Finally, no mention is made of the distribution of patients between the 3 hospitals. Were the patients studied evenly distributed between the different centers? Was more surgery done in the evening at one or another of the hospitals? Was the complication rate the same at each of the hospitals?

That the incidence of complications in the patients having surgery in the off-hours was not even greater than that reported in this study is somewhat reassuring. Emergencies happen and off-hours surgery is frequently required.

Minimizing the differences in these complication rates is, though, important. As mentioned by the authors, surgeons do not typically work in shifts. Although with increasing limitations of work hours for residents in all subspecialties being suggested by the Accreditation Council for Graduate Medical Education (ACGME), residents may increasingly be required to do so. Potential complications related to this requirement—such as greater frequency of transfer of care and lack of continuity of care–have yet to be quantified. Only through identification and study of the complications associated with extended work hours and their restriction in any medical subspecialty can systems be developed to improve upon them.

C. A. Lien, MD

References

1. Taffinder NJ, McManus IC, Gul Y, Russell RC, Darzi A. Effect of sleep deprivation on surgeons' dexterity on laparoscopy simulator. *Lancet.* 1998;352:1191.
2. Henriques JP, Haasdijk AP, Zijlstra F, Zwolle myocardial infarction study group. Outcome of primary angioplasty for acute myocardial infarction during routine duty hours versus during off-hours. *J Am Coll Cardiol.* 2003;41:2138-2142.
3. Kahol K, Leyba MJ, Deka M, et al. Effect of fatigue on psychomotor and cognitive skills. *Am J Surg.* 2008;195:195-204.
4. Grantcharov TP, Bardram L, Funch-Jensen P, Rosenberg J. Laparoscopic performance after one night on call in a surgical department: prospective study. *BMJ.* 2001;323:1222-1223.

Alarming Levels of Carboxyhemoglobin in Banked Blood

Ehlers M, Labaze G, Hanakova M, et al (Albany Med Ctr, NY)

J Cardiothorac Vasc Anesth 23:336-338, 2009

Objective.—To determine the level of carboxyhemoglobin found in banked blood in the Albany, NY region.

Design.—A retrospective descriptive analysis of carboxyhemoglobin (COHb) levels in a series of packed red blood cell (PRBC) units.

Setting.—The blood bank of a university tertiary care hospital in Albany, NY.

Participants.—All PRBC units considered for possible use in pediatric cardiac surgery were first analyzed for levels of COHb.

Interventions.—Only those units with COHb levels of <1.5% were deemed acceptable for use during pediatric cardiac surgery.

Measurements and Results.—A sample of blood drawn from the sample side arm of each PRBC unit was analyzed on a Chiron 855 Blood Gas Analyzer (Chiron Inc, Emeryville, CA, now Siemens/Bayer RapidLab 865) to determine the level of COHb. The average COHb level was 0.78% (standard deviation ± 1.48%), and out of the 468 units tested, 48 (10.3%) had COHb levels of 1.5% or greater. The highest recorded COHb level was 12%.

Conclusions.—The transfusion of PRBC units may artificially elevate readings of COHb and cause confusion over possible causes. Certain high-risk

populations (eg, cyanotic neonates undergoing cardiopulmonary bypass) may be especially at risk. Although levels of COHb in the US blood supply are dropping, institutions may want to consider analyzing COHb levels in their PRBC units before transfusion in these high-risk populations.

▶ This is 1 of 7 reports of carboxyhemoglobin levels in banked blood since 1980.[1-6] Anyone can have carboxyhemoglobin levels up to 1%, but people who smoke are likely to have higher levels. Blood donors include cigarette smokers and nonsmokers. All published studies have found that banked blood may have elevated levels of carboxyhemoglobin. In one study, 49% of the blood tested had carboxyhemoglobin levels >1.5%.[5] Once blood levels reach 20%, symptoms of organ ischemia, such as seizures, occur.

Consequences of administering carboxyhemoglobin contaminated blood to patients remain to be determined. Its half-life after transfusion is not known, and whether or not carboxyhemoglobin may be beneficial in certain patient populations is debated. Transfusion of large amounts of carboxyhemoglobin contaminated blood to pediatric patients or patients with cyanotic heart disease may put them at additional risk of tissue hypoxia—the very problem clinicians are trying to avoid through transfusion.

The authors of this article checked the levels of carboxyhemoglobin in blood set aside for pediatric heart surgeries over a period of time of more than 1½ years. Interestingly, 10% of the banked blood that was tested had carboxyhemoglobin levels <1.5%. Carboxyhemoglobin levels ranged from 0% to 12%, and the average carboxyhemoglobin concentration any month was <1%. Based on these results, to avoid inadvertently administering blood contaminated with carboxyhemoglobin to patients at risk, units should be checked for it and labeled as they are obtained. There are, though, no national standards for checking for carboxyhemoglobin in banked blood.

Also of interest, over the 19-month period of time over which the units were checked, average carboxyhemoglobin levels per month were decreasing. Whether or not this was reflective of a changing donor population in the area, changing smoking habits, or an ongoing trend is not known but could be useful in determining future handling of blood in at-risk populations.

C. A. Lien, MD

References

1. Ehlers M, McCloskey D, Devejian NS. Alarming levels of carboxyhemoglobin in a unit of banked blood. *Anesth Analg*. 2003;97:289-290.
2. Uchida I, Tashiro C, Koo YH, Mashimo T, Yoshiya I. Carboxyhemoglobin and methemoglobin levels in banked blood. *J Clin Anesth*. 1990;2:86-90.
3. Aker J. Carboxyhemoglobin levels in banked blood: a comparison of cigarette smokers and non-smokers. *AANA J*. 1987;55:421-426.
4. Poulton TJ. Carboxyhemoglobin levels in banked blood. *Chest*. 1985 Mar;87: 408-409.
5. Aronow WS, O'Donohue WJ Jr, Freygang J, Sketch MH. Carboxyhemoglobin levels in banked blood. *Chest*. 1984;85:694-695.
6. Spiess W, Weisshaar D, Vojdanovski B. Carboxyhaemoglobin concentrations in the recipients of banked blood (author's transl) [in German]. *Anasth Intensivther Notfallmed*. 1980;15:486-493.

10 Obstetric Anesthesia

Analgesia for Labor

Neuraxial techniques for labor analgesia should be placed in the lateral position

Tsen LC (Harvard Med School, Boston, MA)

Int J Obstet Anesth 17:146-149, 2008

Many consider spinal and epidural insertion to be an art rather than a science, and believe there are no scientific reasons to favor one technique over another. Maternal position is a case in point, where the mother is commonly placed sitting with the belief that evidence to support a particular maternal position is lacking. However, the scientific literature demonstrates clear advantages of the lateral position. Its use optimizes the overall experience and outcome for all three participants: mother, fetus and anesthesiologist.

▶ This review represents the first half of a pro-con debate regarding the use of the lateral position for administration of neuraxial analgesic/anesthetic techniques in laboring women. The author noted that "for the mother, the lateral position is less physiologically demanding and reduces the need to abandon the technique due to vagal reflexes." Further, the author stated that "the lateral position enables the provision of neuraxial analgesia (and anesthesia) in the event of a cord prolapse, fetal head entrapment, or complex presentation, and may subsequently avoid a general anesthetic." Finally, the author concluded that, for the anesthesiologist, a more comfortable patient, and a reduction in inadvertent vessel cannulation, dural puncture, epidural catheter movement, hypotension and the subsequent use of general anesthesia are all observed. The author's opinions are similar to my own, although I acknowledge that use of the sitting position is often advantageous in obese parturients, and in situations when time is of the essence. In my judgment, anesthesiology trainees should obtain experience in the administration of neuraxial analgesic/anesthetic techniques in both the lateral and the sitting position.

D. H. Chestnut, MD

Neuraxial techniques for labor analgesia should be placed in the lateral position

Polley LS (Univ of Michigan Health System, Ann Arbor)
Int J Obstet Anesth 17:149-152, 2008

In my view, the disadvantages of the lateral position far outweigh any theoretical advantages. My argument is based on the following advantages of the sitting position: the technical ease of insertion, superior patient comfort, possible improved analgesia for combined spinal epidural (CSE), and decreased aortocaval compression.

▶ This review represents the second half of a pro-con debate regarding the use of the lateral (vs sitting) position for administration of neuraxial analgesic/anesthetic techniques in laboring women. The author of this review offers arguments in favor of the use of the sitting position. She noted that "advantages of the sitting position include easy identification of the midline, symmetric distribution of adipose tissue without obscuring the midline, faster insertion times, and fewer difficulties with catheter passage." The author opined that "patient comfort is increased with the sitting position, particularly for overweight women." Further, she noted that "the sitting position enhances distribution of intrathecal hypobaric opioids and decreases the potential for aortocaval compression from the tight fetal curl used with lateral positioning." She acknowledged that "the sitting position may increase the risk of epidural vein puncture, but she stated that there are other available clinical strategies to minimize this complication." I encourage readers to read both of these reviews in order to obtain a balanced perspective on this subject. In my judgment, anesthesiology trainees should obtain experience in the administration of neuraxial analgesic/anesthetic techniques in both the lateral and the sitting position.

D. H. Chestnut, MD

Urinary catheterization in labour with high-dose *vs* mobile epidural analgesia: a randomized controlled trial

Wilson MJA, on behalf of the COMET Study Group (UK) (Royal Hallamshire Hosp, Sheffield, UK; et al)
Br J Anaesth 102:97-103, 2009

Background.—Dense perineal block from epidural analgesia increases the risk of urinary catheterization in labour. Mobile epidurals using low-dose local anaesthetic in combination with opioid preserve maternal mobility and may reduce the risk of bladder dysfunction. We conducted a three-arm randomized controlled trial to compare high-dose epidural pain relief with two mobile epidural techniques.

Methods.—A total of 1054 primparous women were randomized to receive high-dose bupivacaine, epidural analgesia (Control), combined spinal epidural (CSE), or low-dose infusion (LDI). The requirement for urinary catheterization during labour and postpartum was recorded. Both end points were pre-specified secondary trial outcomes. Women were evaluated by postnatal interview, when their bladder function had returned to normal.

Results.—Relative to Control, more women who received mobile epidural techniques maintained the ability to void urine spontaneously at any time (Control 11%, CSE 31% and LDI 32%) and throughout labour (Control 3.7%, CSE 13% and LDI 14%), for both mobile techniques $P<0.01$. There was no difference in the requirement for catheterization after delivery. Women in the CSE group reported a more rapid return of normal voiding sensation, relative to high-dose Control ($P=0.02$).

Conclusions.—Relative to conventional high-dose block, mobile epidural techniques encourage the retention of normal bladder function and reduce the risk of urinary catheterization in labour.

▶ In this study, the authors evaluated the effect of epidural analgesia technique on the requirement for maternal urinary bladder instrumentation both during and after labor; specifically, the authors evaluated this effect as a secondary outcome of a study performed earlier, the Comparative Obstetric Mobile Epidural Trial (COMET).[1] In that study, the authors observed that mobile (ambulatory or low dose) epidural analgesia during labor was associated with a reduction in the incidence of instrumental vaginal delivery, when compared with a traditional high-dose technique. In this secondary analysis, the authors observed that mobile epidural analgesia reduced the risk of urinary catheterization during labor, when compared with a higher dose technique. The results of this study illustrate a fundamental principle, namely, that epidural analgesia during labor is not a generic procedure.

D. H. Chestnut, MD

Reference

1. The COMET Study Group UK. The Comparative Obstetric Mobile Epidural Trial. Effect of low-dose mobile versus traditional epidural techniques on mode of delivery. *Lancet.* 2001;358:19-23.

Ambulation in labour and delivery mode: a randomised controlled trial of high-dose vs mobile epidural analgesia

Wilson MJA, MacArthur C, Cooper GM, et al (Royal Hallamshire Hosp, Sheffield, UK; Univ of Birmingham, UK; et al)
Anaesthesia 64:266-272, 2009

Compared to high-dose epidurals where mobility is impossible, mobile epidurals have been shown to reduce instrumental vaginal delivery rates. The mechanism for this benefit may depend on women walking or adopting upright postures during labour. We investigated maternal motor power and ambulation of 1052 primparous women randomised to high-dose epidural (Control), Combined Spinal Epidural (CSE) or Low-Dose Infusion (LDI) as a pre-specified, secondary outcome of the Comparative Obstetric Mobile Epidural Trial. Modified Bromage power scores and the level of mobility a woman actually achieved were recorded each hour after epidural placement during first and second stage, until delivery. Relative to control, significantly more women maintained normal leg power throughout labour in both mobile groups and significantly more women with CSE maintained superior leg power for longer than with LDI. Observational analysis did not demonstrate an association between the level of ambulation a woman actually achieved after epidural placement and delivery mode.

▶ The previously published Comparative Obstetric Mobile Epidural Trial (COMET) demonstrated a decreased instrumental vaginal delivery rate with either combined spinal-epidural (CSE) or a low-dose epidural infusion, when compared with a "high-dose" epidural technique, in laboring nulliparous women.[1] This article includes the analysis of a predefined secondary outcome of the COMET trial, namely the effect of the 2 "mobile techniques on maternal motor power and ambulation in labour." When compared with the control (high dose) group, significantly more women maintained normal leg power throughout labor in both mobile groups. Further, among the 3 groups, CSE analgesia followed by intermittent epidural bolus injections of low-dose solution appeared to offer the greatest potential for parturients to retain the potential to walk during labor, without compromise of the quality of analgesia. However, the authors observed that "women who attained a greater level of mobility during the first stage in either mobile (low dose) group were no more likely to progress to spontaneous vaginal delivery." Thus, the authors concluded that their data "do not support the assertion that ambulation in the first stage of labor per se has a specific beneficial impact on delivery mode."

D. H. Chestnut, MD

Reference

1. The COMET Study Group UK. The Comparative Obstetric Mobile Epidural Trial: Effect of low-dose mobile versus traditional epidural techniques on mode of delivery. *Lancet*. 2001;358:19-23.

Pregnancy Increases Excitability of Mechanosensitive Afferents Innervating the Uterine Cervix

Liu B, Tong C, Eisenach JC (Wake Forest Univ School of Medicine, Winston-Salem, NC)

Anesthesiology 108:1087-1092, 2008

Background.—Labor pain derives primarily from stimulation of afferents innervating the uterine cervix and lower uterine segment. The authors have previously shown that the excitability of these afferents is regulated by sex hormones and test in this study whether pregnancy also alters their excitability.

Methods.—After animal care committee approval, SpragueDawley rats (nonpregnant, pregnant days 17 and 21) were anesthetized, and two metal rods were placed through the cervix for distension. The right hypogastric nerve was dissected and carefully teased until recording from a single unit was obtained. Spontaneous activity and the response to a graded distension (20–80 g) were recorded for off-line analysis.

Results.—A total of 151 fiber units were recorded. Pregnancy was associated with an increase In spontaneous nerve activity in the absence of a mechanical stimulus (median of 0.98 and 1.56 Hz from pregnant days 17 and 21, respectively, compared with 0.45 Hz in nonpregnant; $P < 0.01$). The proportion of fibers responding to the weakest stimulus (20 g) was significantly greater in pregnant than in nonpregnant animals. The response to graded distension differed significantly among groups, with day 21 > day 17 > nonpregnant.

Conclusions.—Afferents that innervate the uterine cervix sprout into this tissue during late pregnancy, and estrogen increases excitability of these mechanosensitive afferents. Here, the authors show that excitability also increases during pregnancy. These data suggest that, close to the onset of labor, there is an increased input to the spinal cord from cervical distension and an increased depolarization of afferent terminals in the cervix, effects that could influence pain and the progress of labor.

▶ The results of this laboratory animal study complement anatomic studies, suggesting that physiologic changes during late pregnancy enhance pain during labor. This helps explain the clinical observation that "uterine contractions of similar intensity to those in early labor occur in many women throughout pregnancy, but these contractions before late pregnancy are usually painless." The authors speculated that "increased afferent traffic in late pregnancy could contribute to the labor process in addition to increasing pain perception."

D. H. Chestnut, MD

Elevation of Uterine Basal Tone and Fetal Heart Rate Abnormalities After Labor Analgesia: A Randomized Controlled Trial

Abrão KC, Francisco RPV, Miyadahira S, et al (São Paulo Univ, Brazil)
Obstet Gynecol 113:41-47, 2009

Objective.—To estimate the effects of combined spinal–epidural and traditional epidural analgesia on uterine basal tone and its association with the occurrence of fetal heart rate (FHR) abnormalities.

Methods.—Seventy-seven laboring patients who requested pain relief during labor were randomly assigned to combined spinal–epidural ($n = 41$) or epidural analgesia ($n = 36$). Uterine contractions and FHR were recorded 15 minutes before and after analgesia. Uterine tone was evaluated with intrauterine pressure catheter. Primary outcomes were the elevation of baseline uterine tone and occurrence of FHR prolonged decelerations or bradycardia after analgesia. The influence of other variables such as oxytocin use, hypotension, and speed of pain relief were estimated using a logistic regression model.

Results.—The incidence of all outcomes was significantly greater in the combined spinal–epidural group compared with epidural: uterine hypertonus (17 compared with 6; $P = .018$), FHR abnormalities (13 compared with 2; $P < .01$), and both events simultaneously (11 compared with 1; $P < .01$). Logistic regression analysis showed the type of analgesia as the only independent predictor of uterine hypertonus (odds ratio 3.526, 95% confidence interval 1.21–10.36; $P = .022$). For the occurrence of FHR abnormalities, elevation of uterine tone was the independent predictor (odds ratio 18.624, 95% confidence interval 4.46–77.72; $P < .001$). Regression analysis also found a correlation between decrease on pain scores immediately after analgesia and the estimated probability of occurrence of hypertonus and FHR abnormalities.

Conclusion.—Combined spinal–epidural analgesia is associated with a significantly greater incidence of FHR abnormalities related to uterine hypertonus compared with epidural analgesia. The faster the pain relief after analgesia, the higher the probability of uterine hypertonus and FHR changes.

Clinical Trial Registration.—Umin Clinical Trials Registry, http://www.umin.ac.jp/ctr/index.htm, UMIN000001186.

Level of Evidence.—I.

▶ In this study an intrauterine pressure catheter was used to assess uterine tone in all study subjects, and cardiographic records were evaluated by 2 maternal-fetal medicine physicians who were blinded to the group assignment. The investigators observed a transient elevation of uterine tone in almost half of the patients in the combined spinal-epidural (CSE) group, and among those 17 patients, 11 (65%) had fetal heart rate (FHR) abnormalities during the first 15 minutes after intrathecal injection of bupivacaine with sufentanil. Thus, the authors concluded that these observations support the conclusions of others, namely that the rapid onset of intrapartum intrathecal analgesia likely causes an abrupt decline in circulating concentrations of catecholamines, especially epinephrine. This predisposes to an increase in uterine tone, which in turn predisposes to FHR abnormalities, including prolonged decelerations and bradycardia. The authors recommended that all women receiving CSE analgesia during labor "should be carefully monitored" during the first 30 minutes after intrathecal injection of analgesic drugs.

D. H. Chestnut, MD

Early Compared With Late Neuraxial Analgesia in Nulliparous Labor Induction: A Randomized Controlled Trial

Wong CA, McCarthy RJ, Sullivan JT, et al (The Northwestern Univ Feinberg School of Medicine, Chicago, IL)

Obstet Gynecol 113:1066-1074, 2009

Objective.—To determine whether early initiation of neuraxial analgesia (anesthetic[s] placed around the nerves of the central nervous system) compared with systemic opioid analgesia, followed later in labor by epidural analgesia, increases the rate of cesarean delivery in nulliparas undergoing induction of labor.

Methods.—Nulliparas undergoing induction of labor who requested analgesia when cervical dilation was less than 4 cm participated in the study. Patients were randomized to neuraxial (early) or systemic opioid (late) analgesia at the first analgesia request. Patient-controlled epidural analgesia was initiated in the early group at the second analgesia request and in the late group at cervical dilation of 4 cm or greater or at the third analgesia request. The primary outcome was the rate of cesarean delivery.

Results.—The rate of cesarean delivery was not different between groups (neuraxial [early] 32.7% compared with systemic [late] 31.5%, 95% confidence interval of the difference −3% to 6%, $P = .65$). A sample size of 30,500 would be required to detect a difference at the observed rate. There were no differences in the mode of vaginal delivery or Apgar scores. Pain scores were significantly lower (median 1 compared with 5 on a 0–10 scale, $P < .001$) and labor duration shorter (median 528 minutes compared with 569 minutes, $P = .047$) in the early group. The incidence of reassuring fetal heart rate tracings after analgesia was not different between groups.

Conclusion.—Early-labor neuraxial analgesia does not increase the cesarean delivery rate compared with late epidural analgesia in nulliparas undergoing induction of labor.

▶ This study complements the authors' earlier study in which they observed that there was no difference in the rate of cesarean delivery in nulliparous women in spontaneous labor who were randomly assigned to receive early-labor neuraxial analgesia when compared with similar women randomly assigned to receive early-labor systemic opioid analgesia followed later by neuraxial analgesia.[1] Likewise, both of these authors' studies complement similar studies that we performed at the University of Iowa over a decade ago, in which we observed that there was no difference in the cesarean delivery rate among nulliparous women in either spontaneous labor or who were undergoing oxytocin induction of labor, who were randomly assigned to receive early-labor epidural analgesia when compared with similar women who received early-labor systemic opioid analgesia followed later by epidural analgesia.[2,3]

D. H. Chestnut, MD

References

1. Wong CA, Scavone BM, Peaceman AM, et al. The risk of cesarean delivery with neuraxial analgesia given early versus late in labor. *N Engl J Med.* 2005;352: 655-665.
2. Chestnut DH, Vincent RD, McGrath JM, et al. Does early administration of epidural analgesia affect obstetric outcome in nulliparous women who are in spontaneous labor? *Anesthesiology.* 1994;80:1201-1208.
3. Chestnut DH, Vincent RD, McGrath JM, Choi WW, Bates JN. Does early administration of epidural analgesia affect obstetric outcome in nulliparous women who are receiving intravenous oxytocin? *Anesthesiology.* 1994;80:1193-1200.

Success of Spinal and Epidural Labor Analgesia: Comparison of Loss of Resistance Technique Using Air versus Saline in Combined Spinal-Epidural Labor Analgesia Technique

Grondin LS, Nelson K, Ross V, et al (Univ of Vermont/Fletcher Allen Health Care, Burlington, VT; Wake Forest Univ School of Medicine, Winston-Salem, NC)

Anesthesiology 111:165-172, 2009

Background.—Comparison of air *versus* saline for loss of resistance technique (LORT) in combined spinal epidural labor analgesia (CSE) has not been evaluated, and neither has the relation between CSE characteristics (the presence/absence of initial spontaneous clear fluid return or upon aspiration) and spinal/epidural analgesia outcomes. The authors hypothesized that there is no difference in the spinal analgesia success or epidural catheter efficacy between using air *versus* saline LORT for CSE.

Methods.—A total of 360 patients were randomized to air or saline LORT for CSE. Primary outcome was spinal analgesia success as defined by verbal pain score of no more than 3 at 15 min after spinal dose administration. Secondary outcomes were CSE characteristics, catheter replacement, and average hourly epidural drug consumption.

Results.—Results from 345 patients were analyzed. Spinal analgesia success, epidural catheter replacement, and drug consumption were not different between using air or saline LORT and were also independent of the presence/absence of fluid return on aspiration if initial spontaneous fluid returned to the spinal needle. However, epidural catheters inserted in absence of initial fluid return had a significantly higher catheter replacement rate (28.6%) than the 4.1% among those with initial fluid return ($P < 0.03$).

Conclusions.—Spinal analgesia success rate and epidural efficacy are independent of whether air or saline is used for LORT during CSE. Practice of aspiration for fluid after observing initial fluid return may be unnecessary because this practice does not alter spinal/epidural analgesia outcomes. However, epidural catheters inserted with the absence of initial fluid returned to spinal needle may pose a high failure risk.

▶ For many years I used air—or a combination of saline and air—for the loss of resistance technique (LORT) in the identification of the epidural space for administration of "traditional" epidural analgesia. I converted to the use of the saline LORT after reading reports of a higher incidence of unblocked segments (and less effective epidural analgesia) following the use of the air LORT. Another potential disadvantage of the air LORT is the potential risk of pneumocephalus and early onset headache in patients who experience unintentional dural puncture. However, some anesthesiologists have continued to advocate the use of the air LORT during administration of combined spinal epidural (CSE) labor analgesia, claiming that the use of the saline LORT might "cause 'confusion' with cerebrospinal fluid (CSF) or dural tenting during the needle-through-needle CSE technique and ... result in spinal analgesia failure." However, in this study, the authors noted that "given the very similar success rate of spinal analgesia and epidural efficacy between [the] Air and Saline groups, it is evident that 3 mL of saline injected epidurally did not seem to cause misidentification of spinal fluid return from [the] intrathecal space when [the] spinal needle was inserted during a CSE procedure." The authors also noted that "the absence of initial spontaneous fluid return after insertion of [the] spinal needle in a CSE procedure may potentially indicate a high risk of failure [if] the epidural catheter [is] inserted without repeating the epidural procedure," and they suggested that the epidural space should be reidentified at a different angle or interspace in such situations.

D. H. Chestnut, MD

Second-stage labor duration in nulliparous women: relationship to maternal and perinatal outcomes

Rouse DJ, for the *Eunice Kennedy Shriver* National Institute of Child Health and Human Development Maternal-Fetal Medicine Units Network (Univ of Alabama at Birmingham; et al)

Am J Obstet Gynecol 201:357.e1-7, 2009

Objective.—The purpose of this study was to assess maternal and perinatal outcomes as a function of second-stage labor duration.

Study Design.—We assessed outcomes in nulliparous laboring women who were enrolled in a trial of fetal pulse oximetry.

Results.—Of 5341 participants, 4126 women reached the second stage of labor. As the duration of the second stage increased, spontaneous vaginal delivery rates declined, from 85% when the duration was <1 hour to 9% when it was ≥5 hours. Adverse maternal outcomes that were associated significantly with the duration of the second stage of labor included chorioamnionitis (overall rate, 3.9%), third- or fourth-degree perineal laceration (overall rate, 8.7%), and uterine atony (overall rate, 3.9%). Odds ratios for each additional hour of the second stage of labor ranged from 1.3–1.8. Among individual adverse neonatal outcomes, only admission to a neonatal intensive care unit was associated significantly with second stage duration (odds ratio, 1.4).

Conclusion.—The second stage of labor does not need to be terminated for duration alone.

▶ This study represents a secondary analysis of a clinical trial of fetal pulse oximetry at 14 academic health centers that are members of the highly respected National Institute of Child Health and Human Development Maternal Fetal Medicine Units Network. Of interest, 95% of women in the study cohort received epidural analgesia. The authors concluded that "the duration of the second stage of labor is associated principally with adverse maternal as opposed to adverse neonatal outcomes." Further, they concluded that "extending the duration of the second stage of labor will allow some women to achieve vaginal delivery successfully, even those few women in whom the second stage has lasted 5 hours. These vaginal deliveries, however, have a cost that includes higher rates of significant perineal trauma, infectious morbidity, and uterine atony." In my judgment, obstetric anesthesia providers should strive to provide effective analgesia—but not total anesthesia—during the second stage of labor.

D. H. Chestnut, MD

When to stop pushing: effects of duration of second-stage expulsion efforts on maternal and neonatal outcomes in nulliparous women with epidural analgesia

Le Ray C, Audibert F, Goffinet F, et al (Univ of Montréal, QC, Canada; Université Paris-Descartes, France)

Am J Obstet Gynecol 201:361.e1-361.e7, 2009

Objective.—The purpose of this study was to assess the influence of the duration of active second-stage labor on maternal and neonatal outcomes.

Study Design.—Secondary analysis of the Pushing Early Or Pushing Late with Epidural trial that included 1862 nulliparous women with epidural analgesia who were in the second stage of labor. According to duration of active second-stage labor, we estimated the proportion of spontaneous vaginal deliveries (SVD) with a newborn infant without signs of asphyxia (5-minute Apgar score ≥7 and arterial pH > 7.10). We also analyzed maternal and neonatal outcomes according to the duration of expulsive efforts.

Results.—Relative to the first hour of expulsive efforts, the chances of a SVD of a newborn infant without signs of asphyxia decreased significantly every hour (1- to 2-hour adjusted odds ratio, 0.4; 95% confidence interval [CI], 0.3–0.6; 2- to 3-hour adjusted odds ratio, 0.1; 95% CI, 0.09–0.2; >3-hour adjusted odds ratio, 0.03; 95% CI, 0.02–0.05). The risk of postpartum hemorrhage and intrapartum fever increased significantly after 2 hours of pushing.

Conclusion.—Faced with a decreasing probability of SVD and increased maternal risk of morbidity after 2 hours, we raise the question as to whether expulsive efforts should be continued after this time.

▶ This represents a secondary analysis of the Pushing Early Or Pushing Late with Epidural (PEOPLE) trial.[1] The results suggest that "in the context of continuous fetal surveillance during the second stage of labor, a prolonged second stage does not increase the risk of adverse neonatal outcome." However, after 2 hours of pushing, the risk of maternal intrapartum fever and postpartum hemorrhage increased significantly.

D. H. Chestnut, MD

Reference

1. Fraser WD, Marcoux S, Krauss I, Douglas J, Goulet C, Boulvain M. Multicenter, randomized, controlled trial of delayed pushing for nulliparous women in the second stage of labor with continuous epidural analgesia: the PEOPLE (Pushing Early or Pushing Late with Epidural) Study Group. *Am J Obstet Gynecol*. 2000; 182:1165-1172.

Epidural Analgesia in the Latent Phase of Labor and the Risk of Cesarean Delivery: A Five-Year Randomized Controlled Trial

Wang F, Shen XF, Guo XR, et al (Nanjing Med Univ, China)

Anesthesiology 111:871-880, 2009

Background.—The optimal timing of epidural analgesia has been a controversial issue, and how early women can benefit from epidural analgesia is still debated. The objective of this trial was to test the hypothesis that patient-controlled epidural analgesia given at cervical dilation of 1.0 cm or more does not increase the risk of prolonged labor or Cesarean delivery.

Methods.—After institutional review board approval and patient consent, 12,793 nulliparous patients requesting neuraxial analgesia were enrolled and randomized to an early epidural (cervical dilation at least 1.0 cm) or delayed epidural (cervical dilation at least 4.0 cm) group. A 15-ml epidural analgesic mixture consisting of 0.125% (1.25 mg/ml) ropivacaine plus 0.3 μg/ml sufentanil was given in a single bolus, followed by patient-controlled pump with a 10-ml bolus without background infusion. Repeatable meperidine (25 mg) was prescribed as being the rescue analgesic to patients in the delayed epidural group. The primary outcome was the rate of Cesarean section.

Results.—The median diameters of cervical dilation were 1.6 cm and 5.1 cm in the early and delayed epidural groups, respectively ($P < 0.0001$). The duration of labor from analgesia request to vaginal delivery was equal in both groups (11.3 ± 4.5 h for early epidural and

TABLE 2.—Major Maternal Outcomes after Epidural Analgesia*

Outcomes	Latent Phase Analgesia (n = 6,394)	Active Phase Analgesia (n = 6,399)	*P* Value
Method of delivery			
Cesarean, n (%, 95% CI)	1,486 (23.2, 18.7–24.5)	1,456 (22.8, 18.7–24.9)	0.51
Instrument-assisted vaginal, n (%, 95% CI)†	753 (11.8, 10.5–14.2)	814 (12.7, 10.3–13.5)	0.10
Indications for cesarean‡			
Arrest of dilation, n (%)	979 (65.9)	935 (64.2)	0.34
Arrest of descent, n (%)	214 (14.4)	205 (14.1)	0.80
Other fetal status, n (%)	293 (19.7)	316 (21.7)	0.18
Other outcomes			
Average cervical dilation before epidural placement, cm			< 0.0001
Median	1.6	5.1	
IQR	1.1–2.8	4.2–5.7	
Length of labor (from analgesia request to vaginal delivery), h§	11.3 ± 4.5	11.8 ± 4.9	0.90
Duration of first stage, min			
Latent phase	479 ± 52	485 ± 58	0.22
Active phase	111 ± 44	128 ± 50	0.68
Duration of second stage, min	63 ± 35	67 ± 36	0.87
Average VAS pain ratings (0 – 100 'mm)‖			
First stage of labor			
Latent phase			0.18#
Median	32	48	
IQR	26–40	33–65	
Active phase			0.80#
Median	28	25	
IQR	20–40	20–45	
Second stage of labor			0.46#
Median	22	20	
IQR	12–36	15–40	
Use of oxytocin after analgesia, n (%)	1,492 (23.3)	1,518 (23.7)	0.60
Meperidine consumption, mg	50 ± 25	75 ± 50	0.48
Maximal oxytocin dose, mU/min			0.07#
Median	15	13	
IQR	10–23	9–20	
Duration of epidural analgesia, h			0.02#
Median	12.6	4.8	
IQR	9.7–17.5	3.1–6.4	
Highest sensory block	T8 (T6–T9)	T8 (T6–T9)	1.0#
Oral temperature during labor, °C	37.4 ± 0.4	37.2 ± 0.3	0.52
Breastfeeding success at 6 weeks, n (%)	4,485 (70.1)	4,977 (77.8)	< 0.0001

(Continued)

TABLE 2. (*continued*)

Outcomes	Latent Phase Analgesia (n = 6,394)	Active Phase Analgesia (n = 6,399)	*P* Value
Maternal overall satisfaction score with analgesia (VAS, 0 – 100 mm)			0.01[#]
Median	84	62	
IQR	65–95	50–75	

VAS = Visual Analog Scale; IQR = interquartile range.
[*]Plus-minus values are means ± standard deviation (SD);
[†]The percentage was calculated with the number of subjects need instrumental delivery to the total number of participants precluded to the Cesarean-delivered ones;
[‡]The percentage was calculated with the number of subjects indicating to need Cesarean section to the total number of participants had Cesarean delivery;
[§]the length of labor indicates the time period from the onset of regular uterine contraction to the time after delivery of placenta;
[||]the VAS system of pain or satisfaction rating with analgesia is a 0- to 100-mm linear gauge in which 0 indicates no pain or dissatisfaction with analgesia and 100 indicates worst pain imaginable or very satisfactory with analgesia;
[#]non-normally distributed data were presented as the medians and interquartile ranges, and corresponding *P* values were calculated with the Mann-Whitney U test. If not indicated, the *P* values were calculated by the chi-square test for categorical data.

11.8 ± 4.9 h for delayed epidural group women, $P = 0.90$). No statistically significant difference in the rate of Cesarean section was observed between the two groups on the intention-to-treat analysis (23.2% *vs.* 22.8% in the early and delayed epidural groups, respectively; $P = 0.51$).

Conclusions.—Epidural analgesia in the latent phase of labor at cervical dilation of 1.0 cm or more does not prolong the progression of labor and does not increase the rate of Cesarean in nulliparous women compared with the delayed analgesia at the cervical dilation of 4.0 cm or more (Table 2).

▶ In this study the primary outcome measure (ie, the cesarean delivery rate) did not differ between the 2 groups (Table 2). In addition, early epidural analgesia did not prolong labor or increase the rate of instrumental vaginal delivery when compared with early intramuscular meperidine followed by delayed epidural analgesia. This article was accompanied by an excellent editorial by Flood.[1] Dr Flood noted that this is the largest randomized controlled trial of intrapartum epidural analgesia ever conducted in a single medical center. Dr Flood also called attention to the strengths and weaknesses of "gargantuan studies" such as this one. The authors measured 29 secondary outcomes, and Flood noted that "a trial this large may detect relatively small differences in secondary outcomes that are clinically trivial or even spurious."[1] For example, in this study, early epidural analgesia was associated with less success with breastfeeding, although the difference between groups was small (ie, 70% success in the early epidural group vs 78% success in the late epidural group). Flood noted that "the physiologic mechanism for breastfeeding problems caused by the difference between 4.8h and 12.6 h of exposure to epidural ropivacaine and sufentanil is difficult to imagine," and she concluded that "this finding should be considered a novel hypothesis... that requires further follow-up as a primary endpoint in a subsequent randomized controlled trial." Another odd secondary finding was the absence of a significant difference in pain scores between groups, despite the fact that maternal satisfaction was significantly higher in the early epidural group. Perhaps the higher satisfaction scores in the early epidural group reflected the decreased incidence of nausea and vomiting in that group, but it remains puzzling that the authors did not detect a significant difference in pain scores between groups. Nonetheless, this study provides additional evidence that early administration of epidural analgesia does not prolong labor or increase the risk of operative delivery in nulliparous women.

D. H. Chestnut, MD

Reference

1. Flood P. Primary versus secondary outcomes in gargantuan studies. *Anesthesiology.* 2009;111:704-705.

A comparison of paracervical block with single-shot spinal for labour analgesia in multiparous women: a randomised controlled trial

Junttila EK, Karjalainen PK, Ohtonen PP, et al (Oulu Univ Hosp, Finland)
Int J Obstet Anesth 18:15-21, 2009

Background.—Epidural and spinal analgesia may be contraindicated or unavailable in labour. This randomised controlled study examined the suitability of paracervical block as an alternative method of labour analgesia.

Methods.—Multiparous women in labour were randomised to receive either paracervical block or single-shot spinal analgesia. Pain was quantified using a numerical rating scale. Subsequent analgesia, progress of labour, and mode of delivery were noted. Fetal heart rate patterns were reviewed. Apgar scores and umbilical artery pH measurements were collected. Parturients' satisfaction and willingness to have the same method of labour analgesia again were recorded.

Results.—122 parturients were randomised with data available on 104. Median pain scores decreased significantly in both groups; this was greater with single-shot spinal analgesia (difference between means 2.7; 95% CI 1.9-3.5; $P_g < 0.001$). Parturients receiving paracervical block received subsequent analgesia more often (23/56 vs. 3/48, $P < 0.001$). Progress of labour, instrumental delivery rates, detected abnormal decelerations in cardiotocography and neonatal outcome were similar between groups. Shivering ($P < 0.04$) and pruritus ($P < 0.001$) were more common with single-shot spinal analgesia. Parturients in the paracervical block group were less satisfied (median 7.0, IQR 3.0–8.0 vs. median 9.0, IQR 8.0–10.0; $P < 0.001$) and less willing (28/55 vs. 39/48, $P = 0.002$) to have the same labour analgesia again.

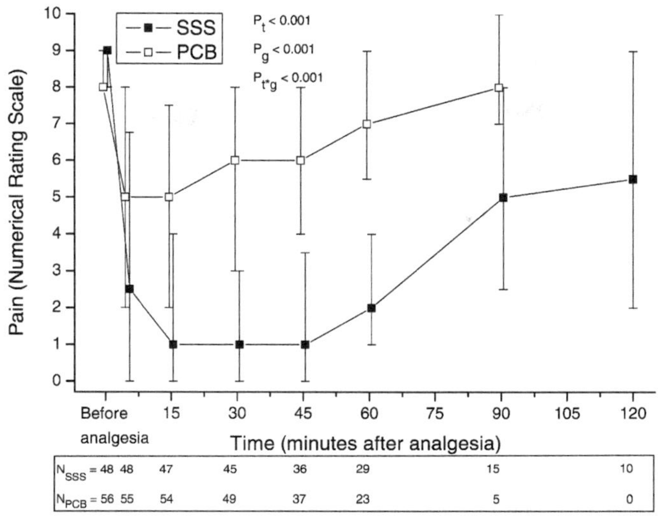

FIGURE 2.—Pain during the study period. Data are median with the 25th–75th percentiles. PCB: paracervical blockade; SSS: single-shot spinal analgesia. Pt = P-time; P_g = P-groups; P_{t*g} = P-time* group. N: number of parturients at the measurement time points. (Reprinted from Junttila EK, Karjalainen PK, Ohtonen PP, et al. A comparison of paracervical block with single-shot spinal for labour analgesia in multiparous women: a randomised controlled trial. *Int J Obstet Anesth.* 2009;18:15-21, with permission from Elsevier Ltd.)

TABLE 2.—Delivery, New Analgesia and Pathological FHR Changes in 90 Minutes After Analgesia

	PCB (n = 56)	SSS (n = 48)	*P*
Delivery within 90 min	28 (50)	29 (60)	0.33
New analgesia within 90 min	21 (38)	2 (4)	<0.001
Abnormal decelerations	4 (7)	4 (8)	>0.9
Late decelerations	1 (2)	3 (6)	0.33
Single prolonged deceleration	3 (5)	1 (2)	0.62
Atypical variable deceleration	0	0	ND

Data are n (%); FHR: fetal heart rate; PCB: paracervical blockade; SSS: single-shot spinal analgesia; ND: not definable.

Conclusions.—Paracervical block was less effective than single-shot spinal analgesia. Both methods were associated with a low incidence of fetal bradycardia but maternal side effects were more common with single-shot spinal analgesia (Fig 2 and Table 2).

▶ In the United States, the use of paracervical block during labor has declined precipitously during the last 3 decades. This decline in the popularity of paracervical block has resulted from both the fear of fetal complications (eg, fetal bradycardia), and the increased popularity and use of neuraxial analgesic techniques. Meanwhile, paracervical block has remained a commonly used intrapartum analgesic technique in Scandinavian countries. The authors of this report noted that in 2004-2005, 17.1% of parturients in Finland received paracervical block during labor, and in 2004, 26.7% of parturients in the authors' labor and delivery unit received paracervical block (compared with 33.7% who received epidural analgesia, and 15.8% who received single-shot spinal analgesia). In this study, paracervical block significantly decreased pain scores, but it was signicantly less effective than single-shot spinal analgesia (Fig 2). Some 27% of women in the paracervical block group received additional analgesia within 1 hour of the performance of paracervical block. Of interest, there were no cases of fetal bradycardia in either group, and there was no difference between groups in the occurrence of abnormal fetal heart rate patterns (Table 2). It is difficult for me to offer enthusiasm for the performance of paracervical block in contemporary obstetric practice in the United States. However, there likely remain some circumstances in which paracervical block is an appropriate intrapartum technique, and careful attention to safety is important.

D. H. Chestnut, MD

Inadequate pain relief with labor epidurals: a multivariate analysis of associated factors

Agaram R, Douglas MJ, McTaggart RA, et al (B C Women's Hosp, Vancouver, Canada)

Int J Obstet Anesth 18:10-14, 2009

Background.—Labor epidural analgesia providing inadequate pain relief may cause maternal dissatisfaction and may fail to produce effective anesthesia when topped up for operative delivery. This study looked at factors associated with inadequate labor epidural analgesia.

Methods.—Data were prospectively collected from 275 parturients receiving labor epidural analgesia. Pain was assessed 30 min after epidural insertion using a verbal pain scale of 0 to 100. A score of 10 or more was considered to represent inadequate pain relief. Sixteen factors chosen by experienced obstetric anesthesiologists for their association with inadequate labor epidural analgesia were studied.

Results.—Fifteen parturients were excluded. Forty-four of the remainder (16.9%) experienced inadequate pain relief. Multiparity, history of a previous failure of epidural analgesia, the use of air for loss of resistance, cervical dilatation >7 cm at insertion all had a statistically significant association with inadequate epidural analgesia ($P < 0.05$). Logistic regression showed that cervical dilatation >7 cm, a history of opioid tolerance, a previous failed epidural and insertion of the epidural by a trainee anesthesiologist increased the odds ratio for inadequate pain relief.

Conclusions.—The final model correctly classified 93% of the epidurals that provided effective analgesia but classified only 9.3% of those providing inadequate pain relief. This information can be used to develop a predictive score and change practice resulting in fewer inadequate epidurals.

► Readers may be surprised by the high number (16.9%) of parturients who experienced "inadequate" pain relief in this study. However, the authors defined "inadequate" analgesia as a verbal pain score of 10 or more (on a scale of 0-100) at 30 minutes after insertion of the epidural catheter. In my experience with the use of pain scores in laboring women this is a strict definition, and I expect that the authors may have overestimated their true incidence of "inadequate" epidural analgesia. Nonetheless, this study suggests that in "real-life situations," inadequate intrapartum epidural analgesia may occur more often than heretofore reported.

D. H. Chestnut, MD

Chronobiology of parturients receiving neuraxial labour analgesia with ropivacaine and fentanyl: a prospective cohort study

Desai S, Leong SB, Yvonne L, et al (KK Women and Children's Hosp, Singapore)

Int J Obstet Anesth 18:43-47, 2009

Background.—The circadian variation in biologic rhythm has been known to affect labour pain. The duration of action of ropivacaine or fentanyl used in treatment of labour pain has been demonstrated to vary with different times of the day. The aim of this study is to find whether the need for epidural supplementation for breakthrough pain is significantly affected by the time of day, in patients who are on a continuous epidural infusion of these drugs.

Methods.—In this prospective cohort study, parturients with spontaneous onset of labour were given a combined spinal-epidural technique with spinal ropivacaine 2 mg + fentanyl 15 μg followed by an epidural infusion of ropivacaine 0.1–0.125% with fentanyl 2 μg/mL at 10 mL/hour. A total of 1657 patients were divided into four groups: (1) morning: analgesia request: 7:01 to 13:00, delivery before 19:00; (2) afternoon: analgesia request: 13:01 to 19:00, delivery before 1:00; (3) evening: analgesia request: 19:01 to 1:00, delivery before 7:00 and (4) night: analgesia request: 1:00 to 7:00, delivery before 13:00. Pain scores before epidural analgesia, need for additional epidural supplementation, side effects and patient satisfaction scores were compared between the groups.

Results.—The pain scores before epidural analgesia were significantly higher in evening and night groups than in morning and afternoon groups (6.95 ± 2.4, 7.38 ± 2.2 compared to 6.67 ± 2.5, 6.49 ± 2.7 respectively,

$P < 0.001$). Incidence of breakthrough pain, side effects and parturient satisfaction scores were not significantly different between groups.

Conclusion.—Parturients with labour onset and neuraxial analgesia request in the evening and night experienced higher pain scores. However, no significant differences in the incidence of breakthrough pain or the quality of analgesia were observed with the provision of commonly used concentrations of ropivacaine with fentanyl via continuous epidural infusion.

▶ The authors cited published evidence regarding the chronobiology of intrapartum pain and analgesia. They suggested 2 reasons why the number of breakthrough pain episodes did not differ between groups, despite higher pain scores in the evening and night groups. First, the initiation of a continuous epidural infusion immediately after the initial spinal dose may have obscured the chronobiologic effect. Second, the dose regimen used in this study may have provided "more than adequate analgesia irrespective of time of the day."

D. H. Chestnut, MD

Analgesia for Labor: Obstetric Outcome and Economic Issues

Effect of food intake during labour on obstetric outcome: randomised controlled trial

O'Sullivan G, Liu B, Hart D, et al (St Thomas' Hosp, London; King's College London; Guy's and St Thomas' NHS Foundation Trust)

BMJ 338:b784, 2009

Objective.—To investigate the effect of feeding during labour on obstetric and neonatal outcomes.

Design.—Prospective randomised controlled trial.

Setting.—Birth centre in London teaching hospital.

Participants.—2426 nulliparous, non-diabetic women at term, with a singleton cephalic presenting fetus and in labour with a cervical dilatation of less than 6 cm.

Intervention.—Consumption of a light diet or water during labour.

Main Outcome Measures.—The primary outcome measure was spontaneous vaginal delivery rate. Other outcomes measured included duration of labour, need for augmentation of labour, instrumental and caesarean delivery rates, incidence of vomiting, and neonatal outcome.

Results.—The spontaneous vaginal delivery rate was the same in both groups (44%; relative risk 0.99, 95% confidence interval 0.90 to 1.08). No clinically important differences were found in the duration of labour (geometric mean: eating, 597 min *v* water, 612 min; ratio of geometric means 0.98, 95% confidence interval 0.93 to 1.03), the caesarean delivery rate (30%*v* 30%; relative risk 0.99, 0.87 to 1.12), or the incidence of vomiting (35% *v* 34%; relative risk 1.05, 0.9 to 1.2). Neonatal outcomes were also similar.

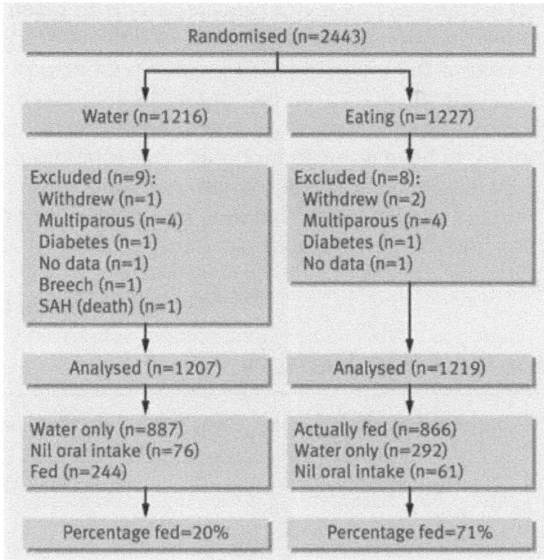

FIGURE 1.—Flow of participants through study. PET = pre-eclamptic toxaemia; SAH = subarachnoid haemorrhage. (Reprinted from O'Sullivan G, Liu B, Hart D, et al. Effect of food intake during labour on obstetric outcome: randomised controlled trial. *BMJ*. 2009;338:b784, with permission from the BMJ Publishing Group.)

Conclusions.—Consumption of a light diet during labour did not influence obstetric or neonatal outcomes in participants, nor did it increase the incidence of vomiting. Women who are allowed to eat in labour have similar lengths of labour and operative delivery rates to those allowed water only.

Trial Registration.—Current Controlled Trials ISRCTN33298015 (Fig 1).

▶ Readers should be aware of the following exclusion criteria for participation in this study: (1) maternal diabetes, (2) presence of a known obstetric or medical complication that would be expected to increase the likelihood of an operative delivery, (3) presence of severe maternal pain, and/or (4) intention to administer parenteral opioids for intrapartum analgesia. Of interest, approximately two thirds of the women in both groups in this study received epidural analgesia. Also, only 71% of women in the eating group, and 20% of women in the water group, ate food during labor (Fig 1). For women in the eating group, "suggested foods included bread, biscuits, vegetables, fruits, low-fat yogurt, soup, isotonic drinks, and fruit juice." The authors concluded that consumption of a light diet during labor did not affect duration of labor or mode of delivery, and it did not affect neonatal outcome. The authors found no evidence of harm, but they acknowledged that "this trial was unable to show evidence of harm as it was not powered to do so given the low prevalence of aspiration, and this question of harm is unlikely to be answered in clinical trials because of the extremely low incidence of acid pulmonary aspiration." The authors stated that in contemporary obstetric practice, "it is the use of regional anesthesia, thereby avoiding intubation, rather than fasting regimens that is likely to have reduced mortality from aspiration." Nonetheless, given the risk of maternal morbidity or mortality associated with aspiration of solid food, I continue to believe that maternal oral intake during labor should be limited to clear liquids, and that consumption of solid food during labor should be discouraged.

D. H. Chestnut, MD

Anesthesia for Cesarean Delivery

Supplementary oxygen for emergency Caesarean section under regional anaesthesia

Khaw KS, Wang CC, Ngan Kee WD, et al (The Chinese Univ of Hong Kong, People's Republic of China)

Br J Anaesth 102:90-96, 2009

Background.—Controversy still exists if the administration of supplementary oxygen to patients having emergency Caesarean section (CS) under regional anaesthesia is beneficial or potentially harmful. Therefore, in a prospective double-blinded study, we randomized patients having emergency CS under regional anaesthesia to receive either air or 60% oxygen until delivery and compared the effects on fetal oxygenation and lipid-peroxidation in the mother and baby.

Methods.—We recruited 131 women having emergency CS under regional anaesthesia. Either 21% (air group) or 60% oxygen (oxygen group) was administered using a Venturi-type facemask until delivery. We compared the oxygen exposure duration, umbilical arterial (UA) and venous (UV) blood gases and oxygen content, and plasma concentration of 8-isoprostane. Subanalysis was performed according to whether or not fetal compromise was considered present.

Results.—Data from 125 patients were analysed. For the oxygen group *vs* the air group, there were greater values for UA Po_2 [mean 2.2 (SD 0.5) *vs* 1.9 (0.6) kPa, $P = 0.01$], UA O_2 content [6.6 (2.5) *vs* 4.9 (2.8) ml dl^{-1}, $P = 0.006$], UV Po_2 [3.8 (0.8) *vs* 3.2 (0.8) kPa, $P < 0.0001$], and UV O_2 content [12.9 (3.5) *vs* 10.4 (3.8) ml dl^{-1}, $P = 0.001$]. There was no difference between the groups in maternal, UA, or UV 8-isoprostane concentration. Apgar scores and UA pH were similar between the groups. Similar changes were observed regardless of whether fetal compromise was considered present ($n = 37$) or not ($n = 88$).

TABLE 2.—Maternal Lipid Peroxide and Neonatal Oxygen and Lipid Peroxide Data for all Cases. Values are Mean (SD)

	Air Group ($n = 64$)	Oxygen Group ($n = 61$)	P-value
O_2 exposure duration (min)	26.7 (11.9)	27.1 (11.4)	0.89
Maternal vein			
Baseline 8-isoprostane (pg ml^{-1})	152.7 (56.0)	138.9 (45.2)	0.20
Delivery 8-isoprostane (pg ml^{-1})	225.7 (102.6)	240.7 (99.2)	0.47
Umbilical artery			
Po_2 (kPa)	1.9 (0.6)	2.2 (0.5)	0.01
Oxyhaemoglobin saturation (%)	24 (14)	31 (11)	0.12
O_2 content (ml dl^{-1})	4.9 (2.8)	6.6 (2.5)	<0.01
8-isoprostane (pg ml^{-1})	457 (222)	473 (193)	0.73
Umbilical vein			
Po_2 (kPa)	3.2 (0.8)	3.8 (0.8)	<0.01
Oxyhaemoglobin saturation (%)	53 (17)	65 (15)	<0.01
O_2 content (ml dl^{-1})	10.4 (3.8)	12.9 (3.5)	<0.01
8-isoprostane (pg ml^{-1})	427 (190)	471 (192)	0.29

Conclusions.—Breathing 60% oxygen during emergency CS under regional anaesthesia increased fetal oxygenation with no associated increase in lipid-peroxidation in the mother or fetus (Table 2).

▶ Some recent studies have questioned the necessity and wisdom of maternal administration of supplemental oxygen during administration of neuraxial anesthesia for elective cesarean delivery. Some evidence has suggested that routine administration of supplemental oxygen may be unnecessary and ineffective, and may even be detrimental in healthy women undergoing elective cesarean delivery. Through normal biologic processes, oxygen is converted to reactive oxygen species, including free radicals, which result in lipid peroxidation. These adverse effects occur with the restoration of perfusion after a period of ischemia (ie, ischemia-reperfusion injury). In this study, maternal administration of 60% oxygen during performance of emergency cesarean delivery under neuraxial anesthesia resulted in increased fetal oxygenation without evidence of increased lipid peroxidation in the mother or fetus (Table 2). Further, the increase in oxygen content was greater in cases of suspected fetal compromise compared with cases in which fetal compromise was not suspected. Although the present study did not demonstrate a difference in clinical outcome associated with administration of supplemental oxygen, the authors concluded that administration of supplemental oxygen during emergency cesarean delivery under neuraxial anesthesia has "potential benefit in terms of improved fetal oxygenation with no evidence for harm from lipid peroxidation." Consensus opinion holds that the emergency cesarean delivery of a compromised fetus should include maternal administration of supplemental oxygen.

D. H. Chestnut, MD

Cesarean by choice? Empirical study of public attitudes

Högberg U, Lynöe N, Wulff M (Umeå Univ, Sweden; Karolinska Institutet, Stockholm, Sweden)

Acta Obstet Gynecol Scand 87:1301-1308, 2008

Objective.—This study examines public attitudes towards maternal requests for cesarean delivery and its association with health care and birth experiences. In addition, this study attempts to ascertain whether gender, age and residence influence these attitudes.

Design.—Cross-sectional population survey with a postal questionnaire.

Setting.—The counties of Stockholm and Vasterbotten in Sweden.

Population.—Equal numbers of women and men between 20 and 80 years of age ($n = 2{,}000$) by population size and gender distribution.

Methods.—Descriptive statistics and content analysis.

Results.—Of the 1,066 women (53%) who responded, two-thirds stated that a cesarean should be decided on for medical reasons and by a doctor. One-third considered that a woman, without persuasion, should decide herself about mode of delivery and should be free to choose a cesarean. These respondents used arguments such as women's rights, bodily integrity and childbirth fear. The results were associated with low trust in health care, women being young or middle aged, urban living and having no children. Low trust in health care was associated with experiences of insecurity, vulnerability and perceived maltreatment.

Conclusion.—Public norms towards women's own decision making on mode of delivery are associated with younger age, lower trust in health care and urban living. Antenatal care will encounter more parents asking for a cesarean and demanding that health professionals provide an ethically appropriate informed consent process. Considering the risk of violating young women's trust if not respecting her wish, it seems reasonable that making decisions whether or not to perform a cesarean is part of shared decision making.

▶ In 2007, the cesarean delivery rate in the United States was 31.8%, which is the highest rate ever recorded in this country. The cesarean delivery rate in the United States has increased by 54% since 1996. During the last several years, one of the most striking changes in obstetric practice has been the increasing performance of cesarean delivery on maternal request. Estimates suggest that cesarean delivery on maternal request accounts for 4% to 18% of all cesarean deliveries performed in the United States, and it seems likely that this number will continue to grow. The 2006 National Institutes of Health State-of-the-Science Conference Statement acknowledged that "there is insufficient evidence to evaluate fully the benefits and risks of cesarean delivery on maternal request compared with planned vaginal delivery." However, the statement noted that "after thorough discussion and review, cesarean delivery on maternal request may be a reasonable alternative to planned vaginal delivery."[1] In my judgment, this permissive statement has "opened the door" to performance of an increasing number of cesarean deliveries without an obstetric or medical indication. I fear that we will see the adverse consequences of the increased performance of cesarean delivery for years to come.

D. H. Chestnut, MD

Reference

1. National Institutes of Health state-of-the science conference statement: cesarean delivery on maternal request, March 27-29, 2006. *Obstet Gynecol.* 2006;107: 1386-1397.

Elective caesarean section increases the risk of respiratory morbidity of the newborn

Borgwardt L, Bach D, Nickelsen C, et al (Copenhagen Univ Hosp, Hvidovre, Denmark)

Acta Paediatr 98:187-189, 2009

Elective caesarean section upon maternal request has become more common during the last decades. Two surveys in the United Kingdom demonstrated that elective caesarean section upon maternal request increased from 1% in the mid 1970s and 1980s, to 30–38% in the 1990s. In Denmark, the overall frequency of caesarean section increased from 11.1% to 20.4% from 1982 to 2004. A Danish study stated that caesarean section upon maternal request is found as one of the main causes to the increase in caesarean section in general.

This study aims to investigate the association among elective caesarean sections, spontaneous vaginal deliveries and neonatal respiratory morbidity in normal pregnancies expecting a normal uncomplicated birth. This is an important issue and has relevance to paediatricians when evaluating the neonatal infants after elective caesarean sections and to obstetricians when counselling mothers in choosing way of delivery.

This is a retrospective study based on information from patient administrative systems and clinical databases at Hvidovre Hospital, Copenhagen University Hospital, Denmark. Information was extracted for all women giving birth in the period 1 January 2003 to 31 December 2005 at Hvidovre Hospital, Copenhagen University Hospital.

▶ In this retrospective study from Denmark, the authors concluded that infants delivered by elective cesarean delivery between 37 and 39 weeks gestation had an increased risk of admission to a neonatal unit compared with infants delivered by spontaneous vaginal delivery. Further, the diagnosis of respiratory morbidity was 10 times more frequent among those delivered by elective cesarean delivery than among those infants delivered vaginally (4.25% vs 0.42%, RR 10.2, $P < .0001$). Similarly, a recent study performed by the Maternal-Fetal Medicine Units Network in the United States demonstrated that elective repeat cesarean delivery performed before 39 weeks gestation was associated with an increased risk of respiratory complications and an increased risk of admission to a neonatal intensive care unit.[1]

D. H. Chestnut, MD

Reference

1. Tita ATN, Landon MB, Spong CY, et al. Timing of elective repeat cesarean delivery at term and neonatal outcomes. *N Engl J Med.* 2009;360:111-119.

Timing of Elective Repeat Cesarean Delivery at Term and Neonatal Outcomes

Tita ATN, Landon MB, Spong CY, et al (Univ of Alabama at Birmingham; Ohio State Univ, Columbus; Eunice Kennedy Shriver Natl Inst of Child Health and Human Development, Bethesda, MD; et al)

N Engl J Med 360:111-120, 2009

Background.—Because of increased rates of respiratory complications, elective cesarean delivery is discouraged before 39 weeks of gestation unless there is evidence of fetal lung maturity. We assessed associations between elective cesarean delivery at term (37 weeks of gestation or longer) but before 39 weeks of gestation and neonatal outcomes.

Methods.—We studied a cohort of consecutive patients undergoing repeat cesarean sections performed at 19 centers of the Eunice Kennedy Shriver National Institute of Child Health and Human Development Maternal–Fetal Medicine Units Network from 1999 through 2002. Women with viable singleton pregnancies delivered electively (i.e., before the onset of labor and without any recognized indications for delivery before 39 weeks of gestation) were included. The primary outcome was the composite of neonatal death and any of several adverse events, including respiratory complications, treated hypoglycemia, newborn sepsis, and admission to the neonatal intensive care unit (ICU).

Results.—Of 24,077 repeat cesarean deliveries at term, 13,258 were performed electively; of these, 35.8% were performed before 39 completed weeks of gestation (6.3% at 37 weeks and 29.5% at 38 weeks) and 49.1% at 39 weeks of gestation. One neonatal death occurred. As compared with births at 39 weeks, births at 37 weeks and at 38 weeks were associated with an increased risk of the primary outcome (adjusted odds ratio for births at 37 weeks, 2.1; 95% confidence interval [CI], 1.7 to 2.5; adjusted odds ratio for births at 38 weeks, 1.5; 95% CI, 1.3 to 1.7; P for trend <0.001). The rates of adverse respiratory outcomes, mechanical ventilation, newborn sepsis, hypoglycemia, admission to the neonatal ICU, and hospitalization for 5 days or more were increased by a factor of 1.8 to 4.2 for births at 37 weeks and 1.3 to 2.1 for births at 38 weeks.

Conclusions.—Elective repeat cesarean delivery before 39 weeks of gestation is common and is associated with respiratory and other adverse neonatal outcomes.

► In 2007 the cesarean delivery rate in the United States was 31.8%, which is the highest rate ever recorded in this country. The cesarean delivery rate in the United States has increased by 54% since 1996. This change reflects, in part, the decreased performance of trial of labor after previous cesarean (and the increased performance of elective repeat cesarean delivery), as well as the increased performance of elective cesarean delivery on maternal request. This study determined that a "high proportion of elective cesarean deliveries in the United States are performed before 39 weeks." The authors noted that this practice "may be driven by several factors, including a woman's desire to give birth once term is attained and an obstetrician's desire to schedule the procedure at a convenient time." Unfortunately, this study demonstrated that "these early deliveries are associated with a preventable increase in neonatal morbidity and admissions to the neonatal ICU, which carry a high economic cost." The authors recommended that elective cesarean delivery should be delayed until 39 weeks gestation.

D. H. Chestnut, MD

Randomised double-blinded comparison of phenylephrine vs ephedrine for maintaining blood pressure during spinal anaesthesia for non-elective Caesarean section

Ngan Kee WD, Khaw KS, Lau TK, et al (The Chinese Univ of Hong Kong, China)

Anaesthesia 63:1319-1326, 2008

In a randomised, double-blinded study, we compared boluses of phenylephrine 100 µg with ephedrine 10 mg for treating hypotension (systolic blood pressure < 100 mmHg) in 204 patients having non-elective Caesarean section under spinal anaesthesia. Umbilical arterial (UA) and venous (UV) pH and base excess were similar between groups. In the ephedrine group, UA lactate concentration was higher (median 2.6 [interquartile range 2.3–3.3] vs 2.4 [1.9–3.0] $mmol.l^{-1}$, $p = 0.002$) and UV lactate concentration was higher (2.5 [2.2–3.2] vs 2.3 [1.9–2.8] $mmol.l^{-1}$, $p = 0.016$) and more patients had nausea or vomiting (12.7% vs 3.9%, $p = 0.02$). Clinical neonatal outcome was similar. Of the protocol-compliant patients ($n = 148$), UA Po_2 and UV Po_2 were lower in the phenylephrine group although oxygen content was similar. We conclude that phenyl-ephrine and ephedrine are both suitable vasopressors for use in non-elective Caesarean sections.

▶ Recent clinical studies have demonstrated the efficacy and safety of the use of phenylephrine for prevention and/or treatment of hypotension during administration of neuraxial anesthesia for cesarean delivery. However, the authors of this report noted that previous studies primarily included patients undergoing elective cesarean delivery, and that few data are available for nonelective cases. The authors suggested that "possible adverse effects of vasopressors on uteroplacental perfusion" may be more likely to occur in nonelective cases with preanesthetic evidence of fetal compromise. In this study, despite small differences between groups in umbilical cord blood lactate concentration and PO_2, there were no differences between groups in fetal acid-base status or neonatal clinical outcome. However, it should be noted that the authors excluded patients with chronic hypertension, pre-eclampsia, and/or severe fetal compromise, and only 24% of the patients in this study had preanesthetic evidence of fetal compromise. Nonetheless, this study adds to the growing body of evidence that both phenylephrine and ephedrine are appropriate vasopressors for treatment of hypotension during administration of neuraxial anesthesia for cesarean delivery.

D. H. Chestnut, MD

Continuous Invasive Blood Pressure and Cardiac Output Monitoring during Cesarean Delivery: A Randomized, Double-Blind Comparison of Low-dose versus High-dose Spinal Anesthesia with Intravenous Phenylephrine or Placebo Infusion

Langesæter E, Rosseland LA, Stubhaug A (Rikshospitalet Univ Hosp, Norway)
Anesthesiology 109:856-863, 2008

Background.—Prevention of hemodynamic instability during cesarean delivery during spinal anesthesia has been the aim of several studies. Noninvasive monitoring has been used in all previous studies. This is the first study in healthy pregnant women with continuous invasive recording of arterial blood pressure, cardiac output, and systemic vascular resistance. The aim of this randomized trial was to compare the effects of two different intrathecal doses of bupivacaine, with or without intravenous phenylephrine infusion, on cardiac output and systolic blood pressure.

Methods.—In this double-blinded study, 80 healthy women scheduled to undergo elective cesarean delivery were randomly assigned to one of four different groups receiving 7 mg spinal bupivacaine with or without a concomitant low-dose infusion of phenylephrine ($0.25\ \mu g \cdot kg^{-1} \cdot min^{-1}$) or 10 mg spinal bupivacaine with or without phenylephrine infusion. All patients had 4 μg sufentanil added to the spinal solution and had cohydration with 750 ml saline, 0.9%.

Results.—The low-dose spinal bupivacaine group with intravenous phenylephrine infusion was the most stable group regarding all hemodynamic variables. The authors found significant differences between this group and the group that was given the high dose of bupivacaine with intravenous placebo infusion regarding cardiac output ($P = 0.005$), systemic vascular resistance ($P < 0.0001$), and systolic blood pressure ($P = 0.012$).

Conclusions.—This study shows that low-dose bupivacaine (with sufentanil), combined with a low-dose infusion of phenylephrine and moderate cohydration, gives the best hemodynamic stability during spinal anesthesia for cesarean delivery.

▶ The authors continuously measured maternal blood pressure using an invasive intra-arterial catheter, and they assessed maternal cardiac output using the LiDCO*plus* (LiDCO Ltd., Cambridge, United Kingdom), which is a "new minimally invasive technique ... based on ...a continuous arterial waveform analysis system (PulseCO) coupled to a single-point lithium indicator dilution calibration system (LiDCO)." The authors stated that the LiDCO*plus* allows continuous assessment of blood pressure and a "beat-to-beat" measurement of cardiac output, stroke volume, and systemic vascular resistance. The authors administered hypobaric spinal bupivacaine rather than the more commonly administered hyperbaric spinal bupivacaine. The 2 doses evaluated in this study were 7 mg and 10 mg of hypobaric bupivacaine, and the authors acknowledged that "using a combined spinal-epidural technique may be advisable when giving lower doses of bupivacaine for spinal anesthesia." Nonetheless, the authors concluded that this study adds to the evidence in support of prophylactic phenylephrine infusion during administration of spinal anesthesia for cesarean delivery.

D. H. Chestnut, MD

Bispectral Index Values During Sevoflurane-Nitrous Oxide General Anesthesia in Women Undergoing Cesarean Delivery: A Comparison Between Women With and Without Prior Labor

Yoo KY, Jeong CW, Kang MW, et al (Chonnam Natl Univ Med School, Gwangju, South Korea)

Anesth Analg 106:1827-1832, 2008

Background.—An end-tidal concentration of 1% sevoflurane (1% ET_{SEVO}) in 50% nitrous oxide (N_2O) during elective cesarean delivery has been associated with bispectral index (BIS) values >60, which are associated with an increased risk of awareness. We hypothesized that BIS values during sevoflurane-N_2O general anesthesia for cesarean delivery would be lower in women with prior labor compared with women without prior labor.

Methods.—Forty patients undergoing cesarean delivery were enrolled in this observational study. One group had urgent surgery after labor (labor group, $n = 20$) and the other had elective surgery without labor (control group, $n = 20$). General anesthesia was induced with thiopental 4 mg/kg, followed by succinylcholine 1.5 mg/kg, and maintained with 1% ET_{SEVO} and 50%N_2O in oxygen. BIS values, systolic arterial blood pressure, heart rate, plasma stress hormone concentrations, Apgar scores, and postoperative analgesia variables were assessed and compared between groups.

Results.—BIS values during the period between intubation and delivery were lower in the labor group than in the control group ($P < 0.001$). Plasma norepinephrine concentrations increased at delivery compared with baseline in both groups. They were higher in the labor group than in the control group both at baseline and at delivery. Systolic arterial blood pressure, heart rate, Apgar scores, surgical characteristics, and plasma concentrations of vasopressin and cortisol were not different between groups. Postoperative visual analog scale pain scores were similar between groups, while the labor group consumed less analgesics ($P < 0.01$) during the first 24 h after the operation.

Conclusions.—Prior labor was associated with lower intraoperative BIS values during sevoflurane/N_2O general anesthesia and reduced postoperative analgesic consumption in women undergoing cesarean delivery compared with women without prior labor.

▶ Published reports have suggested that the incidence of intraoperative awareness and recall seems to be higher in pregnant women receiving general anesthesia for cesarean delivery than in nonpregnant patients receiving general anesthesia for nonobstetric surgery. The authors noted that animal studies have demonstrated that "noxious stimulation activates spinal antinociceptive pathways...[and that] the activation of these pathways may reduce the painful sensation to a second noxious stimulus." The authors also cited human studies that have demonstrated that labor and other stresses result in the release of the endogenous opioid β-endorphin. The authors suggested that "labor pain may activate the spinal inhibitory noradrenergic pathways to elicit antinociception during subsequent cesarean delivery and the immediate postoperative period." In this study, "the difference in bispectral index (BIS) values between groups was observed before (at tracheal intubation) and after the administration of sevoflurane, suggesting that labor affects the BIS response to both thiopental and sevoflurane anesthesia." The authors acknowledged several limitations to their study, including the fact that "the labor group differed from the control group in many aspects, including the presence of anxiety, exhaustion..., nonreassuring fetal status, exposure to various medications, [and] acid-base status. ..." Therefore, additional studies are needed "to elucidate the underlying mechanisms for the observed differences between groups, which may be multifactorial."

D. H. Chestnut, MD

A Survey of Obstetric Perianesthesia Care Unit Standards

Wilkins KK, Greenfield MLVH, Polley LS, et al (Univ of Michigan Health System, Ann Arbor)

Anesth Analg 108:1869-1875, 2009

Background.—Although obstetric patients are generally healthy, population risk is increasing because of increases in maternal age, obesity, and rates of multifetal pregnancies, and complications may occur in the immediate postoperative period. In this study, we sought to identify the current level of recovery care for obstetric patients in North American academic institutions after either general or major neuraxial anesthesia for cesarean delivery.

Methods.—A survey of obstetric anesthesia recovery practices was delivered electronically to 135 obstetric anesthesiology directors of North American academic institutions from June to October, 2007. Surveys were completed electronically and anonymously.

Results.—The response rate was 54.8% (74 of 135). Respondents reported a median of 2550 deliveries per year (interquartile range [IQR] 2000, 4000), with 30% delivered by cesarean delivery (IQR 25.5%, 32.5%) and 5% of cesarean deliveries performed under general anesthesia (IQR 4%, 8%). Most institutions recovered postcesarean patients in either an obstetric perianesthesia care unit or a labor, delivery, and recovery room. Recovery care was staffed solely by perinatal nurses, rather than dedicated perianesthesia care unit nurses in most institutions. Forty-five percent (28 of 62) of institutions had no specific postanesthesia recovery training for nursing staff providing postcesarean care for patients recovering from neuraxial or general anesthesia. Forty-three percent (29 of 67) of respondents rated the recovery care provided to cesarean delivery patients as lower quality than care given to general surgical patients. Respondents who relied solely on perinatal nurses to provide postanesthesia care were most likely to perceive that postanesthetic care for cesarean delivery was of lower quality than that given to general surgery patients ($P = 0.008$).

Conclusions.—Guidelines put forth by the American Society of Anesthesiologists Task Force on Postanesthetic Care and the American Society of PeriAnesthesia Nurses apply to all postoperative patients regardless of their recovery locations. Results from this survey suggest that the level of care provided for postanesthesia recovery from cesarean delivery in North American academic institutions may not meet these guidelines.

▶ The results of this survey suggest that a substantial number of academic health centers are not in compliance with standards and guidelines that state that postanesthesia care for obstetric patients should be equivalent to that provided for nonobstetric patients. It is not likely that a survey of community hospitals would demonstrate a higher level of compliance than that observed in academic health centers. The authors called attention to some of the post-anesthesia problems that may occur in the obstetric population, including postpartum hemorrhage, hypoventilation, and airway obstruction. The authors noted factors that are associated with an increased risk for these and other complications, including advanced maternal age, obesity, and multiple gestations. Of interest, the incidence of each of these factors is on the rise. The authors acknowledged some of the unique factors associated with postanesthesia care of obstetric patients, including the concurrent care of a second patient (ie, the neonate), the mother's desire to initiate breast-feeding, and the presence of family members. The authors concluded their report with a recommendation that "future efforts to enhance patient safety during obstetric postanesthesia recovery should rigorously define the optimal postanesthesia curriculum for perinatal nurses, establish a requirement for basic life support (BLS) certification, evaluate the role of advanced cardiac life support (ACLS) certification, evaluate the costs and benefits of continuous electrocardiography (ECG) monitoring by qualified personnel, and establish environmental and staffing solutions to ensure continuous bedside monitoring during the obstetric postanesthesia recovery."

D. H. Chestnut, MD

Haemodynamic effects of repeated doses of oxytocin during Caesarean delivery in healthy parturients

Langesæter E, Rosseland LA, Stubhaug A (Oslo Univ Hosp – Rikshospitalet, Norway)

Br J Anaesth 103:260-262, 2009

Background.—The haemodynamic effects of oxytocin 5 u have been described previously, but still some authors attribute these effects to the delivery itself. We studied the haemodynamic effects of two repeated doses of oxytocin i.v. in 20 healthy women during spinal anaesthesia for Caesarean delivery.

Methods.—Data were obtained from a randomized controlled study of 80 pregnant women undergoing an elective Caesarean section. All women had an arterial line inserted, and LidCOPlus was used for measuring cardiac output (CO), stroke volume (SV), and systemic vascular resistance (SVR).

Results.—Twenty women required a second bolus of oxytocin 5 u. Both the first and the second doses produced clinically and statistically significant haemodynamic changes, but the haemodynamic changes induced by the second dose were smaller than after the first dose. The mean maximal change in CO after the first and second doses were 94% (CI 70–117) and 42% (CI 33-52), respectively ($P<0.0001$), and for systolic arterial pressure 31% (CI 27–35) and 23% (CI 20–27), respectively ($P=0.003$).

Conclusions.—An initial bolus of oxytocin 5 u produced prominent haemodynamic changes, whereas a second bolus produced smaller

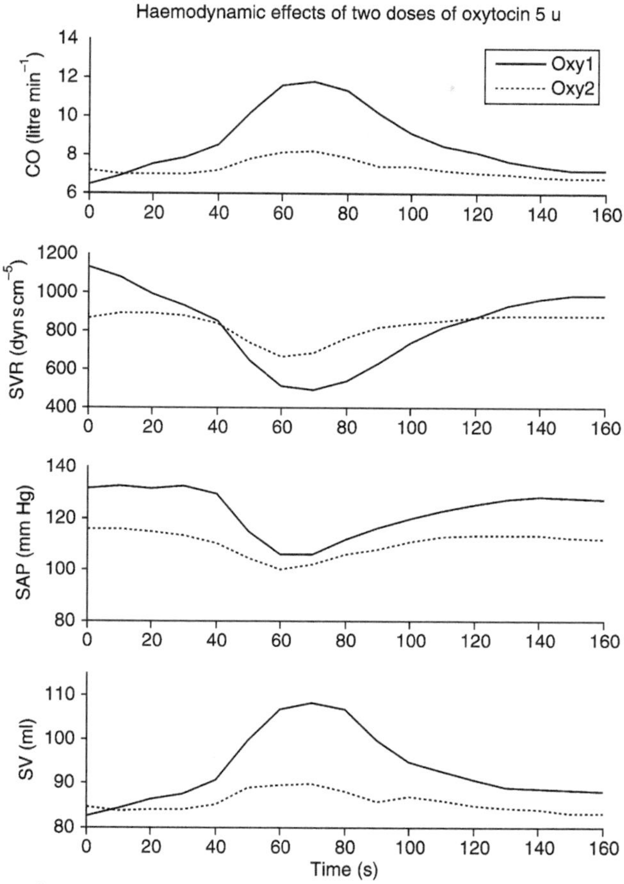

FIGURE 1.—The haemodynamic effects of two doses of oxytocin 5 u i.v. in 20 patients. Injection of oxytocin 5 u is administered at time=30 s. CO, cardiac output; SVR, systemic vascular resistance; SAP, systolic arterial pressure; SV, stroke volume. Oxy1, first dose of oxytocin 5 u. Oxy2, second dose of oxytocin 5 u. (Reprinted from Langesæter E, Rosseland LA, Stubhaug A. Haemodynamic effects of repeated doses of oxytocin during caesarean delivery in healthy parturients. *Br J Anaesth.* 2009;103:260-262, with permission from The Board of Management and Trustees of the British Journal of Anaesthesia, Oxford University Press.)

changes. This could be due to desensitization of endothelial oxytocin receptors (Fig 1).

▶ How many reports of the adverse maternal hemodynamic effects of intravenous bolus administration of oxytocin are needed? In this study, the first intravenous bolus dose of 5 u of oxytocin resulted in a mean maximum decrease in maternal systolic arterial pressure of 31% (Fig 1). And the second dose resulted in a mean maximum decrease in maternal systolic arterial pressure of 23%, but readers should note that the absolute maternal blood pressure was lower after the second dose than after the first dose, because the average maternal blood pressure at the time the second dose was given was lower than the average maternal blood pressure at the time the first dose was given (Fig 1). The authors thankfully concluded that "An implication of the findings reported here is that administration of oxytocin 5 u as a bolus should probably be abandoned because the large hemodynamic effects could be dangerous to vulnerable parturients." The word "probably" should probably be deleted from that conclusion!

D. H. Chestnut, MD

Placental Transfer and Fetal Metabolic Effects of Phenylephrine and Ephedrine during Spinal Anesthesia for Cesarean Delivery

Ngan Kee WD, Khaw KS, Tan PE, et al (The Chinese Univ of Hong Kong)

Anesthesiology 111:506-512, 2009

Background.—Use of ephedrine in obstetric patients is associated with depression of fetal acid-base status. The authors hypothesized that the mechanism underlying this is transfer of ephedrine across the placenta and stimulation of metabolism in the fetus.

Methods.—A total of 104 women having elective Cesarean delivery under spinal anesthesia randomly received infusion of phenylephrine (100 μg/ml) or ephedrine (8 mg/ml) titrated to maintain systolic blood pressure near baseline. At delivery, maternal arterial, umbilical arterial, and umbilical venous blood samples were taken for measurement of blood gases and plasma concentrations of phenylephrine, ephedrine, lactate, glucose, epinephrine, and norepinephrine.

Results.—In the ephedrine group, umbilical arterial and umbilical venous pH and base excess were lower, whereas umbilical arterial and umbilical venous plasma concentrations of lactate, glucose, epinephrine, and norepinephrine were greater. Umbilical arterial Pco_2 and umbilical venous Po_2 were greater in the ephedrine group. Placental transfer was greater for ephedrine (median umbilical venous/maternal arterial plasma concentration ratio 1.13 *vs.* 0.17). The umbilical arterial/umbilical venous plasma concentration ratio was greater for ephedrine (median 0.83 *vs.* 0.71).

Conclusions.—Ephedrine crosses the placenta to a greater extent and undergoes less early metabolism and/or redistribution in the fetus compared with phenylephrine. The associated increased fetal concentrations of lactate, glucose, and catecholamines support the hypothesis that depression of fetal pH and base excess with ephedrine is related to metabolic effects secondary to stimulation of fetal β-adrenergic receptors. Despite historical evidence suggesting uteroplacental blood flow may be better maintained with ephedrine, the overall effect of the vasopressors on fetal oxygen supply and demand balance may favor phenylephrine.

▶ Of interest, the study subjects received no intravenous prehydration before administration of spinal anesthesia. Rather, at intrathecal injection of drug, rapid intravenous fluid infusion (maximum = 2 L) was started, and maternal blood pressure was maintained using an intravenous infusion of either phenylephrine 100 ug/mL or ephedrine 8 mg/mL. The authors made 3 major conclusions. First, "ephedrine crosses the placenta to a greater extent and undergoes less early metabolism and/or redistribution in the fetus" than does phenylephrine. Second, depression of fetal pH and base excess with ephedrine seems to be related to "metabolic effects secondary to stimulation of fetal beta-adrenergic receptors." The authors stated that "although ephedrine may have more favorable effects on fetal oxygen supply compared with phenylephrine, this advantage may be negated by its greater placental transfer and the [subsequent] undesirable effects... on fetal oxygen demand." And third, "the overall effect of the vasopressors on fetal oxygen supply and demand balance may favor phenylephrine" over ephedrine. The weight of contemporary evidence favors the use of phenylephrine as a first-line vasopressor during administration of spinal anesthesia for cesarean delivery.

D. H. Chestnut, MD

Antimicrobial Prophylaxis for Cesarean Delivery Before Skin Incision

Owens SM, Brozanski BS, Meyn LA, et al (Univ of Pittsburgh School of Medicine, PA)

Obstet Gynecol 114:573-579, 2009

Objective.—To estimate the effect of a hospital-wide change in the timing of antimicrobial prophylaxis in cesarean deliveries on maternal and neonatal infections.

Methods.—In November 2004, our institution instituted guidelines recommending that the administration of antimicrobial prophylaxis for cesarean delivery be administered before skin incision rather than after umbilical-cord clamping. We reviewed all cesarean deliveries from two time periods. Group 1 received antibiotics after umbilical-cord clamping (July 2002 to November 2004). Group 2 received antibiotics before skin incision (June 2005 to August 2007). Rates of maternal and neonatal infectious complications were compared between groups.

Results.—There were 4,229 cesarean deliveries in group 1 and 4,781 cesarean deliveries in group 2. Compared with women receiving antimicrobial prophylaxis after umbilical-cord clamping, those administered antimicrobial prophylaxis before skin incision had lower rates of postpartum endometritis (2.2% compared with 3.9%) and wound infection (2.5% compared with 3.6%). After multivariable logistic regression, antimicrobial prophylaxis before skin incision remained associated with lower rates of endometritis (odds ratio [OR] 0.61, 95% confidence interval [CI] 0.47–0.79) and wound infection (OR 0.70, 95% CI 0.55–0.90). Antimicrobial prophylaxis before skin incision had no adverse effect on neonatal infection rates or on the evaluation of the neonate.

Conclusion.—Antimicrobial prophylaxis before skin incision, compared with after cord clamping, resulted in lower rates of maternal infections and

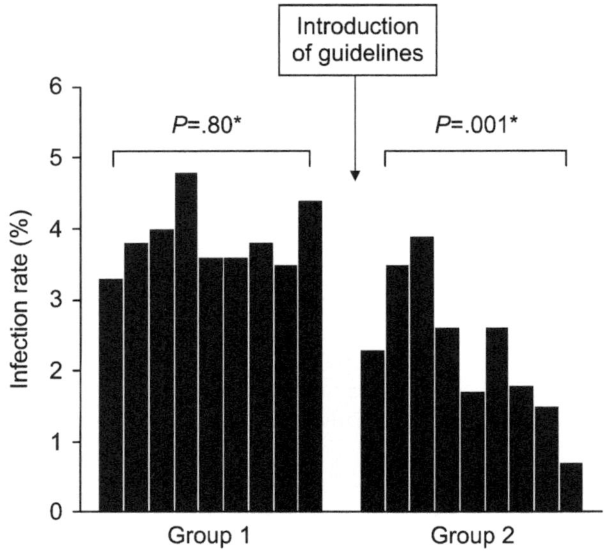

FIGURE 1.—Postpartum endometritis by 3-month intervals. Group 1: July 2002–November 2004, after umbilical-cord clamping. Group 2: June 2005–August 2007, before skin incision. Each bar represents a consecutive 3-month period. **P* from χ^2 for linear trend. Owens. Antimicrobial Prophylaxis in Cesarean Delivery. Obstet Gynecol 2009. (Reprinted from Owens SM, Brozanski BS, Meyn LA, et al. Antimicrobial prophylaxis for cesarean delivery before skin incision. *Obstet Gynecol.* 2009;114:573-579, with permission from The American College of Obstetricians and Gynecologists.)

had no effect on neonatal infections. Antimicrobial prophylaxis for cesarean delivery should occur before skin incision, consistent with basic tenets of surgical antimicrobial prophylaxis.

Level of Evidence.—II. (Fig 1).

▶ This retrospective study adds to the growing body of evidence suggesting that maternal administration of antimicrobial prophylaxis before skin incision for cesarean delivery (as opposed to administration after umbilical cord clamping) is associated with a reduction in the rates of both postcesarean endometritis and postcesarean wound infection (Fig 1). Also in this study, the administration of antimicrobial prophylaxis before skin incision did not have any adverse effect on the rates of neonatal infection evaluation, diagnosis of culture-proven early-onset neonatal infection, or treatment of early-onset presumed neonatal infection. The authors acknowledged the limitations of the retrospective study design, and the authors recommended performance of a large randomized controlled trial that has adequate size (and statistical power) to evaluate neonatal outcomes.

D. H. Chestnut, MD

Hemodynamic Effects of Ephedrine, Phenylephrine, and the Coadministration of Phenylephrine with Oxytocin during Spinal Anesthesia for Elective Cesarean Delivery

Dyer RA, Reed AR, van Dyk D, et al (Univ of Cape Town, South Africa; et al)

Anesthesiology 111:753-765, 2009

Background.—Hemodynamic responses to vasopressors used during spinal anesthesia for elective Cesarean delivery, have not been well described. This study compared the effects of bolus phenylephrine and ephedrine on maternal cardiac output (CO). The hypothesis was that phenylephrine, but not ephedrine, decreases CO when administered in response to hypotension during spinal anesthesia.

Methods.—Forty-three patients were randomized to receive 80 μg of phenylephrine or 10 mg of ephedrine. Both pulse wave form analysis and transthoracic bioimpedance changes were used to estimate stroke volume in each patient. Hemodynamic responses to spinal anesthesia and oxytocin were also recorded. A subgroup of 20 patients was randomized to receive oxytocin compared with oxytocin plus 80 μg of phenylephrine after delivery.

Results.—Mean CO and maximum absolute response in CO were significantly lower during the 150 s after phenylephrine administration than after ephedrine (6.2 *vs.* 8.1 l/min, $P = 0.001$, and 5.2 *vs.* 9.0 l/min, $P < 0.0001$, respectively for pulse wave form analysis, and 5.2 *vs.* 6.3 l/min, $P = 0.01$ and 4.5 *vs.* 6.7 l/min, $P = 0.0001$, respectively for bioimpedance changes). CO changes correlated with heart rate changes. Coadministration of phenylephrine obtunded oxytocin-induced decreases in systemic vascular resistance and increases in heart rate and CO. Trends in CO change were similar using either monitor.

Conclusions.—Bolus phenylephrine reduced maternal CO, and decreased CO when compared with ephedrine during elective spinal anesthesia for Cesarean delivery. CO changes correlated with heart rate changes after vasopressor administration, emphasizing the importance of heart rate as a surrogate indicator of CO. Coadministered phenylephrine obtunded hemodynamic responses to oxytocin.

▶ The authors assessed changes in maternal cardiac output using the LiDCOplus monitor (LiDCO, Cambridge, United Kingdom), which uses pulse waveform analysis calibrated with lithium dilution. They also used a monitor of transthoracic bioimpedance (BioZ, Cardio Dynamics International, San Diego, CA) to assess changes in maternal cardiac output and then compared the results of the 2 methods of assessment. The authors noted that "the limits of agreement between absolute values of cardiac output derived from LiDCOplus and BioZ were outside the recommended acceptable 30% in the current study." However, they suggested that "the agreement between the hemodynamic trends demonstrated by both LiDCOplus and BioZ in this study, in response to both vasopressors and oxytocin, provide further evidence of the usefulness of the pulse waveform monitor as a research tool for the study of acute hemodynamic changes during spinal anesthesia." Perhaps the authors' most important conclusion was that maternal heart rate might be "the best surrogate indicator of cardiac output during spinal anesthesia for cesarean delivery." They suggested that "low-dose phenylephrine, insufficient to cause marked mean arterial pressure (MAP) increases above baseline associated with sinus bradycardia, may be the most appropriate intervention for the initial management of hypotension in most cases to restore systemic vascular resistance (SVR) and cardiac output (CO) to baseline levels."

D. H. Chestnut, MD

Comparison of an equal-dose spinal anesthetic for cesarean section and for post partum tubal ligation

Teoh WHL, Ithnin F, Sia ATH (KK Women's and Children's Hosp, Singapore)
Int J Obstet Anesth 17:228-232, 2008

Background.—We postulated that a spinal dose of hyperbaric bupivacaine 12 mg and morphine 100 μg administered for cesarean section would yield an equivalent sensory block height and provide sufficient analgesia if administered within 48 h of delivery for postpartum tubal ligation.

Method.—20 women undergoing postpartum tubal ligation (PPTL) within 48 h of vaginal delivery and 20 undergoing cesarean section (CS) were recruited. Spinal anesthesia was induced with intrathecal hyperbaric bupivacaine 12 mg and morphine 100 μg at L3/4 with patients in the right lateral position.

Results.—Baseline demographics of groups were comparable, but tubal ligation patients had greater parity, with a mean ± SD 14.5 ± 7.5 h from delivery to spinal anesthesia, and shorter duration of surgery, 21.4 ± 7.6 vs. 35.3 ± 11.3 min. Maximal sensory block was higher in group CS than PPTL, T2 (T1-T4) vs. T3 (T2-T5), $P = 0.001$; time to reach maximal level did not differ significantly, (6.9 ± 3.9 vs. 8.7 ± 2.8 min, $P = 0.091$). There was no difference in time for spinal block to recede two segments or to T10, and for motor block recovery to Bromage 2, all $P > 0.05$. More CS patients were hypotensive (80% vs. 45%, $P = 0.048$) and had intraoperative nausea (25% vs. 0%, $P = 0.047$), but mean phenylephrine and ephedrine usage did not differ significantly.

Conclusion.—An equivalent dose of hyperbaric bupivacaine 12 mg and morphine 100 μg for both CS and PPTL resulted in a higher sensory block, more hypotension and nausea in CS patients. The studied regimen might be appropriate for PPTL, but appears excessive for CS.

▶ The results of this study are not surprising, but some anesthesiologists might disagree with one of the author's conclusions. Intrathecal administration of hyperbaric bupivacaine 12 mg and morphine 0.1 mg represents a common drug and dose regimen when giving spinal anesthesia for cesarean delivery. Readers should take note of 2 details of the study methods and participant demographics. First, spinal anesthesia was performed with patients in the right lateral decubitus position. Some anesthesiologists advocate a reduction in the dose of intrathecal bupivacaine when giving spinal anesthesia with the parturient in the lateral position. And second, participants in the 2 groups had a mean weight of 70 kg and 66 kg, respectively, and thus these subjects were somewhat smaller than most parturients in the United States. The authors stated that they do not advocate the routine use of less than 10 mg of hyperbaric bupivacaine given as part of a single-shot spinal (without the possibility of rescue with an epidural catheter), as it subjects the mother to unnecessary risk of needing general anesthesia.

D. H. Chestnut, MD

Parietal peritoneal closure and persistent postcesarean pain

Shahin AY, Osman AM (Assiut Univ, Egypt)

Int J Gynecol Obstet 104:135-139, 2009

Objective.—To assess the incidence of persistent pain after cesarean delivery.

Methods.—A total of 340 pregnant women with no history of abdominal surgery were randomized to undergo or not undergo parietal peritoneal closure following elective cesarean delivery. Pain scores were recorded on the 1st and 15th postoperative day and the women were followed up every 2 weeks up to 8 months after surgery.

Results.—Overall and epigastric abdominal pain were more frequent in the closure than in the nonclosure group. Pain scores on the 1st and 15th days and after 8 months were higher in the closure group, in which the incidence of persistent postcesarean pain was 17.8% after 8 months.

Conclusion.—Parietal peritoneal closure after cesarean delivery is associated with a higher incidence of early and persistent postoperative pain. A high pain score on the 1st day is a predictor of persistent pain.

► Recent evidence suggests that chronic postcesarean pain is a more common problem than previously realized. This observation has significant implications for public health, given the continued increase in the cesarean delivery rate in the United States and other countries. In this study, parietal peritoneal closure during cesarean delivery was associated with a higher incidence of both early and persistent postoperative pain. Further, a high pain score on postoperative day 1 was a predictor of persistent pain.

D. H. Chestnut, MD

Anaesthesia mode for caesarean section and mortality in very preterm infants: An epidemiologic study in the EPIPAGE cohort

Laudenbach V, Mercier FJ, Rozé J-C, et al (Univ of Rouen, France; Clamart & Univ of Paris XI, France; Univ Hosp, Nantes, France; et al)

Int J Obstet Anesth 18:142-149, 2009

Background.—Little is known about the influence of anaesthesia for caesarean section on outcome in very preterm infants.

Methods.—A prospective, population-based, cohort study (the EPIPAGE cohort) included all births before 33 weeks in nine French regions in 1997. Of 2360 infants live-born between 27 and 32 weeks, 1338 were delivered by caesarean section with general anaesthesia (n = 711, 53.1%), spinal anaesthesia (n = 419, 31.3%), or epidural anaesthesia (n = 208, 15.6%). Neonatal mortality was compared among these three groups using bi- (according to gestational age and to anaesthetic technique) and multivariate analyses.

Results.—Neonatal mortality was 10.1% with general anaesthesia, 12.2% with spinal anaesthesia and 7.7% with epidural anaesthesia. After adjustment for gestational age and characteristics of pregnancy, delivery and neonate, spinal anaesthesia was associated with a higher risk of neonatal death than general anaesthesia (adjusted odds ratio, 1.7; 95% confidence interval 1.1 to 2.6).

Conclusion.—In this population-based study, spinal anaesthesia was associated with an increased risk of neonatal mortality in very preterm infants compared to general anaesthesia (and epidural anaesthesia), independently from gestational age and characteristics of the pregnancies, deliveries and neonates. Although this multivariate analysis does not prove a causal relationship, the results suggest it could exist, particularly if maternal haemodynamics are poorly controlled. With recent significant change in the conduct of spinal anaesthesia, further studies are needed to investigate potential harmful effects of anaesthesia on very preterm infants delivered by caesarean section.

▶ The authors acknowledged that "multivariate analysis does not prove a causal relationship per se, but it suggests that one could exist." The authors also acknowledged several important limitations to their study. First, this study was a secondary analysis of a population-based cohort study, "which collected data on maternal anaesthesia but was not initially designed to address outcome of different anaesthetic techniques. Further, the study was a non-randomized observational design." Second, the infants were delivered in more than 150 maternity hospitals, and "the management of each anaesthetic technique probably varied across institutions." The authors correctly noted that spinal anesthesia "is not a generic procedure." Third, the data were collected on deliveries performed 12 years ago, in 1997. The authors called attention to "marked improvements" in spinal anesthetic technique over the last 12 years, including "the addition of lipophilic opioids that allow a reduction in local anaesthetic dose, colloid, or crystalloid coloading, and the decreasing use of ephedrine with the increasing use of phenylephrine." Finally, the authors acknowledged that "the reduction in anaesthetic maternal morbidity and mortality over recent decades can be largely ascribed to widespread use of neuraxial anaesthesia." They concluded that "the results of [this] study should not cast doubt on the use of spinal anaesthesia itself, but rather the modalities of administration of spinal anaesthesia." Good practice should include "efficacious prevention of severe and sustained hypotension."

D. H. Chestnut, MD

Hetastarch co-loading is as effective as pre-loading for the prevention of hypotension following spinal anesthesia for cesarean delivery

Carvalho B, Mercier FJ, Riley ET, et al (Stanford Univ School of Medicine, CA; A. Beclere Hosp, Clamart, France; et al)

Int J Obstet Anesth 18:150-155, 2009

Background.—Pre-loading with hetastarch decreases the incidence and severity of hypotension after spinal anesthesia for cesarean delivery. However, pharmacokinetic studies with crystalloid predict that fluid loading should be more efficacious if rapidly administered immediately after induction of spinal anesthesia. The aim of this study was to compare pre- and co-loading of hetastarch for the prevention of hypotension following spinal anesthesia for cesarean delivery.

Methods.—Forty-six healthy term parturients scheduled for cesarean delivery were randomized to receive 500 mL of 6% hetastarch intravenously, either slowly before spinal anesthesia (pre-loading) or as quickly as possible immediately after spinal anesthesia (co-loading). Systolic blood pressure was maintained at or above 90% of baseline with intravenous vasopressor boluses (ephedrine 5 mg/mL + phenylephrine 25 μg/mL). The primary outcome was the volume of vasopressor mix required. Secondary outcomes included blood pressure and heart rate changes, time to first vasopressor use, nausea or vomiting, and neonatal outcomes (umbilical artery and vein pH, Apgar scores).

Results.—The pre-loading group used 3.5 ± 2 mL (mean ± SD) of vasopressor mixture compared with 3.2 ± 3 mL in the co-loading group ($P = 0.6$). There were no differences in any important maternal hemodynamic or neonatal outcome values between the two study groups.

Conclusion.—Hetastarch co-loading is as effective as pre-loading for the prevention of hypotension after spinal anesthesia for cesarean delivery. Surgery need not be delayed to allow a predetermined pre-load to be administered before induction of spinal anesthesia.

▶ The authors suggested that intravenous infusion of colloid solution is more effective than infusion of crystalloid solution in preventing maternal hypotension during administration of spinal anesthesia for cesarean delivery. The authors acknowledged that infusion of colloid poses "greater risks, including hypocoagulable changes, pruritus, allergic reactions, and increased costs compared with crystalloid solutions." They further noted that the risk of anaphylactoid/anaphylactic reaction following hetastarch administration is extremely rare with an estimated incidence of 0.007% to 0.047%. In other words, the risk of an anaphylactoid/anaphylacic reaction is low but not zero! The authors concluded: "This study adds to the growing evidence that cesarean delivery need not be delayed to allow a predetermined pre-load to be administered before inducting spinal anesthesia. Conversely, in situations where there is no urgency, a hetastarch loading can be administered before cesarean delivery with similar efficacy."

D. H. Chestnut, MD

Complications in Obstetrics and Obstetric Anesthesia

Severe Obstetric Morbidity in the United States: 1998–2005

Kuklina EV, Meikle SF, Jamieson DJ, et al (Quantell, Inc., Taneytown, MD; Natl Insts of Health, Bethesda, MD; Ctrs for Disease Control and Prevention, Atlanta, GA)

Obstet Gynecol 113:293-299, 2009

Objective.—To examine trends in the rates of severe obstetric complications and the potential contribution of changes in delivery mode and maternal characteristics to these trends.

Methods.—We performed a cross-sectional study of severe obstetric complications identified from the 1998–2005 Nationwide Inpatient Sample of the Healthcare Cost and Utilization Project. Logistic regression was used to examine the effect of changes in delivery mode and maternal characteristics on rates of severe obstetric complications.

Results.—The prevalence of delivery hospitalizations (per 1,000) complicated by at least one severe obstetric complication increased from 0.64% (n = 48,645) in 1998–1999 to 0.81% (n = 68,433) in 2004–2005. Rates of complications that increased significantly during the study period included renal failure by 21% (from 0.23 to 0.28), pulmonary embolism by 52% (0.12 to 0.18), adult respiratory distress syndrome by 26% (0.36 to 0.45), shock by 24% (0.15 to 0.19), blood transfusion by 92% (2.38 to 4.58), and ventilation by 21 % (0.47 to 0.57). In logistic regression models, adjustment for maternal age had no effect on the increased risk for these complications in 2004–2005 relative to 1998–1999. However, after adjustment for mode of delivery, the increased risks for these complications in 2004–2005 relative to 1998–1999 were no longer significant, with the exception of pulmonary embolism (odds ratio 1.30) and blood transfusion (odds ratio 1.72). Further adjustment for payer, multiple births, and select comorbidities had little effect.

Conclusion.—Rates of severe obstetric complications increased from 1998–1999 to 2004–2005. For many of these complications, these increases were associated with the increasing rate of cesarean delivery.

▶ The authors noted that the increased rates of severe obstetric complications were associated with the increasing rate of cesarean delivery. The authors acknowledged that their results "do not establish causality." The authors expressed concern regarding "the independent increase in rates of pulmonary embolism...because...it is the most common direct cause of maternal mortality in the United States." In a recent review of maternal mortality in a large health care delivery system, Clark et al called attention to the potential value of thromboembolism prophylaxis in women undergoing cesarean delivery.[1] Clark et al stated that given the potential for bleeding complications with methods of neuraxial anesthesia commonly used for cesarean delivery, they are in the process of implementing a policy of universal pneumatic compression device use for all women undergoing cesarean delivery in their system.

D. H. Chestnut, MD

Reference

1. Clark SL, Belfort MA, Dildy GA, Herbst MA, Meyers JA, Hankins GD. Maternal death in the 21st century: causes, prevention, and relationship to cesarean delivery. *Am J Obstet Gynecol.* 2008;199:36.e1-36.e5.

Circulatory arrest in late pregnancy: caesarean section a vital decision for both mother and child

Zdolsek HJ, Holmgren S, Wedenberg K, et al (Univ Hosp, Linköping, Sweden; Dept of Obstetrics and Gynaecology, Eskilstuna, Sweden)
Acta Anaesthesiol Scand 53:828-829, 2009

Circulatory arrest during pregnancy is extremely rare and there should be a well-planned strategy for its management in all hospitals. To consider the priority of the mother's life over the child's and an unwarranted preterm delivery may lead to hesitancy and uncertainty and jeopardize both of them. In these situations, speed is a priority. Cardiopulmonary resuscitation should commence immediately. The anaesthesiologist should be well aware of the possible advantage of a caesarean section. Even if the obstetrician is responsible for the decision to perform the operation, the anaesthesiologist should strongly support the action. An 'emergency caesarean kit' with the essential surgical instruments should be immediately available in every labour ward and emergency department.

▶ If initial efforts to restore circulation are unsuccessful in a pregnant woman who has suffered cardiac arrest after 20 weeks' gestation, the physician should consider immediate hysterotomy and delivery of the infant. Extrauterine survival of the infant is unlikely before 24 weeks' gestation; however, the American

Heart Association (AHA) has endorsed performance of an emergency hysterotomy as early as 20 weeks' gestation to enable successful maternal resuscitation.[1] The AHA has concluded: "The best survival rate for infants >24 to 25 weeks' gestation occurs when the delivery of the infant occurs no more than 5 minutes after the mother's heart stops beating. This typically requires that the provider begin the hysterotomy about 4 minutes after cardiac arrest. Emergency hysterotomy ... may seem counterintuitive given that the key to salvage of a potentially viable infant is resuscitation of the mother. But the mother cannot be resuscitated unless venous return and aortic output are restored."[1]

D. H. Chestnut, MD

Reference

1. American Heart Association. Cardiac arrest associated with pregnancy. IV. *Circulation.* 2005;112:150-153.

Respiratory Depression After Neuraxial Opioids in the Obstetric Setting

Carvalho B (Stanford Univ School of Medicine, CA)

Anesth Analg 107:956-961, 2008

Neuraxial opioids have contributed significantly to improved labor and postcesarean delivery analgesia. In the obstetric population, epidural and intrathecal opioids are associated with a very low risk of clinically significant respiratory depression. Although rare, respiratory depression is a serious risk; patients may die or suffer permanent brain damage as a consequence. This review discusses the mechanism and incidence, as well as the prevention, detection, and management of respiratory depression with morphine, extended-release epidural morphine, and lipophilic opioids in the labor and cesarean delivery setting.

▶ This is a concise and well written focused review of this subject. I encourage readers to also review the recently updated American Society of Anesthesiologists practice guidelines for the prevention, detection, and management of respiratory depression associated with neuraxial opioid administration.[1]

D. H. Chestnut, MD

Reference

1. American Society of Anesthesiologists Task Force on Neuraxial Opioids. Practice guidelines for the prevention, detection, and management of respiratory depression associated with neuraxial opioid administration. *Anesthesiology.* 2009;110: 218-230.

Liability Associated with Obstetric Anesthesia: A Closed Claims Analysis

Davies JM, Posner KL, Lee LA, et al (Univ of Washington School of Medicine, Seattle)

Anesthesiology 110:131-139, 2009

Background.—Obstetrics carries high medical liability risk. Maternal death and newborn death/brain damage were the most common complications in obstetric anesthesia malpractice claims before 1990. As the liability profile may have changed over the past two decades, the authors reviewed recent obstetric claims in the American Society of Anesthesiologists Closed Claims database.

Methods.—Obstetric anesthesia claims for injuries from 1990 to 2003 (1990 or later claims; $n = 426$) were compared to obstetric claims for injuries before 1990 ($n = 190$). Chi-square and z tests compared categorical variables; payment amounts were compared using the Kolmogorov-Smirnov test.

Results.—Compared to pre-1990 obstetric claims, the proportion of maternal death ($P = 0.002$) and newborn death/brain damage ($P = 0.048$) decreased, whereas maternal nerve injury ($P < 0.001$) and maternal back pain ($P = 0.012$) increased in 1990 or later claims. In 1990 or later claims, payment was made on behalf of the anesthesiologist in only 21% of newborn death/brain damage claims compared to 60% of maternal death/brain damage claims ($P < 0.001$). These payments in both groups were associated with an anesthesia contribution to the injury ($P < 0.001$) and substandard anesthesia care ($P < 0.001$). Anesthesia-related newborn death/brain damage claims had an increased proportion of delays in anesthetic care ($P = 0.001$) and poor communication ($P = 0.007$) compared to claims unrelated to anesthesia.

Conclusion.—Newborn death/brain damage has decreased, yet it remains a leading cause of obstetric anesthesia malpractice claims over time. Potentially preventable anesthetic causes of newborn injury included delays in anesthesia care and poor communication between the obstetrician and anesthesiologist.

► The authors stated that "the major finding of this closed claims review is that, compared with pre-1990 obstetric claims, the proportion of maternal death and newborn death/brain damage decreased in obstetric claims from 1990 or later, whereas the proportion of claims for maternal nerve injury increased." The authors attributed the decrease in maternal respiratory events to the "use of respiratory system monitors" in contemporary anesthesia practice, the decreased use of general anesthesia in obstetric practice, and the "enhanced awareness" of the risk of pulmonary aspiration of gastric contents in obstetric patients. The authors attributed the reduction in claims for newborn death and brain damage to the growing recognition that "most cases of newborn brain damage are due to antenatal factors, and only a minority are related to intrapartum hypoxia. ..." However, the authors observed that "anesthesia-related claims for newborn death/brain damage were associated with anesthesia delay, poor communication, and substandard anesthesia care in response to difficult intubation or block-related hypotension." The authors suggested that "neonatal outcome may be improved by better communication between obstetrician and anesthesiologist, particularly concerning the urgency of cesarean section." The authors also noted that "delays in diagnosis and resuscitation of high neuraxial block were preventable causes of maternal death/brain damage."

D. H. Chestnut, MD

Overview of Maternal Morbidity During Hospitalization for Labor and Delivery in the United States: 1993–1997 and 2001–2005

Berg CJ, MacKay AP, Qin C, et al (Ctrs for Disease Control and Prevention, Atlanta, GA)

Obstet Gynecol 113:1075-1081, 2009

Objective.—To assess progress toward meeting the U.S. *Healthy People 2010* objective of reducing the rate of maternal morbidity at delivery hospitalization by comparing National Hospital Discharge Survey data from two time periods.

Methods.—Using data from the National Hospital Discharge Survey, we estimated rates of intrapartum morbidity defined by obstetric complications, preexisting medical conditions, and cesarean delivery during 2001–2005 and compared them with rates published for 1993–1997. We calculated and compared the rates for categories of morbidity as well as rates for the summary groups of morbidity.

Results.—Between the two time periods, the rate of obstetric complications remained unchanged at 28.6%; the prevalence of preexisting medical conditions at delivery increased from 4.1% to 4.9%. Rates of chronic hypertension and preeclampsia, gestational and preexisting diabetes, asthma, and postpartum hemorrhage increased, whereas rates of third- and fourth-degree lacerations and various types of infection decreased. The cesarean delivery rate increased from 21.8% to 28.3%.

Conclusion.—Between 1993–1997 and 2001–2005, the rate of intrapartum morbidity associated with obstetric complications was unchanged and the rate of pregnancies complicated by preexisting medical conditions increased.

▶ The authors called attention to the increased prevalence of obesity among pregnant women and in the general population in the United States. The authors also called attention to the steady increase in the percentage of births to women of older ages. Thus, it is not surprising that "between the two time periods of this analysis, the rates of pregnancy-induced hypertension, chronic hypertension, and both preexisting and gestational diabetes, all more common with increasing body mass index (BMI) and with increasing maternal age, have increased among pregnant women." Of special concern is the observed increase in the rate of postpartum hemorrhage. Meanwhile, the cesarean delivery rate in the United States has increased sharply and now exceeds 30%, and I expect the cesarean delivery rate to increase further in the years ahead.

D. H. Chestnut, MD

Factors Associated With Peripartum Hysterectomy

Bodelon C, Bernabe-Ortiz A, Schiff MA, et al (Univ of Washington, Seattle; Universidad Peruana Cayetano Heredia, Lima, Peru; Harborview Injury Prevention and Res Ctr, Seattle, Washington; et al)

Obstet Gynecol 114:115-123, 2009

Objective.—To identify factors associated with peripartum hysterectomy performed within 30 days postpartum.

Methods.—This was a population-based case–control study using Washington State birth certificate registry (1987–2006) linked to the Comprehensive Hospital Abstract Reporting System. Cases underwent hysterectomy within 30 days postpartum. Controls were frequency matched 4:1. Exposures included factors related to hemorrhage, delivery method, multiple gestations, and infection. Incidence rates of peripartum hysterectomy and maternal and neonatal morbidity and mortality were assessed. Adjusted odds ratios (aORs) by maternal age, parity, gestational age, year of birth, and mode of delivery and 95% confidence intervals (CIs) were computed.

Results.—There were 896 hysterectomies. Incidence rates ranged from 0.25 in 1987 to 0.82 per 1,000 deliveries in 2006 (χ^2 for trend, $P < .001$). Factors related to hemorrhage were strongly related to peripartum hysterectomy. Placenta previa (192 cases compared with 23 controls; aOR 7.9, 95% CI 4.1–15.0), abruptio placenta (71 compared with 55; aOR 3.2, 95% CI 1.8–5.8), and retained placenta (214 compared with 28; aOR 43.0, 95% CI 19.0–97.7) increased the risk of hysterectomy, as did uterine atony, uterine rupture, and thrombocytopenia. Having multiple gestations did not. As compared with vaginal delivery, vaginal delivery after cesarean (27 cases compared with 105 controls; aOR 1.9, 95% CI 1.2–3.0), primary cesarean (270 compared with 504; aOR 4.6, 95% CI 3.5–6.0), and repeat cesarean (296 compared with 231; aOR 7.9, 95% CI 5.8–10.7) increased the risk of peripartum hysterectomy. Among the 111 women who had hysterectomy on readmission (12.8% of cases), hemorrhage- and infection-related factors were still strongly associated with peripartum hysterectomy.

Conclusion.—Incidence rates of peripartum hysterectomy are increasing over time. The most important risk factor for peripartum hysterectomy is hemorrhage, most notably caused by uterine rupture, retained placenta, and atony of uterus (Fig 1).

▶ The authors observed "an increasing trend in the incidence rates of peripartum hysterectomy from 1987-2006" (Fig 1). The authors also noted that contributing factors may include the increased cesarean delivery rate and

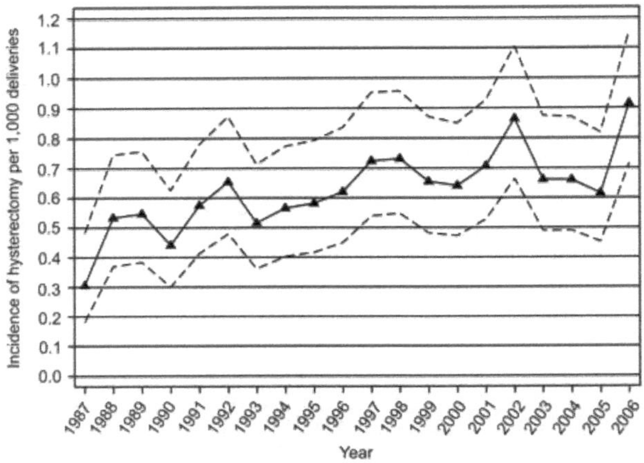

FIGURE 1.—Trends of peripartum hysterectomy in Washington State from 1987 to 2006. The *dashed lines* represent the 95% confidence intervals. Bodelon. Factors Related to Peripartum Hysterectomy. Obstet Gynecol 2009. (Reprinted from Bodelon C, Bernabe-Ortiz A, Schiff MA, et al. Factors associated with peripartum hysterectomy. *Obstet Gynecol.* 2009;114:115-123. Copyright 2009, with permission from The American College of Obstetricians and Gynecologists.)

other factors such as abnormal placentation. The authors suggested that "uterine scarring, especially with [the] increasing number of previous cesarean deliveries, increases the risk of peripartum hysterectomy, even in the absence of placenta previa." Readers of this article should note that the group of patients with abnormal placentation included patients with placenta previa, placental abruption, and/or retained placenta. Further, the group of patients with retained placenta included patients with placenta accreta, placenta increta, and/or placenta percreta. Thus, the coding for retained placenta limited the authors' ability to distinguish placenta accreta, placenta increta, and placenta percreta from other forms of retained placenta. The authors made the following observation: "With today's imaging capabilities, knowledge of abnormal placentation can lead clinicians to prepare for delivery with interventional radiologists, uterotonics, uterine balloon compression devices, transfusion services, and the optimal surgical team available." The authors then concluded that "having all potentially life-saving devices ready and assembling the appropriate team before delivery in at-risk situations could potentially decrease the maternal and neonatal morbidity and mortality associated [was] peripartum hysterectomy that was observed in the last 2 decades in Washington State."

D. H. Chestnut, MD

The Frequency and Complication Rates of Hysterectomy Accompanying Cesarean Delivery

Shellhaas CS, for the Eunice Kennedy Shriver National Institutes of Health and Human Development (NICHD) Maternal–Fetal Medicine Units Network (MFMU) (Ohio State Univ, Columbus; et al)

Obstet Gynecol 114:224-229, 2009

Objective.—To estimate the frequency, indications, and complications of cesarean hysterectomy.

Methods.—This was a prospective, 2-year observational study at 13 academic medical centers conducted between January 1, 1999, and December 31, 2000, on all women who underwent a hysterectomy at the time of cesarean delivery. Data were abstracted from the medical record by study nurses. The outcomes included procedure frequency, indications, and complications.

Results.—A total of 186 cesarean hysterectomies (0.5%) were performed from a cohort of 39,244 women who underwent cesarean delivery. The leading indications for hysterectomy were placenta accreta (38%) and uterine atony (34%). Of the hysterectomy cases with a diagnosis recorded as accreta, 18% accompanied a primary cesarean delivery, and 82% had a prior procedure ($P < .001$). Of the hysterectomy cases with atony recorded as a diagnosis, 59% complicated primary cesarean delivery, whereas 41% had a prior cesarean ($P < .001$). Major maternal complications of cesarean hysterectomy included transfusion of red blood cells (84%) and other blood products (34%), fever (11%), subsequent laparotomy (4%), ureteral injury (3%), and death (1.6%). Accreta hysterectomy cases were more likely than atony hysterectomy cases to require ureteral stents (14% compared with 3%, $P = .03$) and to instill sterile milk into the bladder (23% compared with 8%, $P = .02$).

Conclusion.—The rate of cesarean hysterectomy has declined modestly in the past decade. Despite the use of effective therapies and procedures to

TABLE 3.—Indications for Cesarean Hysterectomy

Indication	Overall Number (n = 186)	Primary Cesarean Deliveries (n = 80)	Repeat Cesarean Deliveries (n = 106)
Accreta	71 (38.2)	13 (16.3)	58 (54.7)
Atony	64 (34.4)	42 (52.5)	22 (20.8)
Cervical cancer	13 (7.0)	9 (11.3)	4 (3.8)
Uterine rupture	10 (5.4)	2 (2.5)	8 (7.5)
Leiomyomas	9 (4.8)	6 (7.5)	3 (2.8)
Extension	2 (1.1)	2 (2.5)	0 (0.0)
Other*	17 (9.1)	6 (7.5)	11 (10.4)

Data are n (%).

*Extensive adhesions, patient desire, uterine artery laceration, inability to close uterus, diffuse uterine hemorrhage, or uncontrolled bleeding.

TABLE 4.—Complications of Cesarean Hysterectomy

Complication	n (%)	95% Confidence Interval
Transfusion		
Packed or whole red blood cells	156 (83.9)	(77.9–88.6)
Fresh frozen plasma	59 (31.7)	(25.1–38.9)
Cryoprecipitate	22 (11.8)	(7.6–17.3)
Platelets	28 (15.1)	(10.2–20.7)
Postoperative fever	21 (11.3)	(7.4–16.4)
Ileus	10 (5.4)	(2.7–9.3)
Exploratory laparotomy	7 (3.8)	(1.8–7.6)
Hospital readmission	7 (3.8)	(1.8–7.6)
Urinary tract infection	6 (3.2)	(1.4–6.7)
Cuff abscess	5 (2.7)	(1.1–5.8)
Maternal death	3 (1.6)	(0.4–4.6)
Bowel injury	2 (1.1)	(0.2–3.8)
Wound dehiscence	2 (1.1)	(0.2–3.8)
Septic pelvic thrombophlebitis	1 (0.5)	(0.03–2.7)
Confirmed deep vein thrombosis	1 (0.5)	(0.03–2.7)

control hemorrhage at cesarean delivery, a small proportion of women continue to require hysterectomy to control hemorrhage from both uterine atony and placenta accreta.

Level of Evidence.—II (Tables 3 and 4).

▶ This study includes data from 184 387 deliveries performed at 13 academic health centers, and the study was performed by members of the highly respected National Institute of Child Health and Human Development (NICHD) Maternal-Fetal Medicine Units Network. Several findings deserve emphasis. First, placenta accreta was the most common reason for hysterectomy, accounting for 38% of the cases, and uterine atony was the second most common reason for hysterectomy, accounting for 34% of the cases (Table 3). Second, among the patients with uterine atony only 4% required hysterectomy, whereas 71% of the patients with placenta accreta required hysterectomy. Of interest, the authors stated that "the condition of accreta may have been underdiagnosed ... [in part because] some cases of atony may have actually been complicated by focal areas of accreta leading to hemorrhage." And third, some 84% of the patients undergoing cesarean hysterectomy received one or more units of red blood cells (Table 4).

D. H. Chestnut, MD

Severe maternal morbidity for 2004–2005 in the three Dublin maternity hospitals

Murphy CM, Murad K, Deane R, et al (Rotunda Hosp, Dublin, Ireland; Natl Maternity Hosp, Dublin, Ireland; Coombe Women's Hosp, Dublin, Ireland; et al)
Eur J Obstet Gynecol Reprod Biol 143:34-37, 2009

Objective.—To assess the prevalence and causes of severe maternal morbidity in Dublin over a two year period from 2004 to 2005.

Study Design.—A prospective cohort study from January 2004 to December 2005 was undertaken in the three large maternity hospitals in Dublin, which serve a population of 1.5 million people. All are tertiary referral centres for obstetrics and neonatology and have an annual combined delivery rate of circa 23,000 births. Cases of severe maternal morbidity were identified. A systems based classification was used. The primary cause of maternal morbidity and the number of events experienced per patient was recorded.

Results.—We identified 158 women who fulfilled the definition for severe maternal morbidity, giving a rate of 3.2 per 1000 maternities. There were two maternal deaths during the time period giving mortality to morbidity ratio of 1:79. The commonest cause of severe morbidity was vascular dysfunction related to obstetric haemorrhage. Eclampsia comprised 15.4% of cases. Intensive care or coronary care admission occurred in 12% of cases.

Conclusion.—The prevalence of severe maternal morbidity in this population is 3.2/1000 maternities. Obstetric haemorrhage was the main cause of severe maternal morbidity (Table 1a).

▶ Given the decline in the maternal mortality rate in developed countries over the last several decades, the authors stated that "maternal mortality can no longer act as a sole marker for quality of care for a pregnant woman." In this study, the most common cause of severe maternal morbidity was "vascular dysfunction related to haemorrhage," which the authors defined as "hypovolaemia requiring more than 5 units of blood" (Table 1a). Uterine atony and genital tract injury were the 2 most common causes of severe obstetric hemorrhage. There were 16 cases of emergency peripartum hysterectomy, for a rate of 0.3 per 1000 maternities. The authors noted that the incidence of admission to an intensive care unit may not be an accurate surrogate marker for severe maternal morbidity, in part because intensive care unit admission depends on the availability of intensive care unit beds. The authors encouraged the use of "skills and drills sessions" to prepare obstetric providers for management of obstetric hemorrhage and other obstetric emergencies. As an aside, I should note that the maternal mortality rate in the United States has increased slightly in the last several years—a disturbing trend that may reflect several factors, including the increased prevalence of obesity and the increased cesarean delivery rate.

D. H. Chestnut, MD

TABLE 1a.—Classification of Severe Maternal Morbidity

Cause of Morbidity (System-Based)	Definition	Total Number of Severe Events ($n = 211$)[a]	Rate Per thousand Maternities[b]
Vascular dysfunction	Hypovolaemia requiring more then five units red cells	74	1.5
Coagulation dysfunction	Acute thrombocytopenia requiring platelet transfusion	30	0.6
Cardiac dysfunction	Pulmonary oedema—requiring frusemide iv or intubation	8	0.2
	Cardiac arrest	1	
Metabolic dysfunction	Thyroid crisis	0	0.06
	Diabetic ketoacidosis blood glucose > 15 mmol/l, pH < 7.1	3	
Cerebral dysfunction	Coma > 12 h	0	0.6
	Subarachnoid or intracerbral haemorrhage	3	
	Eclampsia (seizure in the presence of pre-eclampsia)	24	
	Status epilepticus	1	
Acute renal dysfunction	Creatinine > 400 or urea > 15 mmol/l, or oliguria, 400 ml/24 h	4	0.04
Acute liver dysfunction	Acute onset of biochemical disturbance andAST/ALT > 200 mmmol/l	2	0.02
Respiratory dysfunction	Intubation and ventilation > 1 h other than for general anaesthetic	6	0.3
	Radiologically proven pulmonary embolism	11	
Immunological dysfunction	Emergency hysterectomy for sepsis	2	0.04
	Septic shock requiring ICU admission	0	
	Anaphylactic shock (an allergic reaction resulting in collapse with hypotension, dyspnoea and rash)	0	
Intensive care unit admission for any reason		21	0.4
Cardiac intensive care admission		3	0.06
Anaesthetic complications	Failed/difficult intubations requiring reversal	2	0.02
	High spinal causing hypotension < 90 mmHg > 60 min	0	
Peri-partum hysterectomy		16	0.3
Totals		211	n/a

[a]Number of occurrences of a particular morbidity, noting that 45 patients experienced more than one event.
[b]Number of severe morbidity events per thousand maternities (all pregnancies including ectopics and miscarriages) not mutually exclusive categories (noting that 45 patients experienced more than one event).

Introduction of cell salvage to a large obstetric unit: the first six months

King M, Wrench I, Galimberti A, et al (Royal Hallamshire Hosp, Sheffield, UK)

Int J Obstet Anesth 18:111-117, 2009

Background.—We introduced red-cell salvage to our obstetric unit following a two-month period of training and education. We report a service evaluation of the first six months of activity from May to October 2007.

Methods.—The indications for using cell salvage were: placenta praevia, suspected placental abruption, multiple pregnancy, multiple repeat caesarean, previous history of post partum haemorrhage, refusal of blood transfusion, caesarean section at full dilatation, low preoperative haemoglobin and at the discretion of the theatre team.

Results.—The cell saver was used for 46 patients with a blood loss (median; range) of 800 (200–2000) mL and a heterologous transfusion rate of 22% (10 cases). Blood was processed and returned in 19 cases of which nine were emergency and 10 elective. The median volume (range) of blood returned was 390 (200–800) mL. For the unit as a whole the percentage of all theatre cases who received a heterologous transfusion fell from 10.2% for the equivalent time period in the preceding year to 7.9% during the six month period that cell salvage was in use ($P = 0.126$, χ^2). There were no adverse reactions following the administration of processed blood.

Conclusion.—We have successfully introduced cell salvage to our unit in a relatively short period of time and have used it for the largest series of patients reported in the UK.

► This report reflects the more liberal use of intraoperative blood salvage in obstetric patients in the United Kingdom. Intraoperative blood salvage during cesarean delivery is widely regarded as safe in the United Kingdom and is gaining acceptance in the United States, although its practical utility remains a matter of some dispute. The American Society of Anesthesiologists Practice Guidelines for Obstetric Anesthesia recommend that "in cases of intractable hemorrhage when banked blood is not available or the patient refuses banked blood, intraoperative cell salvage should be considered if available."[1] In contrast, the authors of this report decided to use cell salvage during cesarean delivery "whenever the blood loss was likely to necessitate blood transfusion." The authors practice in an obstetric unit with 7200 deliveries per year, and their hospital "does not contain any of the specialties that commonly use cell salvage." Therefore, they wanted to use blood salvage sufficiently often to facilitate staff training and maintenance of staff skills. Despite the liberal use of intraoperative blood salvage, the authors did not observe a significant decline in the rate of heterologous transfusion.

D. H. Chestnut, MD

Reference

1. American Society of Anesthesiologists Task Force on Obstetric Anesthesia. Practice guidelines for obstetric anesthesia. *Anesthesiol.* 2007;106:843-863.

Impact of pelvic arterial embolization for intractable postpartum hemorrhage on fertility

Fiori O, Deux J-F, Kambale J-C, et al (Univ of Pierre et Marie Curie, Paris; Henri Mondor Hosp, Créteil; Tenon Hosp, Paris)

Am J Obstet Gynecol 200:384.e1-384.e4, 2009

Objective.—This study was to determine the long-term outcomes of arterial pelvic embolization for intractable postpartum hemorrhage and particularly its effect on menses, fertility, and outcomes of subsequent pregnancies.

Study Design.—Fifty-six consecutive patients who underwent emergency pelvic arterial embolization for severe postpartum hemorrhage between April 1995 and July 2005 were included in the study. Patients were contacted to obtain information about menses and fertility after pelvic arterial embolization.

Results.—Thirty-four women (61.8%) were successfully contacted. One patient had a hysterectomy. Thirty women (91%) reported regular menses. Thirteen women (38.3%) had a total of 20 spontaneous pregnancies. Eight pregnancies ended during the first trimester. The 12 other pregnancies (60%) were all normal and all patients delivered vaginally healthy babies with normal weight for gestational age.

Conclusion.—The current study suggests that fertility is not adversely affected by arterial pelvic embolization for intractable postpartum hemorrhage and that women can conceive after the procedure with normal pregnancy outcomes.

► In this series, all women resumed menses after uterine artery embolization, and most (91%) women reported that their menses were unchanged. Among the 15 women who desired further pregnancy, only 2 patients attempted to get pregnant but failed to conceive. Among the 12 pregnancies that resulted in liveborn children, recurrence of postpartum hemorrhage occurred in only one case, and bleeding was controlled by intravenous infusion of the prostaglandin E2 analogue sulprostone.

D. H. Chestnut, MD

Impact of a comprehensive patient safety strategy on obstetric adverse events

Pettker CM, Thung SF, Norwitz ER, et al (Yale Univ School of Medicine; et al)
Am J Obstet Gynecol 200:492.e1-492.e8, 2009

Objective.—We implemented a comprehensive strategy to track and reduce adverse events.

Study Design.—We incrementally introduced multiple patient safety interventions from September 2004 through November 2006 at a university-based obstetrics service. This initiative included outside expert review, protocol standardization, the creation of a patient safety nurse position and patient safety committee, and training in team skills and fetal heart monitoring interpretation. We prospectively tracked 10 obstetrics-specific outcome. The Adverse Outcome Index, an expression of the number of deliveries with at least 1 of the 10 adverse outcomes per total deliveries, was analyzed for trend.

Results.—Our interventions significantly reduced the Adverse Outcome Index (linear regression, $r^2 = 0.50$; $P = .01$) (overall mean, 2.50%). Concurrent with these improvements, we saw clinically significant improvements in safety climate as measured by validated safety attitude surveys.

Conclusion.—A systematic strategy to decrease obstetric adverse events can have a significant impact on patient safety.

▶ The authors noted that there is a relative paucity of literature regarding monitoring and preventing obstetric adverse events, despite the fact that childbirth accounts for 4 million hospitalizations every year in the United States. Of interest to anesthesia care providers, the authors initiated a team-training program modeled on crew resource management programs used by the airline and defense industries. Led by their patient safety nurse, "these 4-hour seminars included videos, lectures, and role playing, and always integrated a mix of individuals within the obstetric team." Attendees were given instruction in the "shared mental model for communication," which "is an organized way for team members to conceptualize how a team works and to predict and understand how their team members will behave to improve overall team performance." Attendees also received instruction in "structured communication/debriefing (situation, background, assessment, recommendation), communication key words, the 2-challenge rule, the chain of command, and elements of an effective hand off of care." The authors noted that "initial costs of the program were estimated at $210,000, with ongoing yearly costs of $150,000," but they also noted that "this investment is dwarfed by the average payment ($500,000-1,900,000) for just 1 obstetric liability claim."

D. H. Chestnut, MD

Changing trends in peripartum hysterectomy over the last 4 decades

Flood KM, Said S, Geary M, et al (Royal College of Surgeons in Ireland)

Am J Obstet Gynecol 200:632.e1-632.e6, 2009

Objective.—The purpose of this study was to identify changing trends in peripartum hysterectomy (PH) in a single large obstetric population over the last 40 years.

Study Design.—A retrospective cohort study was performed from 1966-2005 of patients who had PH in any of the 3 Dublin obstetric hospitals. Cases were identified, and details were obtained from the combined patient databases of each hospital.

Results.—There were 872,379 deliveries during the study period, among which 358 women underwent PH (0.4/1000 deliveries). In a comparison of the study decades 1966-1975 with 1996-2005, PH decreased from 0.9 per 1000 deliveries to 0.2 of 1000 deliveries. Although the overall cesarean delivery rate has increased from 6-19% during these 2 decades, the percentage of PH that occurs in the setting of a previous cesarean delivery has increased from 27-57% ($P < .00001$). Indications for PH have changed significantly in this time period, with "uterine rupture" as the indication for PH decreasing from 40.5-9.3% ($P < .0001$) and placenta accreta as the indication increasing significantly from 5.4-46.5% ($P < .00001$).

Conclusion.—PH has decreased over the last 4 decades. However, alongside the rising cesarean delivery rate, there has been a marked increase in the incidence of placenta accreta (Fig 3, Tables 1 and 2).

▶ Readers should note that this retrospective cohort study assessed outcome for 872 379 deliveries over a 40-year period in 3 obstetric hospitals in Dublin,

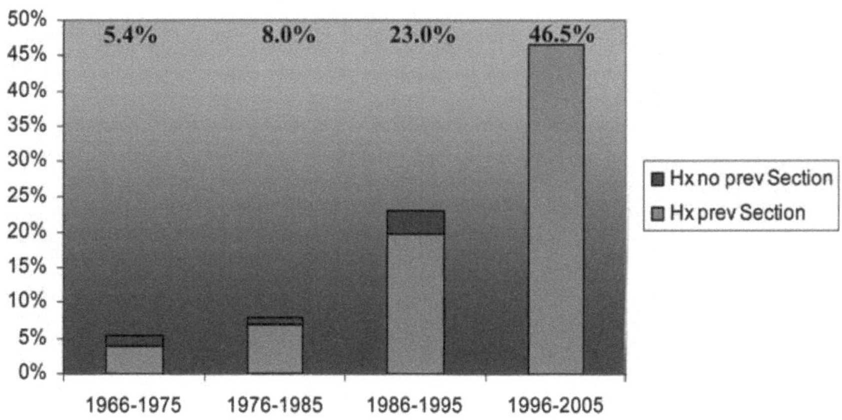

FIGURE 3.—Indication of placenta accreta that is associated with history of cesarean section delivery. *Hx no prev Section*, no history of cesarean section delivery; *Hx prev Section*, history of cesarean section delivery. Flood. Changing trends in peripartum hysterectomy. Am J Obstet Gynecol 2009. (Reprinted from Flood KM, Said S, Geary M, et al. Changing trends in peripartum hysterectomy over the last 4 decades. *Am J Obstet Gynecol.* 2009;200:632.e1-632.e6, with permission from Elsevier.)

TABLE 1.—CS Rate, Incidence of PH, and PH with a History of CS Per Decade

Decade	CS/Total Delivery (%)	PH Incidence (n)	PH with History of CS (n)
1966-1975	6	165 (0.85/1000)	44 (26.7%)
1976-1985	7	104 (0.44/1000)	33 (31.7%)
1986-1995	11	40 (0.2/1000)	18 (45.0%)
1996-2005	19	49 (0.2/1000)	28 (57.1%)
1966-2005	11	358 (0.4/1000)	123 (34.4%)
Comparison of 1966-1975 with 1996-2005	$P < .00001$	$P < .00000$	$P < .00001$

CS, cesarean section delivery; *PH*, peripartum hysterectomy.

TABLE 2.—Peripartum Hysterectomy Indications Per Decade

Decade	Cases: Known Indication (n)	Hemorrhage	Rupture	Accreta	Previa	Cancer	Elective	Other
1966-1975 (%)	148	24	41	5	6	1	14	14
1976-1985 (%)	98	48	26	8	5	1	4	8
1986-1995 (%)	31	41	3	24	13	16	0	3
1996-2005 (%)	43	30	9	47	12	0	0	2
1966-2005 (n)	320	108	90	43	24	8	24	23
Comparison of 1966-1975 with 1996-2005		$P = .24$	$P < .0001$	$P < .00001$				

Ireland. Although the cesarean delivery rate more than tripled over the 4 decades of the study (from 6% in 1966-1975 to 19% in 1996-2005), this rate remains below that in the United States. The authors noted that although the incidence of peripartum hysterectomy (PH) has decreased over the years, the proportion of peripartum hysterectomies performed in women with a history of previous cesarean delivery has increased significantly (Table 1). The authors noted that the association between the rising cesarean delivery rate and the incidence of PH among patients with a history of previous cesarean delivery can be attributed mostly to the occurrence of placenta accreta (Fig 3, Table 2). As in other recent studies, these authors observed that abnormal placentation (ie, placenta previa and/or placenta accreta) constitutes the primary indication for PH in contemporary obstetric practice. The authors expressed concern that with the worldwide increase in cesarean delivery rates, "there will be a significant domino effect involving increased deliveries after [cesarean delivery] and increased morbidly adherent placental cases..., and ... there will be a rise in the number of obstetric hysterectomies required in the future because of placenta accreta alongside significant maternal morbidity."

D. H. Chestnut, MD

Fetal and Neonatal Considerations

Neonatal Outcomes After Elective Cesarean Delivery

Kamath BD, Todd JK, Glazner JE, et al (Univ of Colorado School of Medicine; The Children's Hosp, Denver, CO; Colorado School of Public Health, Denver)
Obstet Gynecol 113:1231-1238, 2009

Objective.—To examine the outcomes of neonates born by elective repeat cesarean delivery compared with vaginal birth after cesarean (VBAC) in women with one prior cesarean delivery and to evaluate the cost differences between elective repeat cesarean and VBAC.

Methods.—We conducted a retrospective cohort study of 672 women with one prior cesarean delivery and a singleton pregnancy at or after 37 weeks of gestation. Women were grouped according to their intention to have an elective repeat cesarean or a VBAC (successful or failed). The primary outcome was neonatal intensive care unit (NICU) admission and measures of respiratory morbidity.

Results.—Neonates born by cesarean delivery had higher NICU admission rates compared with the VBAC group (9.3% compared with 4.9%, $P = .025$) and higher rates of oxygen supplementation for delivery room resuscitation (41.5% compared with 23.2%, $P < .01$) and after NICU admission (5.8% compared with 2.4%, $P < .028$). Neonates born by VBAC required the least delivery room resuscitation with oxygen, whereas neonates delivered after failed VBAC required the greatest degree of delivery room resuscitation. The costs of elective repeat cesarean were significantly greater than VBAC. However, failed VBAC accounted for the most expensive total birth experience (delivery and NICU use).

Conclusion.—In comparison with vaginal birth after cesarean, neonates born after elective repeat cesarean delivery have significantly higher rates of respiratory morbidity and NICU-admission and longer length of hospital stay.

▶ The authors noted that their observations are consistent with other studies that demonstrated higher rates of neonatal respiratory morbidity after elective repeat cesarean delivery, including respiratory distress syndrome, transient tachypnea of the newborn, persistent pulmonary hypertension, and need for supplemental oxygen. The authors hypothesized that "the catecholamine surge that occurs during labor likely plays an important role in both clearance of fetal lung fluid and glycemic control after birth." The authors cautioned that "given the increasing rates of primary cesarean delivery and the concomitant decrease in vaginal birth after cesareans (VBACs) ..., we must consider the risks that primary cesarean delivery places on a woman's subsequent deliveries and subsequent neonates." They concluded that "this argues for greater selectivity in performing a cesarean delivery in the first place, and certainly a greater need for counseling before a primary elective cesarean delivery."

D. H. Chestnut, MD

Anesthesia for Cesarean Delivery and Learning Disabilities in a Population-based Birth Cohort

Sprung J, Flick RP, Wilder RT, et al (Mayo Clinic, Rochester, MN)
Anesthesiology 111:302-310, 2009

Background.—Anesthetics administered to immature brains may cause histopathological changes and long-term behavioral abnormalities. The association between perinatal exposure to anesthetics during Cesarean delivery (CD) and development of learning disabilities (LD) was determined in a population-based birth cohort.

Methods.—The educational and medical records of all children born to mothers residing in five townships of Olmsted County, Minnesota from 1976–1982 and remaining in the community at age 5 were reviewed to identify those with LDs. Cox proportional hazards regression was used to compare rates of LD between children delivered vaginally and *via* CD (with general or regional anesthesia).

Results.—Of the 5,320 children in this cohort, 497 were delivered via CD (under general anesthesia n = 193, and regional anesthesia n = 304). The incidence of LD depended on mode of delivery ($P = 0.050$, adjusted for sex, birth weight, gestational age, exposure to anesthesia before age 4 yr, and maternal education). LD risk was similar in children delivered by vagina or CD with general anesthesia, but was reduced in children receiving CD with regional anesthesia (hazard ratio = 0.64, 95% confidence interval 0.44 to 0.92; $P = 0.017$ for comparison of CD under regional anesthesia compared to vaginal delivery).

Conclusion.—Children exposed to general or regional anesthesia during CD are not more likely to develop LD compared to children delivered vaginally, suggesting that brief perinatal exposure to anesthetic drugs does not adversely affect long-term neurodevelopmental outcomes. The risk of LD may be lower in children delivered by CD whose mothers received regional anesthesia.

▶ Recent reports have highlighted the possible long-term effects of anesthesia on central nervous system structure and function, especially in patients exposed to anesthesia at the extremes of age. Studies performed in vitro and in laboratory animals have demonstrated that some anesthetic drugs can cause apoptosis and other degenerative changes in the young immature brain. The authors of this study recently demonstrated that "repeated, but not single, exposure to anesthesia before the age of 4 yrs is associated with an approximately 2-fold increase in the incidence of learning disabilities (LD)."[1] The authors acknowledged that their data "could not distinguish whether exposure to anesthesia itself increases the risk of LD, or whether the need for anesthesia represents a marker for unidentified confounders that promote LD." It is reassuring that, in this study, children exposed to either general or regional anesthesia during cesarean delivery (CD) were not more likely to develop LD compared with children delivered vaginally, "suggesting that brief perinatal exposure to anesthetic drugs does not adversely affect long-term neurodevelopmental outcomes." An unexpected finding was evidence suggesting that the risk of LD was lower in children delivered via CD under regional anesthesia compared with children delivered vaginally. The authors appropriately cautioned that "such a result from an observational study can only be viewed as hypothesis generating and needs to be confirmed (or refuted) [in a subsequent study], especially considering the possibility that undergoing CD with regional analgesia is simply a marker for unidentified confounders that may explain the differential risk for LD between groups."

D. H. Chestnut, MD

Reference

1. Wilder RT, Flick RP, Sprung J, et al. Early exposure to anesthesia and learning disabilities in a population-based birth cohort. *Anesthesiology.* 2009;110:796-804.

Special Situations in Obstetric Anesthesia

In vitro effects of propofol on gravid human myometrium

Thind AS, Turner RJ (Prince of Wales Hosp, Sydney, New South Wales, Australia)

Anaesth Intensive Care 36:802-806, 2008

The aim of this study was to evaluate the direct effect of propofol (di-isopropyl phenol) on the contractile properties of gravid human uterine muscle.

Six specimens of uterine muscle were obtained from term parturients undergoing elective lower segment caesarean section. Small strips (1×2×12 mm) of muscle were prepared and suspended in an organ bath containing oxygenated Kreb's solution at 36.5°C. Following preparation, spontaneous regular contractions developed at a rate of one contraction every six to 10 minutes. Force of contraction was recorded continuously using an isometric tension transducer. Following baseline measurements, propofol was introduced into the bath at concentrations corresponding to 2 μg/ml, 5 μg/ml and 8 μg/ml. The specimens were also exposed to intralipid in concentrations equivalent to that found in the 8 μg/ml solution of propofol to determine whether this additive influenced uterine contractility. Contractility (defined as area under the tension/time curve) was decreased to 89 ± 6.5% of control at 2 μg/ml, 53 ± 4.3% at 5 μg/ml and 45 ± 4.1% at 8 μg/ml. This decrease in contractility was statistically significant at concentrations >2 μg/ml. Intralipid did not significantly affect uterine contractility. The results of this study show that propofol decreases isolated human uterine muscle contractility in a dose-dependent manner.

▶ The authors noted that the mechanism by which propofol decreases isolated human uterine muscle contractility remains unclear. The authors also noted that "propofol seems to cause a lesser reduction in uterine contractility than the volatile anaesthetics, because sevoflurane causes a decrease in contractility to

50% of control at 0.94 minimum alveolar concentration (MAC), and at 3.5 minimum alveolar concentration it abolishes all uterine activity." Finally, and perhaps most important, the authors acknowledged that this was an in vitro study, and they "do not know what the effects of plasma [protein] binding will have on the effect of contractility in vivo."

D. H. Chestnut, MD

Relationship Between Malpractice Litigation Pressure and Rates of Cesarean Section and Vaginal Birth After Cesarean Section

Yang YT, Mello MM, Subramanian SV, et al (George Mason Univ, Fairfax, VA; Harvard School of Public Health, Boston, MA; et al)

Med Care 47:234-242, 2009

Background.—Since the 1990s, nationwide rates of vaginal birth after cesarean section (VBAC) have decreased sharply and rates of cesarean section have increased sharply. Both trends are consistent with clinical behavior aimed at reducing obstetricians' exposure to malpractice litigation.

Objective.—To estimate the effects of malpractice pressure on rates of VBAC and cesarean section.

Research Design, Subjects, Measures.—We used state-level longitudinal mixed-effects regression models to examine data from the Natality Detail File on births in the United States (1991–2003). Malpractice pressure was measured by liability insurance premiums and tort reforms. Outcome measures were rates of VBAC, cesarean section, and primary cesarean section.

Results.—Malpractice premiums were positively associated with rates of cesarean section ($\beta = 0.15$, $P = 0.02$) and primary cesarean section ($\beta = 0.16$, $P = 0.009$), and negatively associated with VBAC rates ($\beta = -0.35$, $P = 0.01$). These estimates imply that a $10,000 decrease in premiums for obstetrician-gynecologists would be associated with an increase of 0.35 percentage points (1.45%) in the VBAC rate and decreases of 0.15 and 0.16 percentage points (0.7% and 1.18%) in the rates of cesarean section and primary cesarean section, respectively; this would correspond to approximately 1600 more VBACs, 6000 fewer cesarean sections, and 3600 fewer primary cesarean sections nationwide in 2003. Two types of tort reform—caps on noneconomic damages and pretrial screening panels—were associated with lower rates of cesarean section and higher rates of VBAC.

Conclusions.—The liability environment influences choice of delivery method in obstetrics. The effects are not large, but reduced litigation pressure would likely lead to decreases in the total number cesarean sections and total delivery costs.

▶ The authors observed that states with relatively high liability insurance premiums had lower rates of vaginal birth after cesarean delivery (VBAC) and higher rates of cesarean delivery than states with lower liability insurance premiums. Further, 2 types of tort reform—caps on noneconomic damages and pretrial screening panels—were associated with higher rates of VBAC and lower rates of cesarean delivery. However, the predicted effects of a $10 000 reduction in liability insurance premiums were somewhat modest. The authors listed several limitations to their study. They acknowledged that they could not account for the increased patient demand for elective cesarean delivery, and they acknowledged that patient demand for elective cesarean delivery is "reportedly growing as women increasingly seek convenience, predictability, and avoidance of rare but catastrophic risks associated with normal childbirth." Also, they acknowledged that 1 possible challenge to their conclusions is that VBAC may have been attempted too often in states with low liability insurance premiums, and that "malpractice pressure may actually have pushed clinicians in high-liability states toward improved quality of care." However, they also stated that there is little published evidence that cesarean delivery is "underused."

D. H. Chestnut, MD

A Randomized Controlled Trial of Pudendal Nerve Block for Pain Relief After Episiotomy

Aissaoui Y, Bruyère R, Mustapha H, et al (Centre Hospitalier d'Auxerre, France; et al)

Anesth Analg 107:625-629, 2008

Background.—Pain from episiotomy or perineal tears during childbirth is associated with significant pain in the postpartum period. We performed this randomized, double-blind, controlled trial to investigate the efficacy of nerve stimulator-guided unilateral pudendal nerve block for pain relief after episiotomy.

Methods.—Forty women who gave birth vaginally with mediolateral episiotomy were randomized to receive pudendal nerve block with 15 mL of either ropivacaine 7.5 mg/mL (pudendal group) or normal saline (control group) after repair of the episiotomy. Episiotomy pain was assessed with a visual analog scale at rest at 3, 6, 12, 24, and 48 h postepisiotomy and during activities (walking and sitting). Breakthrough pain (visual analog scale >30 mm) was treated with niflumic acid suppositories 700 mg every 12 h. The primary outcome variables were pain scores at rest and during activities over 48 h postpartum.

Results.—Demographic and obstetric characteristics were not different between groups. Successful pudendal nerve stimulation was achieved in all patients. Patients in the pudendal group reported significantly lower pain scores at rest than those in the control group at 3, 6, 12, 24, and 48 h after delivery ($P < 0.05$). They also reported better analgesia while sitting and walking ($P < 0.05$). Additional analgesia was required by three patients (15%) in the pudendal group versus 17 patients (85%) in the placebo group ($P < 0.001$).

Conclusion.—This study demonstrates that nerve stimulator-guided unilateral pudendal nerve block with ropivacaine 7.5 mg/mL is associated with decreased pain and need for additional analgesics during the first 48 h postepisiotomy.

► Pudendal nerve block (PNB) is often performed before vaginal delivery in patients who do not have neuraxial anesthesia, although its efficacy varies and the failure rate is high. The authors of this study stated that the efficacy of PNB is improved by the use of nerve stimulation. Readers should note 2 important methodologic details of this study. First, all enrolled patients underwent a mediolateral episiotomy; thus, these patients received a unilateral PNB. Second, all of the study subjects received epidural analgesia for delivery, and the PNB was performed after repair of the episiotomy. The authors stated that "surprisingly... the duration of pain relief in the pudendal group exceeded the expected duration of ropivacaine (16-18 h)." Further, the authors observed a difference between groups in pain scores as late as 48 hours after delivery. The authors suggested that "the observed duration of postoperative analgesia may have resulted from prevention of peripheral and central hyperalgesia by adequate treatment of pain." The authors then suggested that future studies should assess whether PNB might prevent chronic postpartum perineal pain.

D. H. Chestnut, MD

Outcomes following cholecystectomy in pregnant and nonpregnant women

Kuy S, Roman SA, Desai R, et al (Yale Univ School of Medicine, New Haven, CT; Med College of Wisconsin, Madison)

Surgery 146:358-366, 2009

Background.—This study is the first population-based measurement of outcomes after cholecystectomy during pregnancy.

Methods.—We identified all pregnant women who underwent cholecystectomy in the Healthcare Cost and Utilization Project-Nationwide Inpatient Sample, 1996–2006. Outcomes were fetal, maternal, and surgical complications, length of stay (LOS), and hospital cost. Pregnant and nonpregnant women were compared to examine the effects of pregnancy on laparoscopic cholecystectomy outcomes.

Results.—A total of 9,714 pregnant women underwent cholecystectomy (laparoscopic, 89%). Maternal and fetal complication rates were 4.3% and 5.8%, respectively. Pregnant women who underwent laparoscopic cholecystectomy compared to pregnant women who underwent open procedures had higher rates of surgical (19% vs 10%), maternal (9% vs 4%), and fetal (11% vs 5%) complications; longer LOS (6 vs 4 days); and higher cost ($13,198 vs $9,229), all $P < .0001$. High-volume surgeons were associated with lower rates of surgical (10% vs 13%; $P < .05$), maternal (1% vs 14%), and fetal (4% vs 10%) complications; shorter

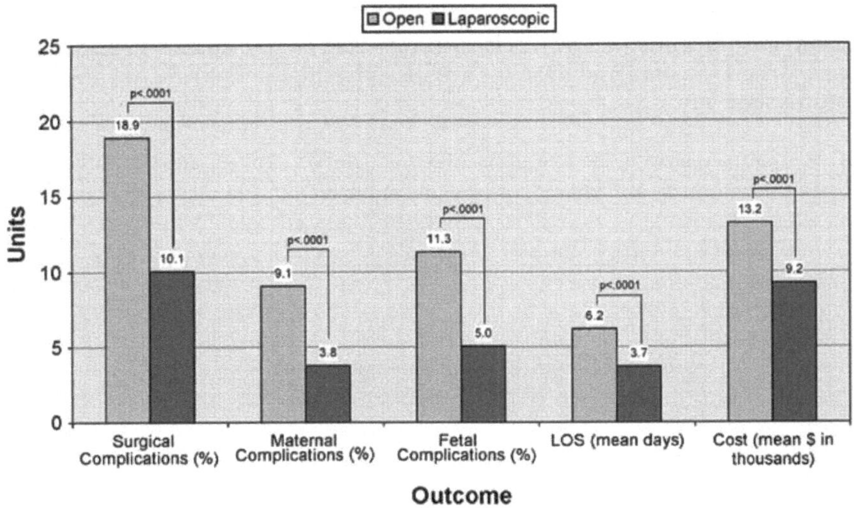

FIGURE 1.—Outcomes after cholecystectomy in pregnant women based on type of procedure. *LOS*, Length of stay. (Reprinted from Kuy S, Roman SA, Desai R, et al. Outcomes following cholecystectomy in pregnant and nonpregnant women. *Surgery.* 2009;146:358-366, with permission from Elsevier.)

TABLE 2.—Significant Predictors of Outcome in Pregnant Women after Cholecystectomy

	Surgical Complications OR (95% CI)	Maternal Complications OR (95% CI)	Fetal Complications OR (95% CI)	Adjusted LOS OR (95% CI)	Adjusted Cost OR (95% CI)
Variable					
Type of cholecystectomy					
Open	2.1 (1.8,2.5)	1.9 (1.4,2.47)	1.9 (1.5,2.4)	1.5 (1.5,1.6)	1.3 (1.2,1.4)
Laparoscopic*	1	1	1	1	1
Surgeon volume					
<75th percentile*	—	1	1	1	1
≥75th percentile	—	0.06 (0.04,0.09)	0.4 (0.3,0.5)	0.9 (0.8,0.9)	0.9 (0.8,0.9)
Insurance					
Private/HMO*	1	—	1	1	1
Medicaid	1.4 (1.2,1.6)	—	1.2 (1.0,1.5)	1.1 (1.1,1.1)	1.1 (1.0,1.1)
No. of biliary diagnoses					
1*	1	—	—	1	1
2	1.4 (1.2–1.6)	—	—	1.4 (1.3–1.4)	1.3 (1.3–1.4)
≥3	3.5 (2.3–5.3)		—	1.7 (1.5–1.9)	1.7 (1.4–1.9)

OR, Odds ratio; *CI*, confidence interval; *LOS*, length of stay.
*Reference groups = laparoscopic, surgeon volume < 75th percentile, private/HMO insurance, 1 biliary diagnosis.

LOS (4 vs 5 days); and lower cost ($8,365 vs $10,350), all $P < .0001$. Patients with Medicaid coverage were associated with higher rates of surgical complications (13% vs 9%), longer LOS (4.3 vs 3.7 days), and higher cost ($10,403 vs $9,037), all $P < .0001$. On multivariable analysis, these factors remained independent predictors of outcome. Pregnancy was associated with longer LOS and higher cost.

Conclusion.—Complications of cholecystectomy during pregnancy are significant, with disparities based on modifiable variables (Fig 1 and Table 2).

► This publication illustrates the importance of reading the entire article. Unfortunately, the abstract incorrectly states that women who underwent laparoscopic cholecystectomy had higher rates of surgical, maternal, and fetal complications than those who underwent open cholecystectomy. However, the opposite was true (Fig 1, Table 2)! In this study, "pregnant women undergoing open cholecystectomy were more likely to have surgical, maternal, and fetal complications, longer length of stay (LOS), and higher hospital costs than pregnant women undergoing laparoscopic procedures." The authors concluded that "data from this large population-based study show [that] open cholecystectomy during pregnancy is an independent predictor for worse outcomes." The authors acknowledged that they could not identify the reasons for choosing an open approach, such as "history of previous surgery, gangrenous gallbladder, or trimester of pregnancy." The authors cited guidelines published by the Society of American Gastrointestinal and Endoscopic Surgeons (SAGES), which states that "laparoscopic cholecystectomy is the treatment of choice in the pregnant patient with gallbladder disease, regardless of trimester."

For further reading on this subject I suggest an article by SAGES.[1]

D. H. Chestnut, MD

Reference

1. Society of American Gastrointestinal and Endoscopic Surgeons. Guidelines for diagnosis, treatment, and use of laparoscopy for surgical problems during pregnancy, http://www.sages.org; 2007.

11 Pain Management

Acute Pain Management

Cost sharing and the initiation of drug therapy for the chronically ill

Solomon MD, Goldman DP, Joyce GF, et al (Stanford Univ School of Medicine, CA)

Arch Intern Med 169:740-748, 2009

Background.—Increased cost sharing reduces utilization of prescription drugs, but little evidence demonstrates how this reduction occurs or the factors associated with price sensitivity.

Methods.—We conducted a retrospective cohort study of older adults with employer-provided drug coverage from 1997 to 2002 from 31 different health plans. We measured the time until initiation of medical therapy for 17 183 patients with newly diagnosed hypertension, diabetes, or hypercholesterolemia.

Results.—For all study conditions, higher copayments were associated with delayed initiation of therapy. In survival models, doubling copayments resulted in large reductions in the predicted proportion of patients initiating pharmacotherapy at 1 and 5 years after diagnosis: for hypertension, 54.8% vs 39.9% at 1 year and 81.6% vs 66.2% at 5 years ($P < .001$); for hypercholesterolemia, 40.2% vs 31.1% at 1 year and 64.3% vs 53.8% at 5 years ($P < .002$); and for diabetes, 45.8% vs 40.0% at 1 year and 69.3% vs 62.9% at 5 years ($P < .04$). However, patients' rate of initiation and sensitivity to copayments strongly depended on their prior experience with prescription drugs. Those without prior drug use (26.1%, 10.4%, and 12.9%) initiated later (833, >1170, and >1402 days later in median time until initiation) and were far more price sensitive (increase of 34.5%, 20.1%, and 27.2% remaining untreated after 5 years when copayments doubled) than those with a history of drug use among patients with newly diagnosed hypertension, hypercholesterolemia, and diabetes, respectively. These results were robust to a wide range of sensitivity analyses.

Conclusions.—High cost sharing delays the initiation of drug therapy for patients newly diagnosed with chronic disease. This effect is greater among patients who lack experience with prescription drugs. Policy makers and physicians should consider the effects of benefits design on patient behavior to encourage the adoption of necessary care.

▶ One of the things that I learned by questioning my mother-in-law who lives in an area with a lot of retired folks in Florida is that many of them do not start their medicines, even when they have Part D drug coverage, if there is a co-pay involved. Many of them wait until they have enough money or wait to see if the doctor asks them about it on the next visit—and many of them ask for larger doses of the same medicine, and then split them in half to take them in a more efficient way. Even when I looked at the Cleveland Clinic drugs costs in our own retirees, and started questioning some of the retirees, even those who only have to pay $4.00 in a co-pay often don't start their medicines very promptly, which increases hospitalization rates. Yes, even when the co-pay is as small as $4.00, and especially when it is much more for non-generic drugs. This helps explain to me why so many pharmaceutical companies have started advertising that the first prescription is at a discount. We are getting patients involved in websites that increase adherence to drug use. This is obviously a major problem for society, as a lot of our hospitalization costs may be, in fact, due to not taking prescribed medicines.

M. F. Roizen, MD

Chest Tube–Delivered Bupivacaine Improves Pain and Decreases Opioid Use After Thoracoscopy

Demmy TL, Nwogu C, Solan P, et al (Univ of New York, Buffalo)

Ann Thorac Surg 87:1040-1047, 2009

Background.—This study compared a simplified method of intrapleural bupivacaine administration with traditional analgesic therapy to decrease postoperative pain and opioid usage in patients after thoracoscopy.

Methods.—Thirty patients who had non-rib-spreading thoracoscopic operations under general anesthesia were prospectively randomized to no local anesthetic infusion (control), intermittent bolus (30 mL every 6 hours), or continuous infusion (5 mL/h). Bupivacaine (0.25%) was delivered through the pleural infusion channel of a specially designed single silicone 28F chest tube. Total intravenous fentanyl patient-controlled analgesia (boluses with basal rate) infused in the first 24 hours postoperatively was the designated primary study end point. Escalations of analgesic therapy, including ketorolac administration, were standardized across all groups. Nurses assessed pain control at onset and every 6 hours by visual analog pain scales (VAPS, 100 mm). VAPS were repeated 10 minutes later to assess any opioid or bupivacaine bolus effects.

Results.—No study-related adverse events occurred. Compared with controls, pooled VAPS scores and 24-hour fentanyl consumption were significantly lower for the intermittent and continuous administration groups (1753 vs 1180 vs 1177 μg/24 h, respective median; $p = 0.04$)

Early (6-hour) VAPS analgesic responses were more certain for intermittent (10 of 10) and continuous (10 of 10) patients than controls (7 of 10, $p = .04$). Five continuous patients successfully maintained VAPS scores below 20 mm throughout the study vs 3 intermittent and 2 controls ($p = .045$).

Conclusions.—Intermittent or continuous intrapleural bupivacaine infused through the chest tube reliably reduces postoperative pain and 24-hour opioid usage in thoracoscopy patients.

▶ Interpleural bupivacaine has been shown to provide effective analgesia for patients who have undergone thoracotomy or upper abdominal incisions. Among thoracotomy patients, the presence of blood or effusions in the pleural space may interfere with the analgesic effect of the local anesthetic. This technique has therefore been largely supplanted by paravertebral or epidural blocks. However, for thoracoscopy it appears to be a reasonable alternative that, in this study, was associated with significant reduction in opioid use. For patients undergoing other types of thoracic and upper abdominal procedures, it is still a good choice for patients for whom epidural analgesia may be impractical or contraindicated.

S. E. Abram, MD

Lack of Analgesia by Oral Standardized Cannabis Extract on Acute Inflammatory Pain and Hyperalgesia in Volunteers

Kraft B, Frickey NA, Kaufmann RM, et al (Med Univ of Vienna, Austria; et al)
Anesthesiology 109:101-110, 2008

Background.—Cannabinoid-induced analgesia was shown in animal studies of acute inflammatory and neuropathic pain. In humans, controlled clinical trials with Δ^9-tetrahydrocannabinol or other cannabinoids demonstrated analgesic efficacy in chronic pain syndromes, whereas the data in acute pain were less conclusive. Therefore, the aim of this study was to investigate the effects of oral cannabis extract in two different human models of acute inflammatory pain and hyperalgesia.

Methods.—The authors conducted a double-blind, crossover study in 18 healthy female volunteers. Capsules containing Δ^9- tetrahydrocannabinol–standardized cannabis extract or active placebo were orally administered. A circular sunburn spot was induced at one upper leg. Heat and electrical pain thresholds were determined at the erythema, the area of secondary hyperalgesia, and the contralateral leg. Intradermal capsaicin-evoked pain and areas of flare and secondary hyperalgesia were measured. Primary outcome parameters were heat pain thresholds in the sunburn erythema and the capsaicin-evoked area of secondary hyperalgesia. Secondary measures were electrical pain thresholds, sunburn-induced secondary hyperalgesia, and capsaicin-induced pain.

TABLE 2.—Side Effects

Side Effect	Self-Rated VAS Cannabis	Self-Rated VAS Placebo	Observer VAS Cannabis	Observer VAS Placebo
Drowsiness	57.3 ± 20.8*	33.6 ± 23.4	67.2 ± 16.9*	40.4 ± 20.2
Sedation	79.1 ± 17.2*	12.2 ± 18.4	59.9 ± 26.5*	9.5 ± 11.2
Euphoria	38.2 ± 35.7	1.0 ± 0.8	25.3 ± 23.3	1.9 ± 4.7
Nausea	27.7 ± 30.5	1.6 ± 2.8	20.5 ± 30.3	0.8 ± 1.0
Dry mouth	70.9 ± 23.9*	4.5 ± 6.1	47.9 ± 27.9*	3.6 ± 4.3
Vertigo	65.0 ± 32.3*	2.3 ± 3.0	48.8 ± 31.8*	2.0 ± 4.2

Data are presented as mean (difference from baseline) ±SD for the whole 8-h study period (n = 17).
Placebo = 5 mg diazepam; VAS = visual analog scale (0–100).
*$P < 0.05$.

Results.—Cannabis extract did not affect heat pain thresholds in the sunburn model. Electrical thresholds (250 Hz) were significantly lower compared with baseline and placebo. In the capsaicin model, the area of secondary hyperalgesia, flare, and spontaneous pain were not altered.

Conclusion.—To conclude, no analgesic or antihyperalgesic activity of cannabis extract was found in the experiments. Moreover, the results even point to the development of a hyperalgesic state under cannabinoids. Together with previous data, the current results suggest that cannabinoids are not effective analgesics for the treatment of acute nociceptive pain in humans (Table 2).

► In this well-designed, placebo-controlled human study, oral cannabinoids had no analgesic or antihyperalgesic effects on experimentally induced pain (Figs 2-5 in the original article). These results are at odds with several animal studies and may reflect species differences. Some studies of the analgesic effect of oral, sublingual, and smoked cannabinoids in patients with chronic pain have shown beneficial effects. On the other hand, there is almost no way to blind participants of controlled studies, given the unique psychopharmacology of these substances. As the authors have suggested, first-pass metabolism of some of the components of the cannabis extract may have affected the result, which may be different for sublingual or smoked preparations. Nevertheless, there was substantial uptake of drug, as indicated by the fairly high incidence of side effects compared with placebo (Table 2). The high incidence of nausea is surprising given the antiemetic properties of cannabis.

S. E. Abram, MD

Morphine With Adjuvant Ketamine vs Higher Dose of Morphine Alone for Immediate Postthoracotomy Analgesia

Nesher N, Ekstein MP, Paz Y, et al (Tel Aviv Univ, Israel)

Chest 136:245-252, 2009

Background.—Thoracotomy is associated with severe pain. We hypothesized that the concomitant use of a subanesthetic dose of ketamine plus a two-third–standard morphine dose might provide more effective analgesia with fewer side effects than a standard morphine dose for early pain control.

Methods.—We conducted a 6-month randomized, double-blind study in patients undergoing thoracotomy for minimally invasive direct coronary artery bypass or for lung tumor resection. After extubation, when objectively awake (≥ 5/10 visual analogue scale [VAS]) and complaining of pain (≥ 5/10 VAS), patients were connected to patient-controlled IV analgesia delivering 1.5 mg of morphine plus saline solution (MO) or 1.0 mg of morphine plus a 5-mg ketamine bolus (MK), with a 7-min lockout time. Rescue IM diclofenac, 75 mg, was available. Follow-up lasted 4 h.

Results.—Forty-one patients completed the study. MO patients ($n = 20$) used 6.8 ± 1.9 mg/h (mean ± SD) and 5.5 ± 3.6 mg/h of morphine during the first and second hours, respectively; MK patients ($n = 21$) used 3.7 ± 1.2 mg/h and 2.8 ± 2.3 mg/h, respectively ($p < 0.01$). The 4-h activation rate of the device was double in the MO patients than in the MK patients (66 ± 54 vs 28 ± 20, $p < 0.001$). The maximal self-rated pain score was 5.6 ± 1.0 for the MO group vs 3.7 ± 0.7 for the MK group ($p < 0.01$). Four MO patients vs one MK patient required diclofenac; 6 MO patients but no MK patients had oxygen saturation by pulse oximetry < 94% on a fraction of inspired oxygen of 0.4 ($p < 0.01$); two MO patients required reintubation. $PaCO_2$ was higher in the MO group (40 ± 6 mm Hg vs 33 ± 5 mm Hg, $p < 0.05$). Heart rate, BP, and incidence of nausea/vomiting were similar; no ketamine-related hallucinations were detected.

Conclusions.—Subanesthetic ketamine combined with a 35%-lower morphine dose provided equivalent pain control compared to the standard morphine dose alone, with fewer adverse side effects and a 45% reduction in morphine consumption.

Trial Registration.—ClinicalTrials.gov Identifier: NCT00625911.

▶ While the pre-emptive effects of ketamine and other N-methyl-D-aspartate (NMDA) antagonists in reducing postoperative pain and opioid requirements are varied, the ability of low-dose ketamine to produce postoperative analgesia is unquestioned. This study indicates that the addition of ketamine to a postoperative morphine regimen reduced pain levels (Fig 2 in the original article) while simultaneously decreasing opioid requirements and overall side effects. While the benefits in terms of improved patient comfort in this study were modest, the benefits of low-dose ketamine in patients on chronic preoperative opioids can be dramatic. The risks of adding small amounts of ketamine to a patient-controlled IV analgesia (PCIA) regimen are miniscule. Nevertheless, many hospital pharmacy and therapeutics committees are reluctant to allow the use of ketamine outside of ICU environments.

S. E. Abram, MD

Adding Gabapentin to a multimodal regimen does not reduce acute pain, opioid consumption or chronic pain after total hip arthroplasty

Clarke H, Pereira S, Kennedy D, et al (Toronto General Hosp, Ontario; Sunnybrook Health Sciences Centre, Toronto, Ontario; et al)

Acta Anaesthesiol Scand 53:1073-1083, 2009

Background.—Gabapentin (GPN) is effective in reducing post-operative pain and opioid consumption, but its effects with regional anesthesia for total hip arthroplasty (THA) are not known. We designed this study to determine whether (1) gabapentin administration reduces pain and opioid use after THA using a multimodal analgesic regimen including spinal anesthesia; (2) pre-operative administration of gabapentin is more effective than post-operative administration.

Methods.—After REB approval and informed consent, 126 patients were enrolled in a double-blinded, randomized-controlled study. Patients received acetaminophen 1 g per os (p.o.), celecoxib 400 mg p.o. and dexamethasone 8 mg intravenously, 1–2 h pre-operatively. Patients were randomly assigned to one of three treatment groups (G1: Placebo/Placebo; G2: GPN/Placebo; G3: Placebo/GPN). Patients received gabapentin 600 mg (G2) or placebo (G1 and G3) 2 h before surgery. All patients had spinal anesthesia [15 mg (3cc) of 0.5% hypobaric bupivacaine with 10 μg of fentanyl]. In the post-anesthetic care unit, patients received gabapentin 600 mg (G3) or placebo (G1 and G2). On the ward, patients received acetaminophen 1000 mg p.o. q6h, celecoxib 200 mg p.o. q12h and a morphine PCA device. Patients were interviewed 6 months post-surgery to determine the incidence and severity of chronic post-surgical pain.

Results.—Mean ± SD cumulative morphine (mg) consumption (G1 = 49.4 ± 24.8, G2 = 47.2 ± 30.1 and G3 = 56.1 ± 38.2) at 48 h and pain scores at 12, 24, 36 and 48 h post-surgery were not significantly different among the groups [G1 ($n = 38$), G2 ($n = 38$) and G3 ($n = 38$)]. Side effect profiles were similar across groups. Six months after surgery, the number of patients who reported chronic post-surgical pain (G1 = 10, G2 = 12 and G3 = 9) and the severity of the pain (G1 = 4.2 ± 2.9, G2 = 4.1 ± 2.2 and G3 = 4.9 ± 2.2) did not differ significantly among the groups ($P > 0.05$).

Conclusions.—A single 600 mg dose of gabapentin given pre-operatively or post-operatively does not reduce morphine consumption or pain scores in hospital or at 6 months after hip arthroplasty within the context of spinal anesthesia and a robust multimodal analgesia regimen.

▶ Previous studies that demonstrated a preemptive analgesic effect for gabapentin or pregabalin were done in patients undergoing general anesthesia. This study demonstrated that, for patients receiving regional anesthesia plus other dexamethasone, celecoxib, and acetaminophen, gabapentin provided no additional benefit in terms of reduced opioid use (see Fig 2 in the original article) or improved pain scores (see Fig 3 in the original article). This is not surprising, as the gabapentin, whether given preoperatively or postoperatively, was administered at a time when pain sensation was blocked by the spinal anesthetic. It is possible that beginning gabapentin postoperatively and continuing it for the first few postsurgical days might still be of benefit.

S. E. Abram, MD

Intrathecal baclofen for postoperative analgesia after total knee arthroplasty

Sanders JC, Gerstein N, Torgeson E, et al (Univ of New Mexico - School of Medicine, Albuquerque)
J Clin Anesth 21:486-492, 2009

Study Objective.—To determine whether intrathecal baclofen is an effective adjunctive agent to decrease acute and chronic postoperative pain after total knee arthroplasty.

Design.—Prospective, randomized, double-blind controlled trial.

Setting.—Operating room and inpatient units of a university hospital.

Patients.—60 adult, ASA physical status I, II, and III patients presenting for total knee arthroplasty.

Interventions.—Anesthesia was provided by spinal injection of 15 mg of 0.75% hyperbaric bupivacaine combined with either 100 mcg baclofen or saline. Sedation was provided with intravenous midazolam and propofol.

Measurements.—Data were collected on adverse effects, opioid usage, and verbal pain scale (VPS) from 0 to 10. The study period was divided into six discrete time intervals that included the 1st 72-hour postoperative period and a three-month post-discharge follow-up telephone call.

Main Results.—The baclofen group used less morphine in the PACU than the control group (5 mg vs. 9.3 mg; $P = 0.04$). VPS were lower in the baclofen group than the treatment group, but significant differences could be demonstrated only in the time periods 48-72 hours and three months postoperatively. At three months, fewer patients in the baclofen group reported pain than the control group (8/27 vs. 19/29; $P = 0.009$). Regression analysis showed that the baclofen group was 4.5 times less likely to report pain at three months (95% CI: 1.5–16.6).

Conclusions.—IT baclofen used as an adjuvant to spinal anesthesia for total knee arthroplasty allows for less postoperative opioid usage and less chronic pain at three months.

▶ It has been known for many years that intrathecal (IT) baclofen produces profound antinociception in animals at doses that produce little or no motor effects.[1] More recently, IT baclofen has been shown to produce effective analgesia in a number of chronic pain states, including neuropathic pain. This study suggests that there are both immediate and delayed benefits to the addition of baclofen to spinal anesthetic protocols. Given the reduced reporting of pain 3 months after surgery, it would be worthwhile to explore the pre-emptive effects of IT baclofen on surgical procedures that are associated with a high incidence of persistent neuropathic pain, such as limb amputation and hernia repair.

S. E. Abram, MD

Reference

1. Wilson P, Yaksh TL. Baclofen is antinociceptive in the spinal intrathecal space of animals. *Eur J Pharmacol.* 1978;51:323-330.

Chronic Musculoskeletal Pain and the Occurrence of Falls in an Older Population

Leveille SG, Jones RN, Kiely DK, et al (Beth Israel Deaconess Med Ctr, Boston, MA; Inst for Aging Res, Boston, MA; et al)

JAMA 302:2214-2221, 2009

Context.—Chronic pain is a major contributor to disability in older adults; however, the potential role of chronic pain as a risk factor for falls is poorly understood.

Objective.—To determine whether chronic musculoskeletal pain is associated with an increased occurrence of falls in a cohort of community-living older adults.

Design, Setting, and Participants.—The Maintenance of Balance, Independent Living, Intellect, and Zest in the Elderly (MOBILIZE) Boston Study is a population-based longitudinal study of falls involving 749 adults aged 70 years and older. Participants were enrolled from September 2005 through January 2008.

Main Outcome Measure.—Participants recorded falls on monthly calendar postcards mailed to the study center during an 18-month period.

Results.—There were 1029 falls reported during the follow-up. A report of 2 or more locations of musculoskeletal pain at baseline was associated with greater occurrence of falls. The age-adjusted rates of falls per person-year were 1.18 (95% confidence interval [CI], 1.13-1.23) for the 300 participants with 2 or more sites of joint pain, 0.90 (95% CI, 0.87-0.92) for the 181 participants with single-site pain, and 0.78 (95% CI, 0.74-0.81) for the 267 participants with no joint pain. Similarly, more severe or disabling pain at baseline was associated with higher fall rates ($P < .05$). The association persisted after adjusting for multiple confounders and fall risk factors. The greatest risk for falls was observed in persons who had 2 or more pain sites (adjusted rate ratio [RR], 1.53; 95% CI, 1.17-1.99), and those in the highest tertiles of pain severity (adjusted RR, 1.53; 95% CI, 1.12-2.08) and pain interference with activities (adjusted RR, 1.53; 95% CI, 1.15-2.05), compared with their peers with no pain or those in the lowest tertiles of pain scores.

Conclusions.—Chronic pain measured according to number of locations, severity, or pain interference with daily activities was associated with greater risk of falls in older adults.

► It is not clear why chronic pain increases falls. Is it distraction from diversion of attention to pain? Is it that chronic pain causes disturbances of gait and alignment that make falling more likely? Is it that chronic pain sensation suppresses proprioceptive responses? That would be my bet, but we really don't know.

What we do know is that this is another rationale, an important one, for treating chronic pain aggressively—to prevent this disability, and yes, the deaths that are the result of falls in the elderly.

M. F. Roizen, MD

Cost effectiveness of two rehabilitation programmes for neck and back pain patients: A seven year follow-up

Jensen IB, Busch H, Bodin L, et al (Karolinska Inst, Stockholm, Sweden; et al)
Pain 142:202-208, 2009

The cost effectiveness of work-oriented rehabilitation for persons on long-term sick leave needs to be assessed. This prospective observational study presents a follow-up seven years after rehabilitation using two different evidence-based work-oriented regimens. Individuals on sick leave for neck and back pain were referred to two rehabilitation programmes in Sweden. The first programme was a relatively low-intensity programme based on orthopaedic manual therapy and exercise programme (OMTP). The second programme was a full-time multidisciplinary programme (MDP). The primary outcome was sickness absence seven years after intervention. Cost effectiveness was calculated on the basis of loss of production due to sickness absence. The results show that participants referred to MDP and with less than 60 sick days before rehabilitation have reduced sickness absence after intervention as compared to matched controls. This corresponds to a cost reduction of about 94,494 EUR per referred individual. Further, the results indicate that participants of the OMTP who have more than 60 sick days before rehabilitation have a statistically significant increased risk of disability pension. This means increased cost in terms of loss of production of

44,593 EUR per referred individual. The results of this study show that MPD but not OMTP achieves the goal of working life-oriented rehabilitation. A direct comparison between the rehabilitation programmes strengthened the assumption that long-term sickness absence prior to rehabilitation is associated with more days on sick leave after rehabilitation. This analysis also indicated the importance of participants' pain self-efficacy beliefs and recovery beliefs on rehabilitation outcome.

▶ There is substantial evidence that multidisciplinary pain management programs focused on increasing function and developing coping strategies in accordance with cognitive behavioral approaches are effective in improving function and facilitating return to employment. This study compared such a program with one that was based on orthopedic manual therapy, fitness exercise, and job training at the workplace. The 2 programs were comparable in cost. The multidisciplinary program was clearly more effective at returning patients to gainful employment, but only for patients who had been absent from work for less than 2 months (see Figs 2 and 3 in the original article). It is unfortunate that most health care reimbursement systems in the United States no longer fund the type of program shown to be effective in this study. Because behavioral, rehabilitation, and medical costs are often covered by separate insurance systems and are often limited to specific providers, the opportunities for patients to participate in such programs are limited.

S. E. Abram, MD

Continuous Buprenorphine Delivery Effect in Streptozotocine-Induced Painful Diabetic Neuropathy in Rats

Canta A, Chiorazzi A, Meregalli C, et al (Univ of Milan Bicocca, Italy; et al)
J Pain 10:961-968, 2009

Diabetic peripheral neuropathy (DPN) can induce loss of nociception as well as mechanical hyperalgesia and tactile allodynia. Pharmacological and clinical studies have shown that buprenorphine, a low-molecular-weight, lipophilic, opioid analgesic available as a transdermal matrix patch formulation, acts on neuropathic pain. To assess the role of buprenorphine in the treatment of DPN-associated neuropathic pain, we used a well-established experimental rat model of DPN in which buprenorphine at doses of 1.2 and 2.4 μg/kg/h was administered by implantable Alzet osmotic pumps for 3 weeks. After 6 weeks of diabetes, nerve conduction velocity (NCV) and behavioural responses to noxious mechanical and thermal stimuli were assessed. Diabetic rats showed an impairment of NCV, mechanical allodynia, and thermal hypoalgesia. Both doses of buprenorphine significantly reversed the diabetes-induced allodynia up to day 7 of treatment. Buprenorphine did not alter either thermal perception or NCV.

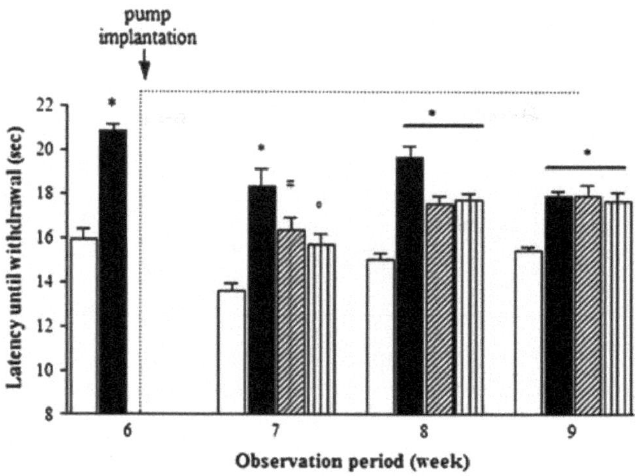

FIGURE 4.—Dynamic plantar analgesiometer paw withdrawal test. Test was performed 6 weeks after streptozotocin (STZ) induction (before pump implantation) and in the following 3 weeks after pump implantation (7, 8, and 9 weeks, respectively, after diabetes induction). Values are mean ± SD. **$P < .0001$ vs CTRL, *$P < .001$ vs CTRL, °$P < .05$ vs CTRL, #$P < .01$ vs CTRL (1-way ANOVA test followed by Tukey-Kramer post-test). CTRL; STZ; STZ + B 1.2; STZ + B 2.4. (Reprinted from Canta A, Chiorazzi A, Meregalli C, et al. Continuous buprenorphine delivery effect in streptozotocine-induced painful diabetic neuropathy in rats. *J Pain.* 2009;10:961-968, with permission from the American Pain Society.)

Perspective.—This study evaluated, through a multimodal approach, the analgesic effect of buprenorphine in an experimental rat model of painful DPN. Our results suggest a possible role for buprenorphine in the management of DPN-associated neuropathic pain (Fig 4).

▶ In this study, animals made diabetic by streptozotocine developed mechanical allodynia, which was evident at 6 weeks when the buprenorphine infusion was begun. The allodynia was diminished during the first week of infusion only, and was not reduced to control animal levels. During the next 2 weeks of infusion there was no significant reduction in allodynia (Fig 4). While these effects may seem disappointing, they may actually be encouraging, because opioid agonists have been shown to produce hyperalgesia and to enhance allodynia in rats with experimentally induced mononeuropathies.[1] In addition, buprenorphine has been shown to provide stronger antihyperalgesic effects in a human experimental pain model.[2] Therefore, there may be a role for buprenorphine in patients with chronic neuropathic and nociceptive pain who have developed tolerance and hyperalgesia from conventional μ-opioid agonists.

S. E. Abram, MD

References

1. Raghavendra V, Rutkowski MD, DeLeo JA. The role of spinal neuroimmune activation in morphine tolerance/hyperalgesia in neuropathic and sham-operated rats. *J Neuroscience.* 2002;22:9980-9989.

2. Koppert W, Ihmsen H, Korber N, et al. Different profiles of buprenorphine-induced analgesia and antihyperalgesia in a human pain model. *Pain*. 2005;118: 15-22.

A randomized double-blind controlled trial of intra-annular radiofrequency thermal disc therapy – A 12-month follow-up

Kvarstein G, Måwe L, Indahl A, et al (Oslo Univ Hosp, Rikshospitalet, Norway; et al)

Pain 145:279-286, 2009

The discTRODE™ probe applies radiofrequency (RF) current, heating the annulus to treat chronic discogenic low back pain. Randomized controlled studies have not been published. We assessed the long-term effect and safety aspects of percutaneous intradiscal radiofrequency thermocoagulation (PIRFT) with the discTRODE™ probe in a prospective parallel, randomized and gender stratified, double-blind placebo-controlled study. Twenty selected patients with chronic low back pain and a positive one-level pressure-controlled provocation discography were randomized to either intra-annular PIRFT or intra-annular sham treatment. A blinded interim analysis was performed when 20 patients had been followed for six months. The 6-month analysis did not reveal any trend towards overall effect or difference between active and sham treatment for the primary endpoint: change in pain intensity (0–10). The inclusion of patients was therefore discontinued. After 12 months the overall reduction from baseline pain had reached statistical significance, but there was no significant difference between the groups. The functional outcome measures (Oswestry Disability Index, and SF 36 subscales and the relative change in pain) appeared more promising, but did not reach statistical significance when compared with sham treatment. Two actively treated and two sham-treated patients reported increased pain levels, and in both groups a higher number was unemployed after 12 months. The study did not find evidence for a benefit of PIRFT, although it cannot rule out a moderate effect. Considering the high number, reporting increased pain in our study, we would not recommend intra-annular thermal therapy with the discTRODE™ probe (Tables 3 and 4).

▶ The use of thermocoagulation of the intervertebral disc for the treatment of discogenic low back pain remains controversial. The 3 therapies introduced for annular thermocoagulation (intradiscal electrothermal therapy (IDET), radiofrequency thermocoagulation (discTRODE), and cooled radiofrequency thermocoagulation [biacuplasty]) have not been conclusively shown to provide substantial benefit in terms of pain control or functional recovery. Controlled trials of IDET show modest benefit at best, and, until this study, there have been no controlled trials of either radiofrequency technique.[1] The lack of substantial benefit with these techniques is not particularly surprising. A study of the effect of IDET on experimentally induced annular tears in

TABLE 3.—Outcome Measurements on Pain Intensity and Pain Interferences on Function (BPI) Among Patients Subjected to Intra-annular Radiofrequency Thermal or Sham Treatment

	Baseline					6 months						12 months					
	Active ($n = 10$)		Sham ($n = 10$)			Active ($n = 10$)		Sham ($n = 9$)				Active ($n = 10$)		Sham ($n = 10$)			
Item	Mean	(SD)	Mean	(SD)	p	Mean	(SD)	Mean	(SD)	p		Mean	(SD)	Mean	(SD)	p	
BPI pain intensity last 24 h*																	
Worst pain	5.4	(2.1)	6.5	(2.2)	0.27	4.4	(2.7)	6.5	(2.0)	0.06		4.0	(3.0)	4.9	(2.7)	0.50	$
Least pain	2.3	(1.4)	2.7	(2.6)	0.68	2.5	(2.0)	3.5	(2.8)	0.36		1.8	(1.3)	3.2	(2.5)	0.14	
Average pain	4.6	(1.8)	5.5	(2.0)	0.30	3.7	(2.2)	5.3	(1.8)	0.09		3.2	(2.3)	4.9	(2.1)	0.12	
Pain now	3.8	(1.5)	5.4	(1.8)	0.046	3.2	(2.2)	5.1	(2.4)	0.08		3.6	(2.6)	4.5	(2.9)	0.47	
BPI pain interference on*																	
General activity	5.5	(2.9)	5.8	(2.1)	0.80	3.7	(2.7)	5.8	(2.4)	0.08		4.2	(3.1)	5.0	(3.0)	0.60	
Mood	5.5	(3.1)	4.4	(2.1)	0.37	3.6	(2.7)	4.3	(2.5)	9.55		3.7	(3.2)	3.8	(2.9)	0.93	
Walking ability	3.4	(3.3)	3.4	(2.9)	1.0	2.0	(1.8)	3.1	(2.6)	0.28		2.0	(1.8)	3.3	(2.6)	0.23	
Work	5.3	(2.5)	6.6	(2.2)	0.27	3.3	(2.4)	5.7	(2.3)	0.06	$	3.3	(3.0)	5.6	(3.0)	0.09	
Relations to others	3.9	(2.4)	3.8	(2.3)	0.91	2.5	(2.6)	3.5	(2.2)	0.52		2.8	(2.9)	3.1	(3.2)	0.83	
Sleep	4.5	(3.4)	4.4	(2.8)	0.97	3.2	(2.7)	4.0	(2.8)	0.71		3.1	(3.0)	4.3	(3.3)	0.39	
Enjoyment of life	5.2	(3.2)	4.3	(3.2)	0.56	3.5	(2.8)	3.2	(2.3)	0.75		2.9	(3.1)	3.1	(3.0)	0.76	$

The groups are compared by Student t-test, and p-values are presented without Bonferroni correction for multiple comparisons. Comparisons to baseline are carried out with the GLM, Repeated measurements; $ means a statistically significant difference from baseline for both groups combined ($p < 0.05$).

*BPI, Brief Pain Inventory; pain intensity and pain interference on function are assessed by numeric 11-graded numeric rating scales. The higher the score, the worse the outcome.

TABLE 4.—Functional and Life of Quality Outcome Measurements Among Patients Subjected to Intra-annular Radiofrequency Thermal or Sham Treatment

	Baseline					6 Months						12 Months					
	Active ($n = 10$)		Sham ($n = 10$)			Active ($n = 10$)		Sham ($n = 9$)				Active ($n = 10$)		Sham ($n = 10$)			
Item	Mean	(SD)	Mean	(SD)	p	Mean	(SD)	Mean	(SD)	p		Mean	(SD)	Mean	(SD)	p	
SF-36**																	
Bodily pain	39.5	(17.9)	32.5	(14.8)	0.35	43.7	(30.1)	35.3	(18.6)	0.46		51.6	(23.8)	39.5	(24.2)	0.29	
Physical functioning	49.0	(20.2)	52.5	(24.2)	0.73	59.0	(23.1)	64.0	(20.4)	0.61	$	65.0	(21.7)	57.5	(21.4)	0.46	
Role physical	27.5	(41.6)	5.0	(10.5)	0.13	27.5	(44.8)	15.0	(24.2)	0.45		41.7	(45.1)	15.0	(31.6)	0.16	
Role emotional	73.3	(43.9)	40.0	(43.9)	0.11	80.0	(35.8)	30.0	(36.7)	0.01#		77.8	(37.3)	46.7	(42.2)	0.11	
Social functioning	60.0	(25.5)	55.0	(25.1)	0.66	68.8	(30.2)	63.8	(23.2)	0.68		73.6	(26.8)	66.3	(28.3)	0.57	
Mental health	66.8	(12.7)	68.0	(13.9)	0.84	71.6	(15.9)	74.8	(12.7)	0.63		76.9	(14.1)	70.0	(14.5)	0.31	
General health	66.4	(19.7)	49.7	(17.7)	0.06	65.9	(20.0)	50.7	(15.2)	0.07		75.2	(10.3)	59.4	(21.2)	0.06	$
Vitality	40.0	(22.2)	30.5	(15.7)	0.28	46.0	(17.9)	39.0	(16.5)	0.38	$	52.8	(22.7)	37.0	(16.7)	0.10	
ODI***	31.6	(10.2)	30.4	(15.3)	0.84	25.2	(14.8)	28.2	(13.1)	0.64		20.0	(16.2)	30.0	(17.1)	0.20	

The p-values are presented without Bonferroni correction for multiple comparisons. Comparisons to baseline are carried out with the GLM, Repeated measurements; $ means statistically significant difference from baseline for both groups combined ($p < 0.05$).

#The groups are compared by Student *t*-test or Mann–Whitney test when not normally distributed.

**SF36, the short form 36 questionnaire subscales range from 0 to 100, and a high level indicates good health.

***ODI, The Oswestry Disability Index score varies from 0 to 100, a high score is associated with a high degree of disability.

sheep demonstrated more severe histologic evidence of injury in those animals treated with thermal annuloplasty.[2] This study showed essentially no benefit in either pain (Table 3) or function (Table 4) at 6- and 12-month follow-up for patients in the treatment group, and worsening of pain in 2 patients from each group; it raises concerns about the safety of probe placement into the disc.

S. E. Abram, MD

References

1. Helm S, Hayek SM, Benyamin RM, Manchikanti L. Systematic review of the effectiveness of thermal annular procedures in treating discogenic low back pain. *Pain Physician*. 2009;12:207-232.
2. Freeman BJ, Walters RM, Moore RJ, Fraser RD. Does intradiscal electrothermal therapy denervate and repair experimentally induced posterolateral annular tears in an animal model? *Spine*. 2003;28:2602-2608.

Comparative Cognitive and Subjective Side Effects of Immediate-Release Oxycodone in Healthy Middle-Aged and Older Adults

Cherrier MM, Amory JK, Ersek M, et al (Univ of Washington, Seattle; Univ of Pennsylvania, Philadelphia; et al)
J Pain 10:1038-1050, 2009

This study measured the objective and subjective neurocognitive effects of a single 10-mg dose of immediate-release oxycodone in healthy, older (> 65 years), and middle-aged (35 to 55 years) adults who were not suffering from chronic or significant daily pain. Seventy-one participants completed 2 separate study days and were blind to medication condition (placebo, 10-mg oxycodone). Plasma oxycodone concentration peaked between 60 and 90 minutes postdose ($P < .01$) and pupil size, an indication of physiological effects of the medication, peaked at approximately 90 to 120 minutes postdose ($P < .01$). Significant declines in simple and sustained attention, working memory, and verbal memory were observed at 1 hour postdose compared to baseline for both age groups with a trend toward return to baseline by 5 hours postdose. For almost all cognitive measures, there were no medication by age-interaction effects, which indicates that the 2 age groups exhibited similar responses to the medication challenge. This study suggests that for healthy older adults who are not suffering from chronic pain, neurocognitive and pharmacodynamic changes in response to a 10-mg dose of immediate-release oxycodone are similar to those observed for middle-aged adults.

Perspective.—Study findings indicate that the metabolism, neurocognitive effects, and physical side effects of oral oxycodone are similar for healthy middle-aged and older adults. Therefore, clinicians should not avoid prescribing oral opioids to older adults based on the belief that

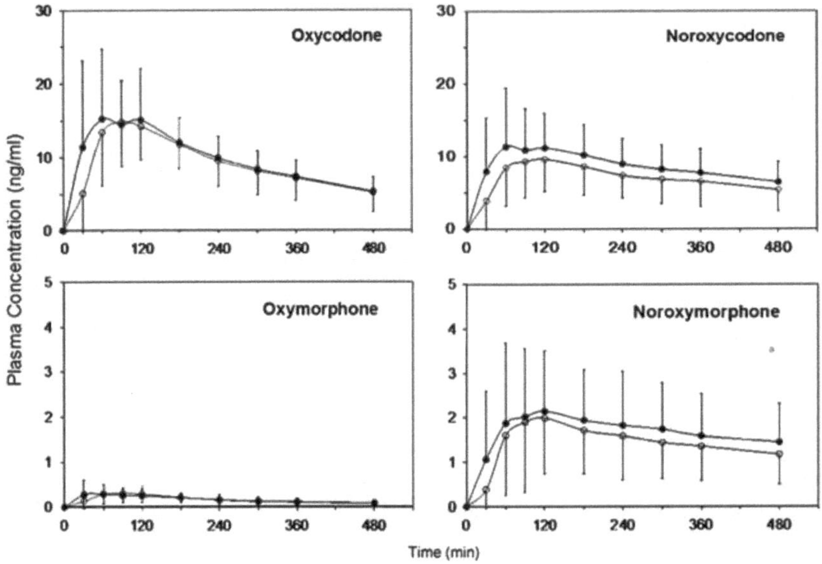

FIGURE 2.—Time course of mean and standard deviations of plasma concentrations of oxycodone and its metabolites noroxycodone, oxymorphone, and noroxymorphone. Older adults are represented by dark circles and middle-aged group by open circles. (Reprinted from Cherrier MM, Amory JK, Ersek M, et al. Comparative cognitive and subjective side effects of immediate-release oxycodone in healthy middle-aged and older adults. *J Pain.* 2009;10:1038-1050, with permission from the American Pain Society.)

older adults are at higher risk for side effects than younger adults (Fig 2, Table 4)

▶ This study helps to dispel the notion that older patients are slower to metabolize and clear opioids, and they have more intense effects on mental functions. It also showed no gender differences for these effects. There were virtually no differences in the time course of plasma levels of oxycodone and its metabolites (Fig 2), and there were minimal differences in cognitive effects (Table 4) between middle-aged and older individuals. Both groups showed some effects on attention tests with modest increases in reaction times. While several studies have shown minimal increases in reaction times for patients on opioids chronically, the effects for opioid naive patients, or for those who use opioids occasionally, are significant, and such patients should be warned against driving within several hours of taking short-acting opioids.

S. E. Abram, MD

TABLE 4.—Neurocognitive Tests. Means and Standard Deviations

	Middle Age Adults			Older Adults		
	Baseline	1 Hour	5 Hours	Baseline	1 Hour	5 Hours
Attention						
Simple reaction time	363.3 (99.7)	**377.97 (92.3)**	368.56 (78)	345.72 (45.5)	**356.04 (60.2)**	331.48 (35.6)
Choice reaction time	554.36 (109.2)	**586.99 (120.9)**	553.81 (88.9)	540.02 (67.4)	**638.90 (138.5)**	622.65 (161.1)
Symbol digit	66.67 (16.1)	**56.17 (12.9)**	**62.06 (13.7)**	60.67 (13.4)	**52.06 (11.1)**	**53.89 (13.7)**
Sustained attention test	463.28 (96.9)	448.06 (109.9)	468.33 (106.1)	406 (96)	**381.11 (108.2)**	402.72 (106)
Working memory						
Alphabet and number sequence	12.28 (2.7)	11.72 (3.1)	12.5 (2.9)	10.33 (3.4)	10.39 (3.5)	10.39 (2.8)
Memory						
Word list test-delay	10.78 (3)	**7.50 (3.9)**	**8.56 (4)**	8.11 (2.5)	**4.67 (3.4)**	**4.72 (2.9)**
Word list-intrusions	.11 (.3)	.33 (.8)	.44 (.8)	.33 (.5)	**1.94 (3.6)**	.50 (.7)

NOTE.—Mean and standard deviation of Neurocognitive tests. **Bold** indicates a significant change from baseline ($P < .01$), with the exception of choice reaction time middle-aged adults at 5 hours which was significant at the $P < .05$ level. Simple and choice reaction time—milliseconds; Digit Symbol—number correct and maximumscore of 132; D2—number correct and maximum score of 182; Numbers and Alphabet Sequencing—number correct and maximum score of 21; Word List Delay—total number of words recalled after a 20-minute delay and maximum score of 15; Word List Intrusions—number of errors or words recalled that were not on the list to be learned.

Even routine painful procedures can be harmful for the newborn

Bellieni CV, Iantorno L, Perrone S, et al (Univ of Siena, Italy)

Pain 147:128-131, 2009

Stressful events can damage neonatal brain through a complexity of events including free radical (FR) generation. We examined whether pain provoked by a routine heel prick can generate an increase in potentially harmful FR in neonatal blood. To this aim, advanced oxidation protein products (AOPP) and total hydroperoxide (TH) concentrations were measured at the beginning (sample A) and at the end (sample B) of each sampling in 64 babies (corrected age: 37.2 ± 2.7 weeks) who underwent heel prick for routine blood tests. We scored pain of every procedure in all newborns. No differences were detected between AOPP and TH blood concentrations at the beginning and at the end of heel prick sampling, considering the whole cohort of babies. Conversely, a significant increase was observed between AOPP and TH blood concentrations considering only those babies who showed the highest pain intensity. When babies' pain was high (ABC score ≥4), mean AOPP and TH blood levels increased significantly; in this case, mean AOPP values increased from 53.5 μm/l (SD = 41.6) to 63.2 μm/l (SD = 44.3) and TH values from 218.3 U Carr (SD = 89.2) to 228.7 U Carr (SD = 93.3), with a significant p value of 0.02 and 0.036, respectively. A significant correlation was also found between AOPP blood levels ratio (sample B/sample A) in each baby, and the correspondent level of pain. These data show that even common routine procedures can be potentially harmful for the newborn if they provoke a high level of pain (Table 3).

▶ The serious consequences of untreated or undertreated pain in newborns has been recognized for only the past 2 decades. Anand and his colleagues[1] demonstrated major adverse effects of surgical interventions performed with little or no analgesia. Fortunately, the mythological notion that neonates experience minimal pain following noxious stimulation has been dispelled. This study showed a correlation between painful heel sticks and increased levels of free radicals, which are known to damage developing nervous systems. Interestingly, the correlation was with the presence of pain, as evaluated by an

TABLE 3.—Changes in Markers of Free Radical Production

	AOPP		TH	
	A	B	A	B
Total group ($n = 64$)	53.1 (SD = 47.3) $p = 0.2$	54.9 (SD = 40.0)	221.0 (SD = 93.5) $p = 0.9$	221.0 (SD = 89.2)
Babies with pain score ≥4 ($n = 34$)	53.5 (SD = 41.6) $p = 0.02$	63.2 (SD = 44.3)	218.3 (SD = 89.2) $p = 0.036$	228.7 (SD = 93.3)
Babies with pain <4	53.8 (SD = 55.3) $p = 0.5$	45.3 (SD = 33.8)	221.4 (SD = 97.3) $p = 0.59$	211.8 (SD = 86.0)

accepted neonatal rating system (Table 3, Fig 1 in the original article). Heel sticks that did not produce pain behaviors were not associated with increases in free radical levels. A variety of measures that reduce the pain and stress of painful interventions are available. This study provides evidence that the time and expense of initiating such measures is justified.

S. E. Abram, MD

Reference

1. Anand KJ, Hickey PR. Pain and its effects in the human neonate and fetus. *N Engl J Med.* 1987;317:1321-1329.

Imaging strategies for low-back pain: systematic review and meta-analysis

Chou R, Fu R, Carrino JA, et al (Oregon Health and Science Univ, Portland; Johns Hopkins Univ School of Medicine, Baltimore, MD)

Lancet 373:463-472, 2009

Background.—Some clinicians do lumbar imaging routinely or in the absence of historical or clinical features suggestive of serious low-back problems. We investigated the effects of routine, immediate lumbar imaging versus usual clinical care without immediate imaging on clinical outcomes in patients with low-back pain and no indication of serious underlying conditions.

Methods.—We analysed randomised controlled trials that compared immediate lumbar imaging (radiography, MRI, or CT) versus usual clinical care without immediate imaging for low-back pain. These trials reported pain or function (primary outcomes), quality of life, mental health, overall patient-reported improvement (based on various scales), and patient satisfaction in care received. Six trials (n = 1804) met inclusion criteria. Study quality was assessed by two independent reviewers with criteria adapted from the Cochrane Back Review Group. Meta-analyses were done with a random effects model.

Findings.—We did not record significant differences between immediate lumbar imaging and usual care without immediate imaging for primary outcomes at either short-term (up to 3 months, standardised mean difference 0·19, 95% CI −0·01 to 0·39 for pain and 0·11, −0·29 to 0·50 for function, negative values favour routine imaging) or long-term (6–12 months, −0·04, −0·15 to 0·07 for pain and 0·01, −0·17 to 0·19 for function) follow-up. Other outcomes did not differ significantly. Trial quality, use of different imaging methods, and duration of low-back pain did not affect the results, but analyses were limited by small numbers of trials. Results are most applicable to acute or subacute low-back pain assessed in primary-care settings.

Interpretation.—Lumbar imaging for low-back pain without indications of serious underlying conditions does not improve clinical outcomes. Therefore, clinicians should refrain from routine, immediate lumbar imaging in patients with acute or subacute low-back pain and without features suggesting a serious underlying condition.

▶ The main outcome of this study is that there is no set pathway to evaluate low back pain by X-ray, CT, MRI, or ultrasound imaging, and nothing appears better than anything else in doing so. A conservative strategy of no imagery appears to be the best approach, unless there is indication of serious underlying condition.

M. F. Roizen, MD

Mortality Risk Associated With Low-Trauma Osteoporotic Fracture and Subsequent Fracture in Men and Women

Bliuc D, Nguyen ND, Milch VE, et al (St Vincent's Hosp, Sydney, Australia)
JAMA 301:513-521, 2009

Context.—There are few data on long-term mortality following osteoporotic fracture and fewer following subsequent fracture.

Objectives.—To examine long-term mortality risk in women and men following all osteoporotic fractures and to assess the association of subsequent fracture with that risk.

Design, Setting, and Participants.—Prospective cohort from the Dubbo Osteoporosis Epidemiology Study of community-dwelling women and men aged 60 years and older from Dubbo, Australia, who sustained a fracture between April 1989 and May 2007.

Main Outcome Measures.—Age- and sex-specific standardized mortality ratios (SMRs) compared with the overall Dubbo population for hip, vertebral, major, and minor fractures.

Results.—In women, there were 952 low-trauma fractures followed by 461 deaths, and in men, 343 fractures were followed by 197 deaths. Age-adjusted SMRs were increased following hip fractures (SMRs, 2.43 [95% confidence interval [CI], 2.02-2.93] and 3.51 [95% CI, 2.65-4.66]), vertebral fractures (SMRs, 1.82 [95% CI, 1.52-2.17] and 2.12 [95% CI, 1.66-2.72]), major fractures (SMRs, 1.65 [95% CI, 1.31-2.08] and 1.70 [95% CI, 1.23-2.36]), and minor fractures (SMRs, 1.42 [95% CI, 1.19-1.70] and 1.33 [95% CI, 0.99-1.80]) for both women and men, respectively. Mortality was increased for all ages for all fractures except minor fractures for which increased mortality was only apparent for those older than 75 years. Increased mortality risk persisted for 5 years for all fractures and up to 10 years for hip fractures. Increases in absolute mortality that were above expected, for 5 years after fracture, ranged from 1.3 to 13.2 per 100 person-years in women and from 2.7 to 22.3 per 100 person-years in men, depending on fracture type. Subsequent fracture was associated with an increased mortality hazard ratio of 1.91 (95% CI, 1.54-2.37) in women and 2.99 (95% CI, 2.11-4.24) in men. Mortality risk following a subsequent fracture then declined but beyond 5 years still remained higher than in the general population (SMR, 1.41 [95% CI, 1.01-1.97] and SMR, 1.78 [95% CI, 0.96-3.31] for women and men, respectively). Predictors of mortality after any fragility fracture for both men and women included age, quadriceps weakness, and subsequent fracture but not comorbidities. Low bone mineral density, having smoked, and sway were also predictors for women and less physical activity for men.

Conclusions.—In a sample of older women and men, all low-trauma fractures were associated with increased mortality risk for 5 to 10 years. Subsequent fracture was associated with increased mortality risk for an additional 5 years.

▶ This was an eye opener to me. When you are going in and doing hip surgery or hip fixation for a low trauma osteoporotic fracture, or giving pain medicine for one of a vertebral fracture or other fracture, realize that man or woman has a substantially increased risk of death not only this year but for the next 10 years. A new fracture in that period just prolongs the problem. Whereas some of my patients used to say oy vey, it appears an osteoporotic fracture in a man isn't as good as poor sperm quality at predicting aging and mortality risk, but does heighten the risk pretty substantially.

M. F. Roizen, MD

Chronic Pain Management

Chronic Pain and Obesity in Elderly People: Results from the Einstein Aging Study

McCarthy LH, Bigal ME, Katz M, et al (Albert Einstein College of Medicine, Bronx, NY)

J Am Geriatr Soc 57:115-119, 2009

Objectives.—To determine the prevalence of chronic pain in elderly people and its relationship with obesity and associated comorbidities and risk factors.

Design.—Cross-sectional.

Setting.—Community.

Participants.—A representative community sample of 840 subjects aged 70 and older.

Measurements.—The prevalence of chronic pain and its relationship with obesity (categories defined according to body mass index (BMI)), other medical risk factors, and psychiatric comorbidities were examined. Chronic pain was defined as pain of at least moderate severity (≥4 on a 10-point scale) some, most, or all of the time for the previous 3 months.

Results.—The sample was mostly female (62.8%), and the average age was 80 (range 70–101). The prevalence of chronic pain was 52% (39.7% in men; 58.9% in women). Subjects with chronic pain were more likely to report a diagnosis of depression (odds ratio (OR) = 2.5, 95% confidence interval (CI) = 1.40–4.55) and anxiety (OR = 2.3, 95% CI = 1.22–4.64). Obese subjects (BMI 30–34.9) were twice as likely (OR = 2.1,

TABLE 2.—Univariate Analysis and Multiple Logistic Regression Model on Chronic Pain

Independent Variable	Univariate Logistic Regression Odds Ratio (95% Confidence Interval)	Multiple Logistic Regression Odds Ratio (95% Confidence Interval)
Age	1.12 (0.83–1.49)	1.02 (0.99–1.05)
Female	2.18 (1.61–2.97)	2.24 (1.63–3.08)
Body mass index, kg/m^2		
<18.5 (underweight)	0.88 (0.25–2.97)	0.56 (0.17–1.85)
18.5–24.9 (normal weight)	Reference	Reference
25.0–29.9 (overweight)	1.17 (0.84–1.61)	1.32 (0.94–1.85)
30.0–34.9 (obese)	2.09 (1.33–3.28)	2.03 (1.27–3.26)
≥35.0 (severely obese)	4.53 (1.85–12.63)	4.12 (1.57–10.82)
Education >12 years	0.74 (0.56–0.98)	0.85 (0.63–1.16)
Depression	2.48 (1.40–4.55)	1.94 (1.03–3.66)
Anxiety	2.33 (1.22–4.64)	2.15 (1.04–4.43)
Diabetes mellitus	1.32 (0.92–1.89)	1.38 (0.92–2.05)
Hypertension	1.41 (1.06–1.88)	1.26 (0.92–1.72)

TABLE 3.—Chronic Pain Location and Obesity

% With Chronic Pain Location	Body Mass Index <30	Body Mass Index ≥30 (Obese)	*P*-Value
Head	3.7	9.4	.003
Face	1.5	0.0	.11
Neck and shoulder	14.9	22.6	.02
Back	21.7	35.9	<.001
Arms and hands	12.9	19.5	.04
Legs and feet	24.1	44.7	<.001
Chest	2.3	5.0	.07
Abdomen and pelvis	6.9	14.5	.002

95%CI = 1.33–3.28) and severely obese subjects (BMI≥35) were more than four times as likely (OR = 4.5, 95% CI = 1.85–12.63) as those of normal weight (BMI 18.5–24.9) to have chronic pain. Obese subjects were significantly more likely to have chronic pain in the head, neck or shoulder, back, legs or feet, and abdomen or pelvis than subjects who were not obese. In multivariate models, obesity (OR = 2.0, 95% CI = 1.27–3.26) and severe obesity (OR = 4.1, 95% CI = 1.57–10.82) were associated with chronic pain after adjusting for age, sex, diabetes mellitus, hypertension, depression, anxiety, and education.

Conclusion.—Chronic pain is common in this elderly population, affects women more than men, and is highly associated with obesity (Tables 2 and 3).

▶ We generally attribute increased pain in obese patients to added load on weight bearing joints (low back, hips, knees), but as the authors point out, non-load-bearing structures are also involved (Table 3). Obesity is known to produce a number of metabolic and inflammatory consequences, including increases in C-reactive proteins and proinflammatory cytokines.[1,2] The association of obesity with chronic pain is robust, independent of other variables, and is related to the severity of the obesity (Table 2). This study provides motivation to test obesity aggressively in middle age. It is not clear from this study whether weight loss in the elderly will reduce pain severity. However, most pain management and primary care physicians have seen improvement in knee, hip, and back pain among patients who have lost large amounts of excess weight.

S. E. Abram, MD

References

1. Herishanu Y, Rogowski O, Polliack A, Marilus R. Leukocytosis in obese individuals: possible link in patients with unexplained persistent neutrophilia. *Eur J Haematol.* 2006;76:516-520.
2. Winkler G, Salamon F, Harmos G, et al. Elevated serum tumor necrosis factor alpha concentrations and bioactivity in Type 2 diabetics and patients with android type obesity. *Diabetes Res Clin Pract.* 1998;42:169-174.

A Prospective Outcome Study on the Effects of Facet Joint Radiofrequency Denervation on Pain, Analgesic Intake, Disability, Satisfaction, Cost, and Employment

Burnham RS, Holitski S, Dinu I (Central Alberta Pain and Rehabilitation Inst, Lacombe, Canada; Univ of Alberta; Lacombe Physiotherapy, Alberta, Canada)
Arch Phys Med Rehabil 90:201-205, 2009

Objective.—To assess the effect of radiofrequency denervation (RFD) on patients with chronic low back pain (LBP) of facet joint origin.

Design.—Prospective cohort study.

Setting.—Interventional pain management program.

Participants.—Consecutive subjects (N = 44; 101 facet joints) over 2 years with chronic refractory mechanical LBP of facet origin established by 2 local anesthetic blocks (medial branch ± intra-articular) resulting in more than 50% pain relief.

Intervention.—RFD of the symptomatic lumbar facet joints.

Main Outcome Measures.—Self-reported pain intensity, frequency, bothersomeness, analgesic intake, satisfaction, disability, back pain–related costs, and employment twice prior to and at 1, 3, 6, 9, and 12 months post-RFD.

Results.—Post-RFD, significant improvements in pain, analgesic requirement, satisfaction, disability, and direct costs occurred. They peaked at 3 to 6 months and gradually diminished thereafter. Satisfaction with medical care and living with current symptoms improved similarly. Overall, satisfaction with the RFD procedure was high, and no complications were reported.

Conclusions.—RFD provides safe and significant short-term improvement in pain, analgesic requirements, function, satisfaction, and direct costs in patients with chronic LBP of facet origin.

▶ This study is of limited value because it lacks a control population. As the authors point out in the introduction, 3 of 5 randomized controlled trials failed to show a significant benefit compared with sham procedures. Another limitation is the rather vague discussion of how medication use was measured and reported. It has been my experience that patients on opioids before radiofrequency denervation (RFD) report improvement in pain levels but rarely reduce their opioid intake following the procedure. As with most outcomes studies involving interventions or medications for chronic pain, there was minimal improvement in employment statistics or other indirect costs. It is difficult to determine whether this therapy is cost-effective. The authors indicate that medical costs diminished following therapy, but a more comprehensive study that accounts for hospitalization for back pain and the cost of the RFD is needed. Another important question is whether repeated RFD procedures provide similar benefits.

S. E. Abram, MD

Financial impact of spinal cord stimulation on the healthcare budget: a comparative analysis of costs in Canada and the United States

Kumar K, Bishop S (Univ of Saskatchewan, Canada)

J Neurosurg Spine 10:564-573, 2009

Object.—Many institutions with spinal cord stimulation (SCS) programs fail to realize that besides the initial implantation cost, budgetary allocation must be made to address annual maintenance costs as well as complications as they arise. Complications remain the major contributing factor to the overall expense of SCS. The authors present a formula that, when applied, provides a realistic representation of the actual costs necessary to implant and maintain SCS systems in Canada and the US.

Methods.—The authors performed a retrospective analysis of 197 cases involving SCS (161 implanted and 36 failed trial stimulations) between 1995 and 2006. The cost of patient workup, initial implantation, annual maintenance, and resources necessary to resolve complications were assessed for each case and a unit cost applied. The total cost allocated for each case was determined by summing across healthcare resource headings. Using the same parameters, the unit cost was calculated in both Canadian (CAD) and US dollars (USD) at 2007 prices.

Results.—The cost of implanting a SCS system in Canada is \$21,595 (CAD), in US Medicare \$32,882 (USD), and in US Blue Cross Blue Shield (BCBS) \$57,896 (USD). The annual maintenance cost of an uncomplicated case in Canada is \$3539 (CAD), in US Medicare \$5071 (USD), and in

TABLE 3.—Summary of Cost Calculations*

Group	Implantation Costs	Annual Maintenance Costs	Mean Cost Per Complication†	Annual Cost/ Complication/ Patient‡	Ratio of Cost/ Complication to Annual Maintenance Cost§	Budgetary Cap¶
Canada (CAD)	$21,595	$3,539	$5,191	$556	1.4	18.9%
US Medicare (USD)	$32,882	$5,071	$9,649	$1,034	2.0	18.5%
US BCBS (USD)	$57,896	$7,277	$21,390	$2,293	2.9	16.5%
mean						18%

*For budgeting purposes, an implanter needs to calculate the initial cost of implantation of an SCS system for a patient at his or her institution, and then add the budgetary cap of 18% for each new patient undergoing implantation of an SCS system.

†Total cost = $327,057 (CAD), $607,857 (Medicare), and $1,347,564 (BCBS) ÷ total number of complications (63).

‡Total cost = $327,057 (CAD), $607,857 (Medicare), and $1,347,564 (BCBS) ÷ number of patients treated (161) ÷ mean follow-up period of 3.65 years.

§The ratio of cost/complication to annual maintenance cost = mean cost/complication ÷ annual maintenance costs.

¶Budgetary cap: cost of annual maintenance + annual cost/complication/patient ÷ implantation cost × 100 (percentage).

BCBS $7277 (USD). The mean cost of a complication was $5191 in Canada (range $136–18,837 [CAD]). In comparison, in the US the figures were $9649 (range $381–28,495) for Medicare and $21,390 (range $573–54,547) for BCBS (both USD). Using these calculations a formula was derived as follows: the annual maintenance cost (a) was added to the average annual cost per complication per patient implanted (b); the sum was then divided by the implantation cost (c); and the result was multiplied by 100 to obtain a percentage (a + b ÷ c × 100). To make this budgetary cap universally applicable, the results from the application of the formula were averaged, resulting in an 18% premium.

Conclusions.—For budgeting purposes the institution should first calculate the initial implantation costs that then can be "grossed up" by 18% per annum. This amount of 18% should be in addition to the implantation costs for the individual institution for new patients, as well as for each actively managed patient. This resulting amount will cover the costs associated with annual maintenance and complications for every actively managed patient. As the initial cost of implantation in any country reflects their current economics, the formula provided will be applicable to all implanters and policy makers alike (Table 3).

▶ This is a must read article for anyone involved in decision-making about the use of spinal cord stimulation. It emphasizes the fact that the total cost of these systems extends well beyond the initial implantation costs and it lists in detail the costs for each type of complication. The article also demonstrates the substantial differences in costs between the Canadian health care system, United States Medicare, and United States private insurance (Table 3), giving us food for thought regarding ways to reduce health care costs in the United States.

S. E. Abram, MD

The Effect of Mesh Removal and Selective Neurectomy on Persistent Postherniotomy Pain

Aasvang EK, Kehlet H (Copenhagen Univ, Denmark)

Ann Surg 249:327-334, 2009

Summary Background Data and Objective.—Persistent pain affects everyday activities in 5% to 8% of patients after groin hernia repair. Because previous reports on the effect of neurectomy and/or mesh removal suffer from methodological problems we performed a detailed prospective trial of the effect of neurectomy and mesh removal on persistent postherniotomy pain.

Methods.—Twenty-one patients with postherniotomy pain >1 year, pain-related impairment of daily activities and a well-defined maximum pain localization where included. Inserted mesh was removed and a selective neurectomy was done in case of macroscopic nerve injury. The primary end point was changes in pain-related impairment of everyday activities assessed by the validated activities assessment scale before surgery and 6 months postoperatively. Quantitative sensory testing was used to evaluate sensory functions pre and postoperatively.

Results.—All patients completed the 6-month follow-up. There was a significant improvement in the activities assessment scale score for the whole group (preoperative vs. 6 months = 27 vs. 13 points, $P = 0.004$), despite 3 patients worsening. Quantitative sensory testing showed a significant postoperative increase in pressure pain detection threshold ($P = 0.045$) and cutaneous detection and pain thresholds (mechanical and warmth) ($P < 0.03$).

Conclusions.—Selective neurectomy and mesh removal may improve pain-related activity impairment in patients with persistent postherniotomy pain. Detailed neurophysiologic assessment is recommended to identify patients who may or may not benefit from reoperation and to allocate patients to specific surgical and/or medical intervention.

▶ Persistent neuropathic pain following herniorrhaphy is a difficult pain management problem with a high rate of treatment failure. This study indicates that 13 of 21 patients experienced improvement in function following surgery, whereas only 3 were worse. The proportion of patients who improved was even higher among patients who did not show evidence of central sensitization (windup) (see Fig 2 in the original article). The results are even more remarkable given the fact that all patients had pain for over a year.

S. E. Abram, MD

Botulinum toxin for diabetic neuropathic pain: A randomized double-blind crossover trial

Yuan R-Y, Sheu J-J, Yu J-M, et al (Taipei Med Univ and Hosp, Taiwan)
Neurology 72:1473-1478, 2009

Background.—Diabetic neuropathy is a common complication in diabetes, with patients typically experiencing diverse sensory symptoms including dysesthesias in the feet and usually accompanied by sleep disturbance. There is still no comprehensive understanding of the underlying biologic processes responsible for diabetic neuropathic pain. Thus, the current symptomatic therapy remains unsatisfactory. Recent experimental evidence suggests that botulinum toxin type A (BoNT/A) may not only inhibit the release of acetylcholine at the neuromuscular junctions, but also modulate afferent sensory fiber firing, thereby relieving neuropathic pain.

Methods.—A double-blind crossover trial of intradermal BoNT/A for diabetic neuropathic pain in 18 patients was conducted to evaluate the effectiveness.

Results.—We find significant reduction in visual analog scale (VAS) of pain by 0.83 ± 1.11 at 1 week, 2.22 ± 2.24 at 4 weeks, 2.33 ± 2.56 at 8 weeks, and 2.53 ± 2.48 at 12 weeks after injection in the BoNT/A group, as compared to the respective findings for a placebo group of 0.39 ± 1.18, −0.11 ± 2.04, 0.42 ± 1.62, and 0.53 ± 1.57 at the same timepoints ($p < 0.05$). Within the BoNT/A group, 44.4% of the participants experienced a reduction of VAS ≥3 within 3 months after injection, whereas there was no similar response in the placebo group. At the 4-week postinjection stage, improvement in sleep quality was measured using the Chinese version of the Pittsburgh Sleep Quality Index.

Conclusions.—This pilot study found that botulinum toxin type A significantly reduced diabetic neuropathic pain and transiently improved sleep quality. Further large-scaled study is warranted.

▶ Intradermal botulinum toxin injected intradermally in the dorsum of both feet provided significantly better pain reduction than placebo at times compatible with the onset and duration of the drug (Figs 2A and B in the original article). The proposed mechanism of action involves reduction in the release of glutamate, substance P, and calcitonin gene-related peptide (CGRP) from the primary afferent nerve terminals as well as effects on the transient receptor potential channel receptor 1 ($TRPV_1$) and adenosine ($P2X_3$) receptors in the periphery. Botulinum toxin has been injected almost everywhere imaginable, and case reports have suggested benefits for most sites of administration. It is of note, however, that (botulinum toxin type A) Botox has not been shown to produce pain relief in patients with myofascial pain syndromes, even when reduced motor endplate activity was documented.[1] At least in that painful condition, there was no evidence of an antinociceptive effect.

S. E. Abram, MD

Reference

1. Qerqma E, Fugelsang-Frederiksen A, Kasch H, Bach FW, Jensen TS. A double-blind, controlled study of botulinum toxin A in chronioc myofascial pain. *Neurology.* 2006;67:241-245.

Efficacy of Steroid and Nonsteroid Caudal Epidural Injections for Low Back Pain and Sciatica: A Prospective, Randomized, Double-Blind Clinical Trial

Sayegh FE, Kenanidis EI, Papavasiliou KA, et al (Aristotle Univ of Thessaloniki-Med School, Greece)

Spine 34:1441-1447, 2009

Study Design.—Prospective, double-blind, randomized, case-control study.

Objective.—To evaluate the efficacy of caudal epidural injections (CEI) containing steroid *versus* nonsteroid preparations when treating patients suffering from low back pain (LBP) and sciatica.

Summary of Background Data.—Literature seems to be deprived of well-designed randomized, controlled studies that evaluate the effectiveness of CEI in the treatment of chronic LBP; hence the value of CEI remains still the subject of controversy.

Methods.—Patients suffering from severe chronic LBP and sciatica were randomly allocated into 2 groups. Steroid-group's patients (n = 93) underwent CEI containing 12 mL of xylocaine 2% and 1 mL of betamethasone dipropionate and betamethasone phosphate (2 + 5) mg/dL. Water for Injection (WFI)-group's patients (n = 90) underwent CEI containing 12 mL of xylocaine 2% and 8 mL of WFI. Both groups were statistically comparable as far as their demographic data and the cause and duration of symptoms were concerned. Patients answered the Oswestry Disability Index questionnaire and underwent physical examination, before and at 1 week, 1 month, 6 months, and 1 year following the CEI.

Results.—Symptoms improved in 132 patients (72.1%) following CEI. The mean Oswestry Disability Index questionnaire score of steroid-group's patients was statistically significant lower than that of the WFI-group at all postinjection re-evaluations. Patients receiving steroid CEI experienced faster relief during the first postinjection week. The Straight Leg Rising test improved in both groups following CEI; this improvement was faster among steroid-group's patients. Fifty-one patients (27.8%), noticed no improvement 1 week post-CEI and underwent a second CEI (with the same preparation) 7 to 14 days later. Nineteen of them reported improvement; 32 (steroid-group:13, WFI-group:19) did not respond well and underwent operative decompression (n = 15) or spinal fusion (n = 17).

Conclusion.—CEI containing local anesthetic and steroids or WFI seems to be effective when treating patients with LBP and sciatica. CEI containing steroid preparations demonstrated better and faster efficacy.

► This study showed some benefit from a moderate volume of caudal epidural injection of local anesthetic and increased response with the addition of betamethasone. The Oswestry Disability Index scores are shown in Fig 1 in the original article. A possible flaw in the design is the difference in volume and concentration of local anesthetic because the nonsteroid group received 8 mL water rather than 1 mL of the steroid. There is controversy over the benefits of high epidural injectate volumes in patients with sciatica related to disc herniation. Most new fluoroscopy-guided techniques use low volumes in an effort to apply higher steroid concentrations at the target neural structures. Studies are needed to determine if higher volumes provide more benefit for some patients.

S. E. Abram, MD

Laparoscopic Uterosacral Nerve Ablation for Alleviating Chronic Pelvic Pain: A Randomized Controlled Trial

Daniels J, Gray R, Hills RK, et al (Birmingham Women's Hosp, UK; Univ of Birmingham, UK; Cardiff Univ, Wales, UK; et al)

JAMA 302:955-961, 2009

Context.—Chronic pelvic pain is a common condition with a major effect on health-related quality of life, work productivity, and health care use. Operative interruption of nerve trunks in the uterosacral ligaments by laparoscopic uterosacral nerve ablation (LUNA) is a treatment option for patients with chronic pelvic pain.

Objective.—To assess the effectiveness of LUNA in patients with chronic pelvic pain.

Design, Setting, and Participants.—Randomized controlled trial of 487 women with chronic pelvic pain lasting longer than 6 months without or with minimal endometriosis, adhesions, or pelvic inflammatory disease, who were recruited to the study by consultant gynecological surgeons from 18 UK hospitals between February 1998 and December 2005. Follow-up was conducted by questionnaires mailed at 3 and 6 months and at 1, 2, 3, and 5 years.

Intervention.—Bilateral LUNA or laparoscopy without pelvic denervation (no LUNA); participants were blinded to the treatment allocation.

Main Outcome Measures.—The primary outcome was pain, which was assessed by a visual analogue scale. Data concerning the 3 types of pain (noncyclical pain, dysmenorrhea, and dyspareunia) were analyzed separately as was the worst pain level experienced from any of these 3 types of pain. The secondary outcome was health-related quality of life, which was measured using a generic instrument (EuroQoL EQ-5D and EQ-VAS).

Results.—After a median follow-up of 69 months, there were no significant differences reported on the visual analogue pain scales for the worst pain (mean difference between the LUNA group and the no LUNA group, −0.04 cm [95% confidence interval {CI}, −0.33 to 0.25 cm]; P=.80), noncyclical pain (−0.11 cm [95% CI, −0.50 to 0.29 cm]; P=.60), dysmenorrhea (−0.09 cm [95% CI, −0.49 to 0.30 cm]; P=.60), or dyspareunia (0.18 cm [95% CI, −0.22 to 0.62 cm]; P=.40). No differences were observed between the LUNA group and the no LUNA group for quality of life.

Conclusion.—Among women with chronic pelvic pain, LUNA did not result in improvements in pain, dysmenorrhea, dyspareunia, or quality of life compared with laparoscopy without pelvic denervation.

Trial Registration.—controlled-trials.com Identifier: ISRCTN41196151

► This is a large, robust controlled trial that demonstrated virtually no reduction in pain at any time period following uterosacral nerve ablation. Previous systematic reviews of the efficacy of the procedure have been inconclusive. While the results are disappointing, they are important, potentially reducing health care costs and patient morbidity.

S. E. Abram, MD

Nortriptyline and gabapentin, alone and in combination for neuropathic pain: a double-blind, randomised controlled crossover trial

Gilron I, Bailey JM, Tu D, et al (Queen's Univ, Kingston, Canada; et al)

Lancet 374:1252-1261, 2009

Background.—Drugs for neuropathic pain have incomplete efficacy and dose-limiting side-effects when given as monotherapy. We assessed the efficacy and tolerability of combined nortriptyline and gabapentin compared with each drug given alone.

Methods.—In this double-blind, double-dummy, crossover trial, patients with diabetic polyneuropathy or postherpetic neuralgia, and who had a daily pain score of at least 4 (scale 0–10), were enrolled and treated at one study site in Canada between Nov 5, 2004, and Dec 13, 2007. 56 patients were randomised in a 1:1:1 ratio with a balanced Latin square design to receive one of three sequences of daily oral gabapentin, nortriptyline, and their combination. In sequence, a different drug was given to each randomised group in three treatment periods. During each 6-week treatment period, drug doses were titrated towards maximum tolerated dose. The primary outcome was mean daily pain at maximum tolerated dose. Analysis was by intention to treat. This trial is registered, number ISRCTN73178636.

Findings.—45 patients completed all three treatment periods; 47 patients completed at least two treatment periods and were analysed for the primary outcome. Mean daily pain (0–10; numerical rating scale) was

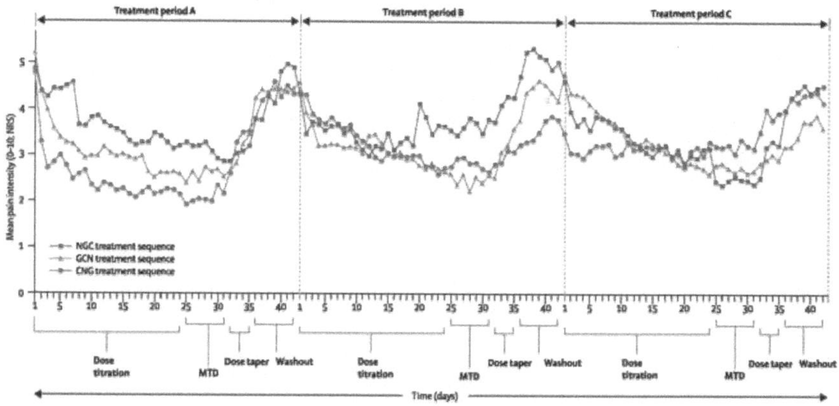

FIGURE 2.—Mean daily pain intensity. Each treatment period contained phases of drug dose titration (24 days), maximum tolerated dose (MTD; 7 days), dose taper (4 days), and washout (7 days). NRS=numerical rating scale. NGC=nortriptyline, gabapentin, and combined nortriptyline and gabapentin. GCN=gabapentin, combined nortriptyline and gabapentin, and nortriptyline. CNG=combined nortriptyline and gabapentin, nortriptyline, and gabapentin. (Reprinted from Gilron I, Bailey JM, Tu D, et al. Nortriptyline and gabapentin, alone and in combination for neuropathic pain: a double-blind, randomised controlled crossover trial. *Lancet*. 2009;374:1252-1261, with permission from Elsevier.)

5·4 (95% CI 5·0 to 5·8) at baseline, and at maximum tolerated dose, pain was 3·2 (2·5 to 3·8) for gabapentin, 2·9 (2·4 to 3·4) for nortriptyline, and 2·3 (1·8 to 2·8) for combination treatment. Pain with combination treatment was significantly lower than with gabapentin (−0·9, 95% CI −1·4 to −0·3, p=0·001) or nortriptyline alone (−0·6, 95% CI −1·1 to −0·1, p=0·02). At maximum tolerated dose, the most common adverse event was dry mouth, which was significantly less frequent in patients on gabapentin than on nortriptyline (p<0·0001) or combination treatment (p<0·0001). No serious adverse events were recorded for any patients during the trial.

Interpretation.—Combined gabapentin and nortriptyline seems to be more efficacious than either drug given alone for neuropathic pain, therefore we recommend use of this combination in patients who show a partial response to either drug given alone and seek additional pain relief. Future trials should compare other combinations to their respective monotherapies for treatment of such pain (Fig 2, Table 4).

► The results of this study in terms of pain reduction were not surprising. As with many other studies, both gabapentin and tricyclic antidepressants show reproducible benefits, with the tricyclics having slightly lower NNT scores. This study goes farther than most, indicating significant further benefit when both drugs are combined (Fig 2). The incidence of side effects, even with the drug combination, was surprisingly low (Table 4). A troublesome side effect of both drugs (ie, weight gain) is usually not evident during the short duration of this study, and is often a reason these drugs are discontinued. Topiramate and zonisamide may be reasonable alternatives to either the tricyclics or

TABLE 4.—Treatment-Emergent Adverse Events in 5% of Patients or More

	During Dose Titration			At Maximum Tolerated Dose		
	Gabapentin (n=54)	Nortriptyline (n=52)	Combined Gabapentin and Nortriptyline (n=52)	Gabapentin (n=46)	Nortriptyline (n=50)	Combined Gabapentin and Nortriptyline (n=50)
Dry mouth	11 (20%)	29 (56%)*	27 (52%)†	8 (17%)	29 (58%)‡	30 (60%)§
Fatigue	7 (13%)	9 (17%)	6 (12%)	2 (4%)	6 (12%)	4 (8%)
Somnolence	9 (17%)	8 (15%)	9 (17%)	1 (2%)	1 (2%)	4 (8%)
Insomnia	3 (6%)	9 (17%)	6 (12%)	0	2 (4%)	2 (4%)
Dizziness	7 (13%)	6 (12%)	6 (12%)	4 (9%)	2 (4%)	4 (8%)
Headache	7 (13%)	5 (10%)	2 (4%)	2 (4%)	2 (4%)	1 (2%)
Constipation	4 (7%)	6 (12%)	5 (10%)	1 (2%)	1 (2%)	1 (2%)
Ataxia	5 (9%)	1 (2%)	5 (10%)	3 (7%)	1 (2%)	5 (10%)
Feeling intoxicated	6 (11%)	1 (2%)	4 (8%)	1 (2%)	0	2 (4%)
Inability to concentrate	6 (11%)	0¶	3 (6%)	2 (4%)	0	2 (4%)
High blood sugar‖	4 (7%)	3 (6%)	4 (8%)	5 (11%)	2 (4%)	3 (6%)
Oedema	5 (9%)	2 (4%)	3 (6%)	4 (9%)	2 (4%)	4 (8%)
Abdominal cramping	5 (9%)	3 (6%)	3 (6%)	0	0	1 (2%)
Urinary retention	2 (4%)	4 (8%)	3 (6%)	1 (2%)	3 (6%)	2 (4%)
Emotional lability	1 (2%)	4 (8%)	1 (2%)	1 (2%)	3 (6%)	0
Difficulty swallowing	0	1 (2%)	0	0	3 (6%)	1 (2%)
Pruritus	0	3 (6%)	0	1 (2%)	1 (2%)	0
Excessive sweating	1 (2%)	3 (6%)	0	2 (4%)	1 (2%)	0
Weight gain	3 (6%)	1 (2%)	3 (6%)	1 (2%)	1 (2%)	0
Blurry vision	3 (6%)	0	0	1 (2%)	0	1 (2%)

Data are number (%).
*p=0·0003 for difference between nortriptyline and gabapentin.
†p=0·001 for difference between combination treatment and gabapentin.
‡p<0·0001 for difference between nortriptyline and gabapentin.
§p<0·0001 for difference between combination treatment and gabapentin.
¶p=0·03 for difference between nortriptyline and gabapentin.
‖Reported by patient home blood glucose monitoring.

gabapentin for patients with this and other side effects, or when neither of these drugs is efficacious. Most studies of the drugs for painful neuropathies are done in patients with diabetic neuropathy or postherpetic neuralgia. The efficacy of these drugs in other neuropathic pain states, particularly traumatic mononeuropathy or radiculopathy, has not been well studied.

S. E. Abram, MD

Incidence of Simultaneous Epidural and Vascular Injection During Cervical Transforaminal Epidural Injections

Smuck M, Tang C-T, Fuller BJ (Stanford Univ, CA; Univ of Michigan, Ann Arbor)

Spine 34:E751-E755, 2009

Study Design.—Prospective, observational *in vivo* study.

Objective.—The aim of this study was to determine the incidence of simultaneous epidural and vascular contrast injection during cervical transforaminal epidural injections.

Summary of Background Data.—In the lumbar spine, vascular contrast patterns are more than twice as likely to appear simultaneous to the anticipated epidural pattern, than they are to occur alone. This is important because practitioners are more likely to miss a vascular pattern when it appears simultaneous to the expected epidural flow. The incidence of intravascular penetration in cervical transforaminal epidural injections is known to exceed than that of lumbar injections, however, no study has determined the incidence of simultaneous epidural and vascular injection in the cervical spine.

Methods.—Contrast patterns were observed with live fluoroscopy during 121 injections performed on 82 patients and categorized as one of the following: epidural only, vascular only, or simultaneous epidural and vascular.

Results.—The incidence of simultaneous epidural and vascular injection during cervical transforaminal epidural injections was 18.9%. The incidence of vascular only injection was 13.9%, for a total vascular injection incidence of 32.8%. There was no correlation between the observed contrast pattern with patients' age, sex, side of injection, needle gauge, or diagnosis. There was a significant correlation between the level of

TABLE 2.—Contrast Patterns by Foraminal Level

Injection Level (n)	C3–C4 (7)	C4–C5 (20)	C5–C6 (43)	C6–C7 (45)	C7–T1 (7)	Total (122)
Epidural only (n)	42.9% (3)	60.0% (12)	58.1% (25)	80.0% (36)	85.7% (6)	67.2% (82)
Vascular only (n)	28.6% (2)	30.0% (6)	11.6% (5)	8.9% (4)	0.0% (0)	13.9% (17)
Simultaneous epidural and vascular (n)	28.6% (2)	10.0% (2)	30.2% (13)	11.1% (5)	14.3% (1)	18.9% (23)
All vascular (n)	57.1% (4)	40.0% (8)	41.9% (18)	20.0% (9)	14.3% (1)	32.8% (40)

injection and the risk of vascular injection. The higher the injection level, the higher the probability of a vascular injection. Fluoroscopy time was significantly increased when a vascular injection was identified.

Conclusion.—Simultaneous epidural and vascular injection accounts for over half of all vascular injections during cervical transforaminal epidural injections. With the risk of severe complications and high incidence of vascular injections in the cervical spine, live fluoroscopy is recommended during contrast injection with specific attention to simultaneous epidural and vascular flow (Table 2).

▶ The very high incidence of intravascular injection of contrast is surprising and concerning. As the authors suggest, it may be more likely that the operator might overlook the vascular spread of dye when a portion of the drug is seen entering the epidural space. Another finding in this study is a higher incidence of intravascular injection at higher cervical levels (Table 2). The authors did not attempt to differentiate between venous and arterial injections or to identify radicular or vertebral artery injections, so it is not known how many of the injections could have produced spinal or cerebellar injuries had particulate steroids been injected. One factor that may have contributed to the high rate of intravascular injection is the use of very small gauge needles.

S. E. Abram, MD

Higher Opioid Doses Predict Poorer Functional Outcome in Patients with Chronic Disabling Occupational Musculoskeletal Disorders

Kidner CL, Mayer TG, Gatchel RJ (PRIDE Res Found, Dallas, TX)

J Bone Joint Surg Am 91:919-927, 2009

Background.—Opioids are frequently used for the postoperative treatment of chronic disabling occupational musculoskeletal disorders. In many such cases, long-term opioid use persists because of patient requests for ongoing pain relief. Little is known about the relationship between chronic opioid use and functional recovery in these patients.

Methods.—A total of 1226 patients with a chronic disabling occupational musculoskeletal disorder were consecutively admitted into an interdisciplinary functional restoration program. They were divided into two groups: 630 patients who reported no opioid use at the time of admission (No group) and 596 patients who reported some opioid use at the time of admission (Yes group). The 516 patients for whom daily opioid doses could be determined were further divided into four subgroups: Low (<30 mg, n = 267), Medium (31 to 60 mg, n = 112), High (61 to 120 mg, n = 78), and Very High (>120 mg, n = 59). During the initial weeks of treatment, patients consented to be weaned from all opioid medications. In addition, the patients were assessed before and after rehabilitation with regard to self-reported measures of pain, function, and depression and were analyzed for change. One year after the termination

TABLE 5.—One-Year Post-Rehabilitation Socioeconomic Outcomes: Opioid Subgroups Controlled for Pre-Rehabilitation Length of Disability (Completers Only)

Variable	No	Low	Medium	High	Very High	P Value*	R^2
Number of patients (% of total) (n = 887)	513 (57.8)	205 (23.1)	75 (8.5)	53 (6.0)	41 (4.6)		
Work return (%)	93.7	88.7	89.5	90.7	75.9	0.05	0.107
Work retention (%)	85.2	70.1	63.0	69.0	55.2	<0.001	0.132
Surgery to same body part (%)	2.1	5.5	2.1	7.7	7.4	NS	
Seeking treatment from new provider (%)	14.0	28.8	36.7	28.2	29.6	0.001	0.052
New injury to same body part (%)	4.4	3.8	13.0	6.3	4.2	NS	
Workers' Compensation case settlement (%)	97.2	98.6	98.0	95.0	100.0	NS	
SSDI or SSI† (%)	1.9	5.7	3.9	4.5	18.5	0.03	0.176

*NS = not significant.
†SSDI = Social Security Disability Income, SSI = Supplemental Security Income.

of treatment, socioeconomic outcomes were assessed to measure work and financial status, healthcare utilization, and recurrent injury-associated pain.

Results.—A higher post-injury opioid dose was associated with a greater risk of program noncompletion, which was anticipated because of the requirement that patients taper opioids. High opioid use was significantly related to important socioeconomic outcomes, such as lower rates of return to work and work retention as well as higher healthcare utilization ($p \leq 0.05$ for all). Moreover, at one year after treatment, the group reporting the highest opioid use was 11.6 times as likely to be receiving Social Security Disability Income/Supplemental Security Income as compared with the group reporting no opioid use at the time of admission into the program.

Conclusions.—Chronic opioid use beginning after a work-related injury is a predictor of less successful outcomes for patients whose final treatment intervention is an interdisciplinary functional restoration program. Higher dose levels are associated with progressively greater indemnity and medical costs for ongoing disability. Physicians involved in the treatment of chronic disabling occupational musculoskeletal disorders should be aware of problems associated with permitting long-term opioid use in patients with a disabling occupational disorder (Table 5).

▶ There is mounting evidence that opioid use, particularly at high doses, is associated with longer periods of disability and a lower likelihood of returning to work. Even when adjusting for severity of injury there appears to be a negative impact of opioid use on recovery from injury. The benefits of using opioids to enable patients with acute pain to successfully participate in therapy may be offset by other effects, such as development of opioid dependence or hyperalgesia. This study indicates that higher disability claims and lower rates of employment are associated with the highest opioid doses (Table 5).

S. E. Abram, MD

Ultrasound of the Lateral Femoral Cutaneous Nerve: Normal Findings in a Cadaver and in Volunteers

Bodner G, Bernathova M, Galiano K, et al (St Bernard's Hosp, Gibraltar, UK; Med Univ Innsbruck, Austria; et al)

Reg Anesth Pain Med 34:265-268, 2009

Objective.—To assess the feasibility of ultrasound (US) in visualizing the lateral femoral cutaneous nerve (LFCN) in a cadaver and 8 volunteers.

Methods.—Ultrasound and US-guided dye injection was performed in 1 cadaver to show the feasibility of detecting the LFCN. We then performed US in 8 volunteers to assess position of the nerve in respect to the anterior iliac spine. We subsequently performed US-guided anesthetic block of the LFCN on both sides with 0.3 mL local anesthetic. Success rate, time to maximum peak blockade, and duration of blockade were noted.

Results.—Ultrasound allowed visualization of the LFCN in the cadaveric specimen on both sides and in all but 1 volunteer. Ultrasound-guided block of the LFCN was successful in all but 1 volunteer. The mean distance of LFCN from the anterior iliac spine was 2.9 cm on the right side and 2.8 cm on the left side. The mean duration of the block was 4.4 hours.

Conclusion.—Ultrasound enables visualization of the LFCN in a cadaver and in volunteers. Ultrasound-guided injection successfully blocked the LFCN.

► It is relatively easy to perform a lateral femoral cutaneous block without the use of ultrasound. However, the use of ultrasound guidance provides for more accurate placement of injectate, such as corticosteroids. In addition, there is considerable variation in the distance of the nerve from the anterior superior iliac spine (ASIS). Ultrasound may also be useful to locate the nerve if pulsed or thermal radiofrequency ablation is contemplated. However, I could find no reference to the use of RF for meralgia paresthetica.

S. E. Abram, MD

Occipital Nerve Blocks: Effect of Symptomatic Medication: Overuse and Headache Type on Failure Rate

Tobin JA, Flitman SS (21st Century Neurology, Phoenix, AZ)

Headache 49:1479-1485, 2009

Objective.—To explore the effect of symptomatic medication overuse (SMO) and headache type on occipital nerve block (ONB) efficacy.

Methods.—We conducted a chart review of all of the ONBs performed in our clinic over a 2-year period.

Results.—Of 108 ONBs with follow-up data, ONB failed in 22% of injections overall. Of the other 78%, the mean decrease in head pain was 83%, and the benefit lasted a mean of 6.6 weeks. Failure rate without SMO was 16% overall, and with SMO was 44% overall ($P < .000$). In those who did respond, overall magnitude and duration of response did not differ between those with and those without SMO. Without SMO, ONB failure rate was 0% for postconcussive syndrome, 14% for occipital neuralgia, 11% for non-intractable migraine, and 39% for intractable migraine. With SMO, failure rate increased by 24% ($P = .14$) in occipital neuralgia, by 36% ($P = .08$) for all migraine, and by 52% ($P = .04$) for non-intractable migraine.

Conclusions.—SMO tripled the risk of ONB failure, possibly because medication overuse headache does not respond to ONB. SMO increased ONB failure rate more in migraineurs than in those with occipital neuralgia, possibly because migraineurs are particularly susceptible to medication overuse headache. This effect was much more pronounced in non-intractable migraineurs than in intractable migraineurs.

▶ The authors of this study indicated that their retrospective study was prompted by the case of a patient who failed occipital block while she was overusing medication; but she later responded after discontinuing her medications. For all headache types, selection of patients for occipital nerve blocks (ONBs) was based on the presence of reproduction of headache symptoms by pressure over the occipital nerve. Their study did not include patients with tension-type headache, a group that had previously been shown to respond poorly to ONB.

S. E. Abram, MD

Financial compensation and vocational recovery: a prospective study of secondary care neck and back patients

Hestbaek L, Rasmussen C, Leboeuf-Yde C (Univ of Southern Denmark, Odense; Hjørring Hosp, Denmark; et al)

Scand J Rheumatol 38:481-487, 2009

Objectives.—Financial compensation has been shown to be a negative prognostic factor for pain and disability in patients with neck or low back pain. It is unclear whether this association is causal and to what extent it hampers return to work. The objective of this study was to assess the direct influence of a financial compensation process on the ability to remain in regular employment in patients with suspected disc herniation.

Methods.—A prospective cohort study with a register-based follow-up at 1, 3, and 5 years after baseline was carried out at two multidisciplinary,

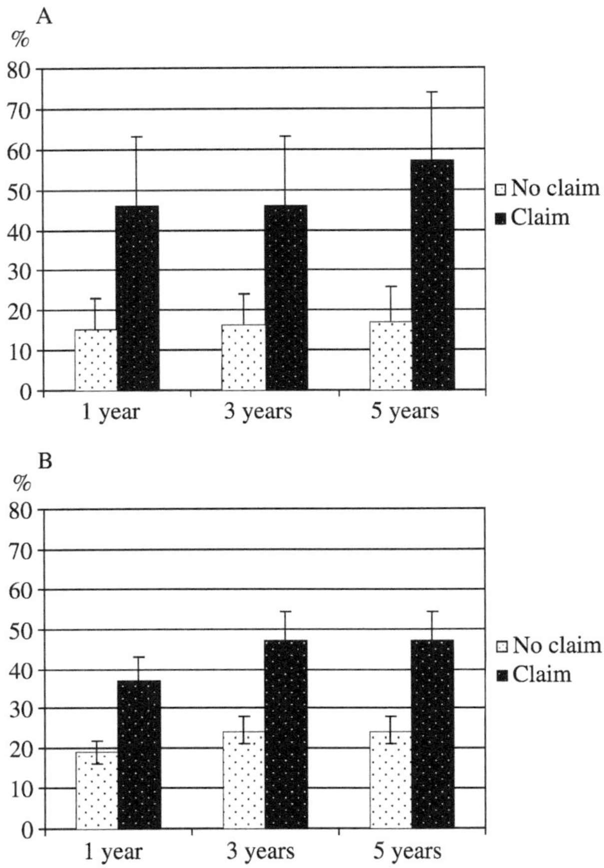

FIGURE 1.—Proportion of patients with (A) neck/arm pain and (B) low back/leg pain who received income substitution at follow-up, by claim status at baseline (95% confidence interval). (Reprinted from Hestbaek L, Rasmussen C, Leboeuf-Yde C. Financial compensation and vocational recovery: a prospective study of secondary care neck and back patients. *Scand J Rheumatol.* 2009;38:481-487.)

non-surgical spine clinics in two public hospitals in Denmark. The study population comprised consecutive patients in regular employment with neck pain radiating to the arm or low back pain radiating to the leg. The exposure variable was any type of claim for financial compensation for the actual low back/leg or neck/arm pain. The outcome measure was receiving income compensation benefits. This information was obtained through national registers. Follow-up points were 1, 3, and 5 years after inclusion.

Results.—The study included 1243 low back pain patients and 202 neck pain patients. The odds ratio, adjusted for relevant confounders, of receiving income compensation benefits in case of baseline financial claim was approximately 2 for low back/leg pain patients and about 4 for neck/arm pain patients at 1, 3, and 5 years.

Conclusions.—In employed patients, a claim for financial compensation for low back or neck pain with radiating pain was found to be independently associated with receipt of income compensation benefits after 1, 3, and 5 years (Fig 1).

► This study indicates that patients with low back or neck pain who file early financial claims for disability are more likely to remain unemployed and will continue receiving unemployment benefits (Fig 1). This effect is independent of other variables. Other studies have indicated that pain levels are higher among patients who receive time loss benefit payments,[1] and patients with high pain ratings are less likely to complete rehabilitation programs and to have low productivity and high health care costs.[2] Whether these data translate to lower success rates for any given therapy is unclear. We found no reduction in success of epidural steroid injections for sciatica among patients receiving financial compensation for their painful condition.[3]

S. E. Abram, MD

References

1. Fulton-Kehoe E, Gluck J, Wu R, Wickizer TM, Franklin GM. Measuring work disability: what can administrative data tell about patient outcomes? *J Occup Environ Med.* 2007;49:651-658.
2. McGeary DD, Mayer TG, Gatchel RJ. High pain ratings predict treatment failure in chronic musculoskeletal disorders. *J Bone Joint Surg Am.* 2006;88:317-325.
3. Abram SE, Anderson RA. Using a pain questionnaire to predict response to steroid epidurals. *Regional Anesthesia.* 1980;5:11-14.

Introduction of low dose transdermal buprenorphine — did it influence use of potentially addictive drugs in chronic non-malignant pain patients?

Skurtveit S, Furu K, Kaasa S, et al (Norwegian Inst of Public Health, Oslo; Norwegian Univ of Science and Technology, Trondheim; et al)

Eur J Pain 13:949-953, 2009

The aim was to study the introduction of the new low dose transdermal buprenorphine (LD-TD-BUP) in Norway, particularly with regard to former use and co-medication with other potentially addictive drugs.

The nationwide Norwegian Prescription Database contains information on all prescription drugs dispensed to individual non-institutionalised patients, and we may follow all individuals who received LD-TD-BUP (Norspan®) after marketing on the Norwegian market on 15/11/05. We studied all prescriptions of opioids and other potentially addictive drugs to patients receiving at least two LD-TD-BUP prescriptions during 2004–2006. Poisson regressions were run with concomitant use of addictive drugs (yes, no) as the endpoint.

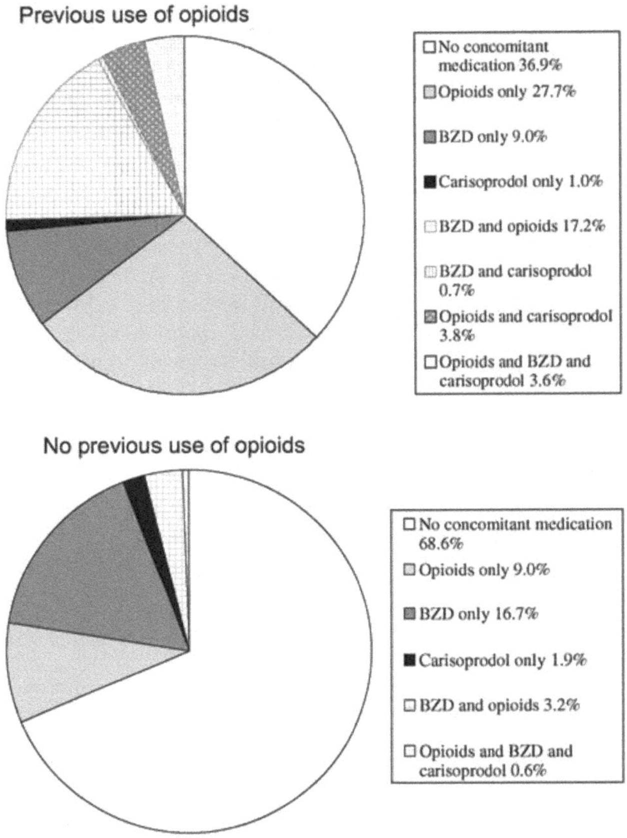

FIGURE 2.—Percentage of patient receiving LD-TD-BUP co-medicated with opioids, benzodiazepines, carisoprodol only or in combination according to (a) previous use of opioids ($N = 1728$) (b) no previous use of opioids ($N = 156$). (Reprinted from Skurtveit S, Furu K, Kaasa S, et al. Introduction of low dose transdermal buprenorphine - did it influence use of potentially addictive drugs in chronic non-malignant pain patients? *Eur J Pain*. 2009;13:949-953, with permission from the European Federation of International Association for the Study of Pain.)

Overall, 1884, non cancer individuals received at least two prescription of LD-TD-BUP. Of these 91.7% received prescriptions of other opioids and 58.6% of them had also been prescribed benzodiazepines/carisoprodol before the prescription of LD-TD-BUP. Of the LD-TD-BUP users who received more than one prescription, 60% co-medicated with at least one other potentially addictive drug, and 24% with at least two. In the multivariate analysis, the variables associated with a higher likelihood of using co-medicated drugs were: previous use of benzodiazepines/carisoprodol relative risk RR = 16.7 (95% CI 10.4–26.9), previous use of opioids RR = 4.0 (1.9–8.7) and younger age 20–40 years RR = 1.9 (1.6–2.3).

So far, it is questionable whether the introduction of LD-TD-BUP actually has stabilised opioids consumption or whether it has complicated and increased the consumption of potentially addictive drugs (Fig 2).

▶ Buprenorphine has been available as a sublingual preparation for use in pain management in Europe since the mid-1990s. It has been marketed in Europe as a moderate to high dose (35-70 mcg/hr) transdermal preparation, also with a pain indication, since 2001. A lower dose preparation (5-20 mcg/hr) was introduced in 2005. In the United States, buprenorphine has been marketed as Subutex (sublingual, 2 or 8 mg) or Suboxone (same doses plus naloxone to discourage IV use) with indications for addiction. This study investigates the effect of low dose transdermal buprenorphine on the use of other addicting drugs in Norway, where there are records of all controlled substance prescriptions. Among patients prescribed the low dose transdermal preparation, a majority of patients continued to be prescribed benzodiazepines and other opioids. Since the study tracks prescriptions and not actual use, and does not track the amount of medications used, it is difficult to determine whether the patients using buprenorphine reduced the use of other drugs. One would anticipate that concomitant opioid use would decline because buprenorphine blocks the effect of opioid agonists. This is dose-related, however, and it is possible to obtain an effect at higher opioid agonist doses. Clearly, patients using opioids before the initiation of the patch were much more likely to continue using opioids subsequently (Fig 2). It is appropriate that the authors included carisoprodol, which is metabolized to meprobamate, in their list of addicting drugs.

S. E. Abram, MD

High cervical spinal cord stimulation after failed dorsal root entry zone surgery for brachial plexus avulsion pain

Lai H-Y, Lee C-Y, Lee S-T (Chang Gung Memorial Hosp and Chang Gung Univ, Kweishan, Taiwan)

Surg Neurol 72:286-289, 2009

Background.—Many patients had intractable pain after brachial plexus avulsion. This article describes a feasible method of high cervical SCS for a patient who failed in DREZ surgery to treat the pain.

> *Case Description.*—A 70-year-old man had right brachial plexus avulsion after a car accident 15 years ago. He complained of chronic spontaneous pain over his right upper limb since then. Two DREZ surgeries failed to relieve the pain. The pain was successfully controlled by high cervical SCS.

Conclusion.—Stimulating the high cervical spinal cord is effective for treating intractable pain after brachial plexus avulsion, which the DREZ surgery failed to relieve.

▶ While a single case report does not justify widespread acceptance of spinal cord stimulation for this condition, it does justify further study. Dorsal root entry zone (DREZ) surgery is extremely invasive and may be associated with serious immediate or delayed complications. A stimulator trial before proceeding with DREZ lesioning may be a reasonable proposition.

S. E. Abram, MD

Altered quantitative sensory testing outcome in subjects with opioid therapy

Chen L, Malarick C, Seefeld L, et al (Massachusetts General Hospital, Boston)
Pain 143:65-70, 2009

Preclinical studies have suggested that opioid exposure may induce a paradoxical decrease in the nociceptive threshold, commonly referred as opioid-induced hyperalgesia (OIH). While OIH may have implications in acute and chronic pain management, its clinical features remain unclear. Using an office-based quantitative sensory testing (QST) method, we compared pain threshold, pain tolerance, and the degree of temporal summation of the second pain in response to thermal stimulation among

TABLE 2.—QST Results by Group.

	Group 1 ($n = 41$)	Group 2 ($n = 41$)	Group 3 ($n = 58$)	ANOVA (F- value; P-value)
CS	27.4 ± 0.4 °C [20.3–31.2 (27.8)]	27.9 ± 0.4 °C [20.7–31.1 (28.5)]	28.2 ± 0.4 °C [14.6–31.5 (28.7)]	0.94; 0.39
WS	35.4 ± 0.3 °C [32.5–40.2 (34.7)]	34.8 ± 0.2 °C [33.1–40.8 (34.5)]	34.9 ± 0.2 °C [32.9–42.6 (34.5)]	1.64; 0.19
CPTh	8.4 ± 1.2 °C [0–25.1 (5.2)]	10.0 ± 1.3 °C [0–26.9 (6.3)]	10.9 ± 1.2 °C [0–27.7 (6.1)]	0.99; 0.38
HPTh	45.3 ± 0.5 °C [36.7–50.8 (45.7)]	45.4 ± 0.4 °C [38.3–49.6 (46.0)]	43.8 ± 0.4 °C [34.3–49.9 (44.5)]	3.91; 0.02*
CPTol	0.5 ± 0.2 °C [0–7.1 (0)]	2.6 ± 0.8 °C [0–23.9 (0)]	3.3 ± 0.7 °C [0–24.8 (0)]	4.32; 0.01*
HPTol	50.1 ± 0.2 °C [47.3–52.9 (49.7)]	49.5 ± 0.3 °C [42.3–53.0 (49.6)]	48.6 ± 0.3 °C [36.3–53.0 (49.0)]	5.85; 0.01*
HPDur	47.6 ± 3.0 s ($n = 35$) [60–60 (60)]	42.4 ± 3.4 s ($n = 35$) [4–60 (60)]	35.2 ± 2.7 s ($n = 54$) [4–60 (41)]	4.25; 0.02*

CS, cold sensation; WS, warm sensation; CPTh, cold pain threshold; HPTh, heat pain threshold; CPTol, cold pain tolerance; HPTol, heat pain tolerance; HPDur, duration of tolerance to supra-threshold heat pain stimulation. The quantitative data are shown as means ± standard error.

*$P < 0.05$, repeated measure one-way ANOVA as compared among three groups. Of note, those numbers shown in a parenthesis under group mean ± standard error represent the range and median number of a QST parameter in each group. For the duration of heat pain tolerance, the number is smaller than the total number of its respective group because a small number of subjects in each group had the heat pain threshold above 47 °C and were not included in this analysis.

TABLE 4.—Clinical Factors Implicated in the Differential Diagnosis of OIH.

Clinical factor	Clinical finding
Temporal summation of second pain	Exacerbated (QST)
Pain threshold (cold or heat)	Decreased (QST) - particularly heat pain
Pain tolerance (cold or heat)	Decreased (QST)
Supra-threshold stimulation	Decreased duration of tolerance (QST)
Average opioid dose	≥75 mg daily morphine equivalent dose
Duration of opioid therapy	≥3 months
Opioid dose escalation	Limited improvement or normalization on QST responses
Opioid dose reduction	Improved opioid analgesia [38]
Pain quality	Burning, diffuse pain, and spontaneous pain similar to those seen with neuropathic pain
Pain location	At and/or beyond the dermatome distribution of a pre-existing pain condition
Pain intensity	Similar or greater than pre-existing pain
Opioid type to be considered	Short-acting vs. long acting; methadone versus other opioid analgesics
Gender	Female vs. male?

Editor's Note: Please refer to original journal article for full references.

three groups of subjects: those with neither pain nor opioid therapy (group 1), with chronic pain but without opioid therapy (group 2), and with both chronic pain and opioid therapy (group 3). We also examined the possible correlation between QST responses to thermal stimulation and opioid dose, opioid treatment duration, opioid analgesic type, pain duration, or gender in group 3 subjects. As compared with both group 1 ($n=41$) and group 2 ($n=41$) subjects, group 3 subjects ($n=58$) displayed a decreased heat pain threshold and exacerbated temporal summation of the second pain to thermal stimulation. In contrast, there were no differences in cold or warm sensation among three groups. Among clinical factors, daily opioid dose consistently correlated with the decreased heat pain threshold and exacerbated temporal summation of the second pain in group 3 subjects. These results indicate that decreased heat pain threshold and exacerbated temporal summation of the second pain may be characteristic QST changes in subjects with opioid therapy. The data suggest that QST may be a useful tool in the clinical assessment of OIH (Tables 2 and 4).

► Several previous studies have documented reduced tolerance to cold water immersion, but minimal changes in pain thresholds or tolerance to other types of experimentally induced pain. In this study, reduced pain heat thresholds and increased temporal summation for thermal pain in chronic pain patients on opioids as compared with chronic pain patients not taking opioids (Table 2 and Fig 1 in the original article). While chronic pain patients on opioids had reduced cold pain thresholds and tolerance compared with control subjects, there were no differences when compared with chronic pain patients not taking opioid. This implies that the presence of chronic pain per se might account for some or all of the differences. The study also found that higher opioid doses were associated with greater differences in heat pain thresholds and exaggerated temporal summation to heat pain. This study supports the notion that opioid administration can increase pain sensitivity, and that pain associated with noxious thermal stimulation is affected to a greater extent than mechanically induced pain. Future clinical investigation should further address ways of detecting hyperalgesia, identifying patients who might improve with opioid reduction or discontinuation, and methods for reversing hyperalgesia in patients who benefit partially from opioid therapy. Table 4 offers some information regarding the differential diagnosis of opioid induced hyperalgesia.

S. E. Abram, MD

Co-morbidity and utilization of medical services by pain patients receiving opioid medications: Data from an insurance claims database

Cicero TJ, Wong G, Tian Y, et al (Washington Univ School of Medicine, St. Louis, MO; Anthem Blue Cross and Blue Shield, St. Louis, MO)

Pain 144:20-27, 2009

We used a large medical insurance claims database to identify three groups: chronic opioid use (>180 therapeutic days, $N = 3726$); acute opioid use (<10 therapeutic days, $N = 37{,}108$); and a non-opioid group ($N = 337{,}366$) who filed at least one insurance claim but none for opioids. Our results showed that although chronic opioid users represented only 0.65% of the total population, they filed 4.56% of all insurance claims, used 45% of all opioid analgesics and had much more physical and psychiatric co-morbidity than the acute opioid or non-opioid samples. Women were substantially over-represented (>63%) in the chronic pain group and used a much greater share of all medical services than males, especially as they grew older. Although our data suggest that chronic pain is optimally managed in a multidisciplinary patient- and gender-specific treatment plan, this was rarely the case with internists being the primary, and often only, physician seen. Moreover, our data suggest that opioids were often used for conditions in which they are generally not indicated (e.g. arthritis and headaches) or contraindicated by co-existing physical ailments (COPD). Finally, we conclude that adherence to the WHO analgesic ladder and other pain treatment guidelines was relatively infrequent: first, opioid extended release preparations which are ideally suited for chronic pain were used only in one in four patients; and, second, the selection of a weak (propoxyphene, codeine, and tramadol) or strong opioid

TABLE 1.—Health Service Utilization by Chronic Opioid, Acute Opioid and Non-opioid Groups

			Chronic Opioid						Acute Opioid						Non-Opioid			
	All $N = 3726$		Male $N = 1370$, 37%		Female $N = 2356$, 63%		All $N = 37,108$		Male $N = 16,654$, 45%		Female $N = 20454$, 55%		All $N = 337,366$		Male $N = 164,596$, 49%		Female $N = 172,770$, 51%	
Average Number	#	SE	#	SE	#	SE	#	SE	#	SE	#	SE	#	SE	#	SE	#	SE
# of insurance claims	169.29	2.25	145.52	3.31	183.12	2.97	57.12	0.34	47.16	0.50	65.23	0.46	28.54	0.08	23.23	0.10	33.60	0.12
Mean of distinct diagnosed ICD-9s	20.66	0.23	17.70	0.35	22.38	0.29	11.61	0.04	9.74	0.06	13.06	0.06	7.79	0.01	6.64	0.01	8.76	0.02
Doctors/providers seen by patient[a]	9.81	0.12	8.57	0.19	10.52	0.15	6.34	0.02	5.46	0.03	7.02	0.03	3.39	0.01	2.68	0.01	4.06	0.01
Office visits	16.91	0.25	14.80	0.38	18.14	0.33	8.67	0.05	7.46	0.07	9.58	0.07	5.06	0.01	4.20	0.02	5.89	0.02
ER visits	0.62	0.03	0.53	0.04	0.67	0.04	0.31	0.00	0.32	0.01	0.30	0.00	0.11	0.00	0.10	0.00	0.11	0.00
Hospital days	1.66	0.09	1.42	0.14	1.80	0.12	0.56	0.02	0.45	0.03	0.64	0.02	0.22	0.01	0.18	0.01	0.26	0.02

[a]Excluding radiologists and pathologists; SAS multiple GLMs (General linear models) procedures were used to specify statistically significant differences (independent variables: groups and female). All estimated parameters were significant at $p < 0.01$. Post hoc tests of group differences were all significant at $p < 0.01$; post hoc tests of gender differences were all significant at $p < 0.05$.

(e.g. morphine and oxycodone) seemed to be driven by numerous factors not necessarily related to the intensity or duration of pain (Table 1).

▶ There is increasing concern that the liberal prescribing of opioids for chronic noncancer pain is associated with increased morbidity, reduced function and increased health care costs. This study demonstrated increased physical and psychiatric comorbidity among patients using opioids chronically. They saw more physicians and had more insurance claims and office, hospital, and ER visits compared with patients who used opioids for acute conditions or who used no opioids (Table 1). While it is possible that it is the painful condition rather than the opioid use that is associated with these differences, there is evidence from other studies that opioid use predicts disability, medical costs, and subsequent surgery independently of other variables.[1,2] The data from this study are particularly compelling given the large numbers of patients in the database. It is of interest that more than three fourths of the patients receiving opioids were being treated by internists and less than 10% of patients with psychiatric comorbidities were treated by a psychiatrist. With the disappearance of the multidisciplinary pain management model, chronic pain management appears to be shifting to opioid prescribing by primary care physicians and to interventional therapies by pain management physicians. A minority of patients receive long-term care from pain management clinics.

S. E. Abram, MD

References

1. Webster BS, Verma SK, Gatchel RJ. Relationship between early opioid prescribing for acute low back pain and disability duration, medical costs, subsequent surgery and late opioid use. *Spine*. 2007;32:2127-2132.
2. Volinn E, Fargo JD, Fine PG. Opioid therapy for nonspecific low back pain and the outcome of work loss. *Pain*. 2009;142:194-201.

Influence of lumbar epidural injection volume on pain relief for radicular leg pain and/or low back pain

Rabinovitch DL, Peliowski A, Furlan AD (Univ of Toronto, Ontario, Canada)
Spine J 9:509-517, 2009

Background Context.—Epidural injections are commonly used to treat low back disorders. It has been proposed that in addition to the anti-inflammatory effects, injected material displaces the dura forward and inward, producing a stretch of the nerve roots that leads to lysis of neural adhesions. Despite this, there are no controlled trials investigating the effect of volume injected with pain as an independent outcome.

Purpose.—Review the existing literature to assess the effect of epidural injection volume on relief of radicular leg and low back pain.

Study Design.—A systematic review of published clinical trials to assess the correlation between volume of epidural injection and relief of radicular leg and low back pain.

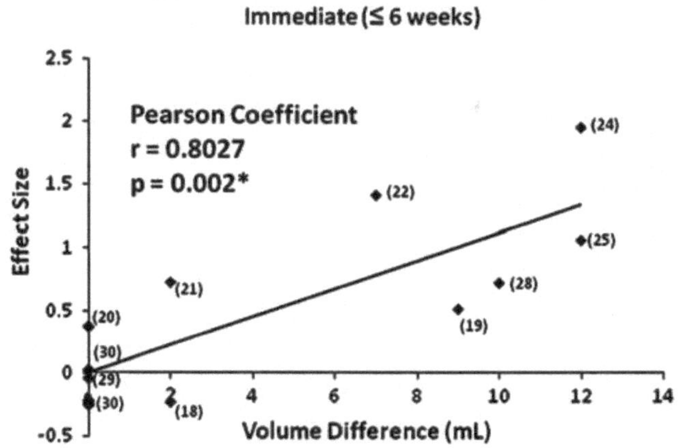

FIGURE 1.—Effect size versus volume difference of epidural injection for the immediate category. (n) represents reference number that corresponds to each study; *p<.05 is statistically significant. (Reprinted from Rabinovitch DL, Peliowski A, Furlan AD. Influence of lumbar epidural injection volume on pain relief for radicular leg pain and/or low back pain. *Spine J*. 2009;9:509-517, with permission from Elsevier Inc.)

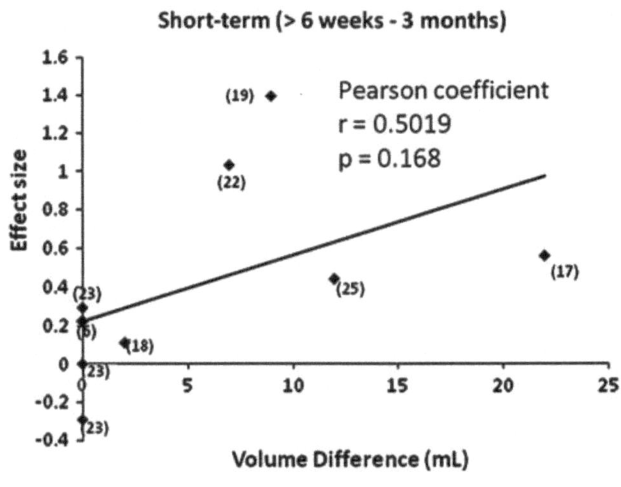

FIGURE 2.—Effect size versus volume difference of epidural injection for the short-term category. (n) represents reference number that corresponds to each study; *p<.05 is statistically significant. (Reprinted from Rabinovitch DL, Peliowski A, Furlan AD. Influence of lumbar epidural injection volume on pain relief for radicular leg pain and/or low back pain. *Spine J*. 2009;9:509-517, with permission from Elsevier Inc.)

Methods.—We searched MEDLINE (1966 to January 2009), EMBASE (1980 to January 2009), The Cochrane Library, and the reference lists of retrieved articles. The literature search was limited to English and Human subjects. Studies were included if they involved the following: 1) a controlled clinical trial; 2) epidural injections in treatment groups compared with control injections; 3) the same approach to epidural

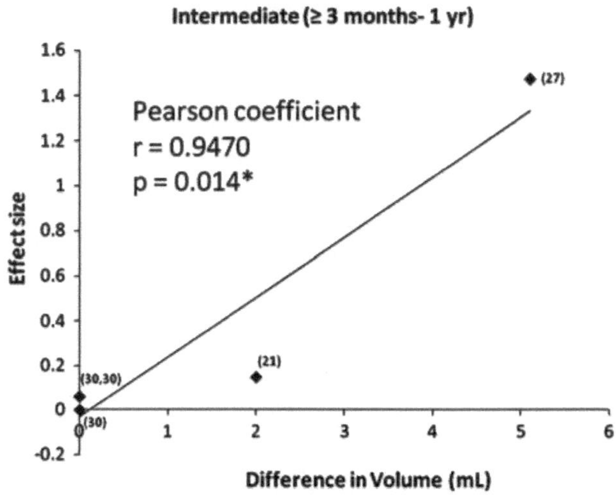

FIGURE 3.—Effect size versus volume difference of epidural injection for the intermediate category. (n) represents reference number that corresponds to each study; *p<.05 is statistically significant. (Reprinted from Rabinovitch DL, Peliowski A, Furlan AD. Influence of lumbar epidural injection volume on pain relief for radicular leg pain and/or low back pain. *Spine J*. 2009;9:509-517, with permission from Elsevier Inc.)

space in both groups; and 4) pain relief as an independent outcome. Trials that measured pain relief for radicular leg and low back pain, before and after epidural injections were included. Using the Cochrane Back Review Group recommendations, pain relief data were extracted independently by two reviewers into four categories: immediate (≤6 weeks); short-term (>6 weeks–3 months); intermediate (≥3 months–1 year); and long-term (≥1 year). Common effect sizes were calculated for each data point. Quality of the trials was assessed (two independent authors) using the 11-item criteria list recommended in the method guidelines for systematic reviews for the Cochrane Back Review Group. The data were analyzed by calculating the following: correlations between volume difference and effect size at each data point; and comparing the average effect sizes in the studies with same volume in both groups to ones with different volumes.

Results.—Fifteen studies fulfilled the inclusion/exclusion criteria. The correlation between volume difference and pain relief was 0.8027 ($p = .002$) for the immediate category, 0.5019 ($p = .168$) for the short-term category, and 0.9470 ($p = .014$) for the intermediate category. Insufficient data were available to calculate the correlation coefficient in the long-term category. There was a statistically significant difference when comparing the mean effect size where the volume injected was the same between the two groups (mean, standard deviation [SD]: 0.07, −0.26) with those where the volumes were different between comparison groups (mean, SD: 0.81, −0.6), irrespective of the medications injected.

Conclusions.—These preliminary results suggest a positive correlation between larger volumes of fluid injected in the epidural space and greater relief of radicular leg pain and/or low back pain. Clinicians should not change their practice, until further high-quality clinical studies confirm these findings (Figs 1-3).

▶ This study showed a correlation between higher injectate volumes and symptomatic improvement during the 6-week to 3-month time period and the 3-month to 1-year time period (Figs 2 and 3), and a nonsignificant trend toward benefit in the under-6-week period (Fig 1). As the authors point out, there are a number of major flaws in the study, including the fact that most of the studies they included were done without fluoroscopy. One postulate is that higher volumes are associated with lysis of epidural adhesions. Another possible explanation might be better spread of drug to target structures distant from the injection site. The use of fluoroscopy with epidurography improves the targeting of the injected drugs. It would be of interest to determine whether the addition of higher volumes might produce added benefit with fluoroscopic guided interlaminar or caudal epidurals. It would seem logical to inject saline or dilute local anesthetic first, followed by a small volume containing steroid subsequently. Very high injectate volumes are associated with adverse effects, (increased intracranial pressure, ophthalmic artery compression, and hypotension) and volumes should probably not exceed 15 to 20 mL. Obviously, better controlled studies are needed before applying the findings of this study to clinical practice.

S. E. Abram, MD

Lacosamide in Painful Diabetic Neuropathy: An 18-Week Double-Blind Placebo-Controlled Trial

Shaibani A, Fares S, Selam J-L, et al (Nerve and Muscle Ctr of Texas, Houston; Univ Clinical Investigators, Inc., Tustin, CA; et al)

J Pain 10:818-828, 2009

The efficacy and tolerability of oral lacosamide (200, 400, and 600 mg/day) was evaluated in patients with painful diabetic neuropathy in a double-blind, randomized, placebo-controlled trial. The primary target dose to be confirmed was lacosamide 400 mg/day. Efficacy was assessed by changes in pain scale scores from baseline, with changes over the last 4 weeks of the 12-week maintenance period regarded as the primary endpoint. Endpoint reductions in mean pain score were higher with all doses of lacosamide, reaching the level of significance with 400 mg/day ($P = .05$). Over the treatment period (titration + maintenance), pain relief was significantly higher than placebo with lacosamide 400 ($P = .02$) and 600 mg/day ($P = .03$). Lacosamide had an early-onset effect with significant reductions over placebo during the titration period. Nonparametric and mixed-model analysis approaches gave similar results, supporting

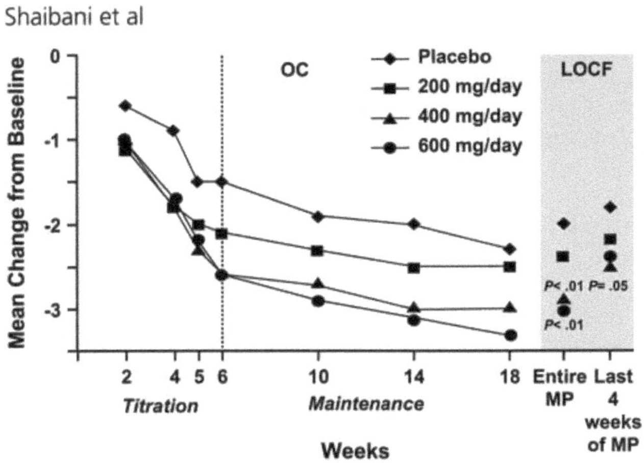

FIGURE 2.—Change in average daily pain score by trial visit week (OC) and at endpoint (ITT-LOCF). Placebo: n = 64, 60, 52, 53, 52, 50, and 47 at weeks 2, 4, 5, 6, 10, 14, and 18, respectively. Lacosamide 200 mg/day: n = 138, 124, 121, 117, 112, 110, and 101 at weeks 2, 4, 5, 6, 10, 14, and 18, respectively. Lacosamide 400 mg/day: n = 120, 110, 96, 96, 91, 81, and 78 at weeks 2, 4, 5, 6, 10, 14, and 18, respectively. Lacosamide 600 mg/day: n = 131, 117, 108, 91, 76, 58, and 49 at weeks 2, 4, 5, 6, 10, 14, and 18, respectively. (OC, observed cases; LOCF, last observation carried forward; MP, maintenance period). (Reprinted from Shaibani A, Fares S, Selam J-L, et al. Lacosamide in painful diabetic neuropathy: an 18-week double-blind placebo-controlled trial. *J Pain.* 2009;10:818-828, with permission from the American Pain Society.)

significant efficacy at 400 mg/day. Secondary criteria such as Patient's Global Impression of Change, responder rates, and pain-free days provided additional support. Adverse events included dizziness, nausea, and headache. Incidence of cognitive and behavioral adverse events was low. This trial suggests that lacosamide has beneficial effects and may be a suitable treatment option for patients with diabetic neuropathic pain.

Perspective.—This study presents efficacy and safety results of a phase 3, double-blind, placebo-controlled trial of the anticonvulsant drug lacosamide in patients with painful diabetic neuropathy. Lacosamide treatment at a dose of 400 mg/day reduced diabetic neuropathic pain with a favorable safety and tolerability profile that may be suitable for patients with diabetes (Fig 2, Table 3).

▶ Lacosamide has the advantage over other sodium channel blockers of selectivity for slow inactivating sodium channels. It should therefore suppress ectopic discharge while producing little effect on normal nerve conduction. This study shows a dose-related reduction in pain of diabetic neuropathy (Fig 2). The incidence of side effects, as with other sodium blocking drugs, was fairly high, particularly at the higher doses (Table 3). It is significant that nearly three fourths of the patients in this trial had failed other medications, such as gabapentin, opioids, and tricyclic antidepressants. This drug may

TABLE 3.—Adverse Events Reported in at Least 5% of Patients in Any Lacosamide Group (Safety Set)

Adverse Event (Preferred Term)	Placebo (N = 65)	Lacosamide 200 mg/day (N = 141)	Lacosamide 400 mg/day (N = 125)	Lacosamide 600 mg/day (N = 137)
	n (%)			
Any event	55 (84.6)	113 (80.1)	99 (79.2)	119 (86.9)
Dizziness	3 (4.6)	8 (5.7)	27 (21.6)	39 (28.5)
Headache	8 (12.3)	14 (9.9)	10 (8.0)	18 (13.1)
Tremor	0	6 (4.3)	12 (9.6)	20 (14.6)
Somnolence	0	7 (5.0)	10 (8.0)	12 (8.8)
Balance disorder	0	4 (2.8)	6 (4.8)	13 (9.5)
Hypoesthesia	0	0	0	7 (5.1)
Nausea	4 (6.2)	14 (9.9)	9 (7.2)	25 (18.2)
Diarrhea	5 (7.7)	9 (6.4)	6 (4.8)	11 (8.0)
Vomiting	0	6 (4.3)	2 (1.6)	9 (6.6)
Flatulence	0	5 (3.5)	0	9 (6.6)
Pruritis	1 (1.5)	6 (4.3)	9 (7.2)	7 (5.1)
Vertigo	1 (1.5)	1 (.7)	1 (.8)	8 (5.8)
Vision blurred	0	2 (1.4)	3 (2.4)	7 (5.1)
Fatigue	2 (3.1)	5 (3.5)	7 (5.6)	6 (4.4)
Sinusitis	2 (3.1)	8 (5.7)	3 (2.4)	1 (.7)
Back pain	2 (3.1)	8 (5.7)	4 (3.2)	5 (3.6)

become a reasonable second- or third-line drug, depending on its side effect profile compared with commonly used anticonvulsants and antidepressants.

S. E. Abram, MD

Ketamine produces effective and long-term pain relief in patients with Complex Regional Pain Syndrome Type 1

Sigtermans MJ, van Hilten JJ, Bauer MCR, et al (Leiden Univ Med Ctr, The Netherlands)

Pain 145:304-311, 2009

Complex Regional Pain Syndrome Type 1 (CRPS-1) responds poorly to standard pain treatment. We evaluated if the N-methyl-D-aspartate receptor antagonist S(+)-ketamine improves pain in CRPS-1 patients. Sixty CRPS-1 patients (48 females) with severe pain participated in a double-blind randomized placebo-controlled parallel-group trial. Patients were given a 4.2-day intravenous infusion of low-dose ketamine ($n = 30$) or placebo ($n = 30$) using an individualized stepwise tailoring of dosage based on effect (pain relief) and side effects (nausea/vomiting/psychomimetic effects). The primary outcome of the study was the pain score (numerical rating score: 0–10) during the 12-week study period. The median (range) disease duration of the patients was 7.4 (0.1–31.9) years. At the end of infusion, the ketamine dose was 22.2 ± 2.0 mg/h/70 kg. Pain scores over the 12-week study period in patients receiving ketamine were significantly lower than those in patients receiving placebo ($P < 0.001$). The lowest pain score was at the end of week 1: ketamine 2.68 ± 0.51, placebo 5.45 ± 0.48. In week 12, significance in pain relief between groups was lost ($P = 0.07$). Treatment did not cause functional improvement. Patients receiving ketamine more often experienced mild to moderate psychomimetic side effects during drug infusion (76% *versus* 18%, $P < 0.001$). In conclusion, in a population of mostly chronic CRPS-1 patients with severe pain at baseline, a multiple day ketamine infusion resulted in significant pain relief without functional improvement. Treatment with ketamine was safe with psychomimetic side effects that were acceptable to most patients.

▶ This study indicates that a 4-day course of intravenous (IV) ketamine produces lasting but not permanent pain reduction in patients with Complex Regional Pain Syndrome Type 1 (CRPS-1). The sampling of ketamine and norketamine blood levels provides useful indicators of levels required to produce pain relief with minimal side effects (Fig 2 in the original article). By the 12th week, there was no residual effect for the 30 patients who received the blinded ketamine (Fig 3 in the original article). However, in an open label study performed subsequently on 20 of those patients, the dissipation of benefit was slower, and there was some residual effect by week 12 (Fig 3 in the original article). This may have been related to an added placebo effect, as patients knew they were receiving active drug, or related to the fact that the procedure was being repeated (perhaps some residual effect from the first infusion), or to selection of patients who performed better in the controlled trial. The lack of functional benefit is discouraging. Perhaps combining the ketamine infusion with an aggressive rehabilitation program might have provided some functional benefit.

A 4-day admission is a hard sell for health care payors, particularly because the benefits were transient. The study does raise the possibility of other protocols, such as a short IV course combined with initiation of a home exercise program, followed by home use of oral ketamine.

S. E. Abram, MD

Duloxetine, a centrally acting analgesic, in the treatment of patients with osteoarthritis knee pain: A 13-week, randomized, placebo-controlled trial

Chappell AS, Ossanna MJ, Liu-Seifert H, et al (Lilly Res Laboratories, Indianapolis, IN; et al)

Pain 146:253-260, 2009

Pain is a common cause of disability in osteoarthritis. Duloxetine, a serotonin and norepinephrine reuptake inhibitor (SNRI), has demonstrated analgesic effects in diabetic peripheral neuropathy and fibromyalgia. Considering its central mechanism of action, duloxetine may be effective in other pain states with evidence of central sensitization. Herein, we report the results of a 13-week, randomized, double-blind, placebo-controlled trial of duloxetine (60–120 mg/day) versus placebo in the treatment of knee pain in 231 patients meeting clinical and radiographic criteria for osteoarthritis of the knee. Duloxetine was superior to placebo on the primary efficacy measure (weekly mean 24-h pain scores) beginning at Week 1 and continuing through the treatment period ($P \leq .05$). There was also a significant improvement in the WOMAC physical functioning subscale and several other secondary outcomes. Adverse-event rates did not differ significantly between treatment groups (49.5% for duloxetine 60–120 mg/day, and 40.8% for placebo).

▶ It has been proposed that the serotonin and norepinephrine reuptake inhibitor (SNRI) type antidepressants are selectively effective for patients with neuropathic pain. Observations and studies in patients with fibromyalgia suggest that this class of drugs may be effective for patients with other types of pain, including those with chronic nociceptive pain. This placebo-controlled study documents significant pain reduction (Fig 3 in the original article) and improved physical function (Fig 4 in the original article) over a 12-week period in patients with osteoarthritis of the knee. A less expensive alternative to duloxetine is venlafaxine, which has been shown to be effective in neuropathic pain trials, and has recently been shown to provide significant pain reduction in a 12-week placebo-controlled trial in osteoarthritis patients.[1]

As with most controlled trials, the duloxetine study did not address the long-term benefit of the drug. It is important to periodically reduce or discontinue drugs prescribed over long periods to determine whether they are still effective.

S. E. Abram, MD

Reference

1. Sullivan M, Bentley S, Fan MY, Gardner G. A single-blind placebo run-in study of venlafaxine XR for activity-limiting osteoarthritis pain. *Pain Med.* 2009;10: 806-812.

Long term clinical outcome of peripheral nerve stimulation in patients with chronic peripheral neuropathic pain

Van Calenbergh F, Gybels J, Van Laere K, et al (Univ Hosp Gasthuisberg, Belgium; et al)

Surg Neurol 72:330-335, 2009

Background.—Chronic neuropathic pain after injury to a peripheral nerve is known to be resistant to treatment. Peripheral nerve stimulation is one of the possible treatment options, which is, however, not performed frequently. In recent years we have witnessed a renewed interest for PNS. The aim of the present study was to evaluate the long-term clinical efficacy of PNS in a group of patients with peripheral neuropathic pain treated with PNS since the 1980s.

Methods.—Of an original series of 11 patients, 5 patients could be invited for clinical examination, detailed assessment of clinical pain and QST examination. The assessments were done both during habitual use of PNS and with the stimulator off.

Results.—Average pain intensity and pain unpleasantness ratings as assessed with visual analog and verbal rating scales showed significant beneficial effects of PNS. Quality of life measures (sleep and daily functioning) also showed positive effects. Quantitative Sensory Testing results did not show significant differences in cold pain and heat pain thresholds between the "ON" and "OFF" conditions.

Conclusion.—In selected patients with peripheral neuropathic pain PNS remains effective even after more than 20 years.

▶ This study indicates that peripheral nerve stimulation can provide many years of improved pain control in some patients. In this small series, 7 of 11 patients had enough benefit to continue using the stimulator for many years. One concern regarding this therapy is the development of fibrosis at the electrode site, reducing efficacy over time. This seems not to be an issue. The devices used were a circumferential electrode developed by Avery Biomedical Devices and a subcutaneous RF receiver with an external power source. These devices are no longer available. All of the patients had upper extremity pain with stimulation of the proximal portion of the nerve supplying the painful region.

The use of surgically implanted electrodes for peripheral nerve stimulation is rare. There is increasing interest in the use of percutaneous leads, but it is not known if the long-term benefits seen in this study will be evident.

S. E. Abram, MD

Intrathecal glycine for pain and dystonia in complex regional pain syndrome

Munts AG, van der Plas AA, Voormolen JH, et al (Leiden Univ Med Ctr, The Netherlands; et al)

Pain 146:199-204, 2009

Since glycinergic neurotransmission plays an important inhibitory role in the processing of sensory and motor information, intrathecal glycine (ITG) administration may be a potential therapy for both pain and movement disorders in patients with complex regional pain syndrome (CRPS). Aims of the current study, which is the first report on ITG in humans, were to evaluate its safety and efficacy. ITG treatment during 4 weeks was studied in CRPS patients with dystonia in the period before they received intrathecal baclofen treatment. Twenty patients were assessed and after exclusion of one patient, the remaining 19 patients were randomized in a double-blind placebo-controlled crossover study. Safety was assessed by clinical evaluation, blood examinations and electrocardiograms. Efficacy measures involved pain (numeric rating scale, McGill pain questionnaire), movement disorders (Burke–Fahn–Marsden dystonia rating scale, unified myoclonus rating scale, tremor research group rating scale), activity (Radboud skills questionnaire, walking ability questionnaire), and a clinical global impression (CGI) and patient's global impression score (PGI). Treatment-emergent adverse events were generally mild to moderate and not different from placebo treatment. During ITG treatment growth hormone levels were slightly increased. Although there was a trend to worsening on the CGI and PGI during ITG treatment, there were no significant differences between ITG and placebo treatment in any of the outcomes. ITG given over 4 weeks was ineffective for pain or dystonia in CRPS. Although no serious adverse events occurred, further studies are required to rule out potential neurotoxicity of ITG.

▶ While negative studies are not terribly exciting they are extremely important in ruling out potentially promising ideas and in identifying pathophysiological mechanisms. While there was no apparent therapeutic benefit in this group of patients, which was composed of very long-term, refractory individuals, there may be a response to intrathecal (IT) glycine in other painful conditions, and there is some preliminary evidence of safety from this study. Another interesting finding was the lack of any detectable placebo response in this population.

S. E. Abram, MD

The treatment of first division idiopathic trigeminal neuralgia with radiofrequency thermocoagulation of the peripheral branches compared to conventional radiofrequency

Huibin Q, Jianxing L, Guangyu H, et al (The Affiliate Stomatology Hosp of Tongji Univ, Shanghai, China)

J Clin Neurosci 16:1425-1429, 2009

The aim of this study was to prospectively evaluate and compare the effects of radiofrequency thermocoagulation of the first division branches of the trigeminal nerve (trigeminal peripheral division radiofrequency thermocoagulation, PRT) versus conventional radiofrequency (CRF) in the treatment of first division idiopathic trigeminal neuralgia (ITN). Fifty patients with first division ITN were randomly divided into two groups. The 20 patients in group 1 were treated with CRF, while the remaining 30 patients in group 2 were treated using PRT. The immediate therapeutic effects, side effects and recurrence rate of idiopathic trigeminal neuralgia were evaluated. The immediate efficacy rates were 95% and 93% in groups 1 and 2, respectively. The recurrence rates of ITN at the 3-year follow-up were 25% and 27% for group 1 and group 2, respectively, and 35% and 40%, respectively, 5 years after treatment. There were no significant differences between groups 1 and 2 at any time. Our study demonstrates that PRT is an effective way to treat first division ITN.

▶ This article provides evidence that peripheral thermal radiofrequency ablation may provide lasting benefit with few complications for patients with trigeminal neuralgia. It may be a reasonable alternative for debilitated patients who are not candidates for microvascular decompression because of serious comorbidities. Unfortunately, the details of the procedure are a bit sketchy. The authors indicate that some patients underwent denervation of second and third divisions at the infraorbital and mental foramina, but it is not clear how many patients in undergoing peripheral denervation had more than 1 division involved. The procedure described involved advancing the radiofrequency (RF) probe about 5 mm into the supraorbital foramen, which may be a difficult proposition given the size of most RF probes (the gauge was not indicated) and the small caliber of the foramen. Another concern is that 3-D CT scan was used to localize foramina, a procedure that is not universally available, and one that uses high levels of radiation.

S. E. Abram, MD

Reduction of allodynia in patients with complex regional pain syndrome: A double-blind placebo-controlled trial of topical ketamine

Finch PM, Knudsen L, Drummond PD (Perth Pain Management Centre, Australia; Murdoch Univ, Perth, Australia)

Pain 146:18-25, 2009

A double-blind placebo-controlled crossover trial was used to determine the effects of topical ketamine, an *N*-methyl-D-aspartate (NMDA) receptor antagonist, on the sensory disturbances in 20 patients with complex regional pain syndrome (CRPS). On two occasions separated by at least one week, sensory tests to light touch, pressure, punctate stimulation, light brushing and thermal stimuli were performed in the symptomatic and contralateral limb and on each side of the forehead before and 30 min after 10% ketamine cream was applied to the symptomatic or healthy limb. Venous blood for the plasma estimations of ketamine and norketamine was obtained 1 h after application of the creams. Ketamine applied to the symptomatic limb inhibited allodynia to light brushing and hyperalgesia to punctate stimulation. Systemic effects of the ketamine are unlikely to account for this as the plasma levels were below detectable limits. As touch thresholds were unchanged, NMDA receptors may contribute to the sensory disturbances in CRPS via actions at cutaneous nociceptors. Allodynia and hyperalgesia were detected in the ipsilateral forehead to a range of stimuli (brushing, pressure, punctate stimulation, cold, heat, and warmth). In several patients, ketamine treatment of the symptomatic limb inhibited allodynia to brushing the ipsilateral forehead, suggesting that the mechanism that mediates allodynia in the symptomatic limb contributed to allodynia at more remote sites. The present study shows promise for the use of topical ketamine as opposed to parenteral and oral forms which often result in undesirable side effects.

▶ Topical ketamine has been available through compounding pharmacies for several years, but evidence for its efficacy has been based on a few case reports. This randomized, placebo-controlled trial reported a significant reduction in allodynia following topical application in patients with complex regional pain syndrome (CRPS) (Fig 1 in the original article), but there was no reduction in baseline pain. Interestingly, pressure pain thresholds were increased after application of both ketamine and placebo (Fig 3 in the original article). Since systemic ketamine provides some reduction in the constant pain associated with CRPS, combinations of systemic (eg, oral) and topical ketamine may be useful. This study helps to differentiate between central and peripheral effects of the drug, suggesting that the antiallodynic effects are at least partially mediated through effects on nerve endings.

S. E. Abram, MD

Outpatient intravenous ketamine for the treatment of complex regional pain syndrome: A double-blind placebo controlled study

Schwartzman RJ, Alexander GM, Grothusen JR, et al (Drexel Univ College of Medicine, Philadelphia, PA)

Pain 147:107-115, 2009

Complex regional pain syndrome (CRPS) is a severe chronic pain condition that most often develops following trauma. The pathophysiology of CRPS is not known but both clinical and experimental evidence demonstrate the important of the NMDA receptor and glial activation in its induction and maintenance. Ketamine is the most potent clinically available safe NMDA antagonist that has a well established role in the treatment of acute and chronic pain. This randomized double-blind placebo controlled trial was designed to evaluate the effectiveness of intravenous ketamine in the treatment of CRPS. Before treatment, after informed consent was obtained, each subject was randomized into a ketamine or a placebo infusion group. Study subjects were evaluated for at least 2 weeks prior to treatment and for 3 months following treatment. All subjects were infused intravenously with normal saline with or without ketamine for 4 h (25 ml/h) daily for 10 days. The maximum ketamine infusion rate was 0.35 mg/kg/h, not to exceed 25 mg/h over a 4 h period. Subjects in both the ketamine and placebo groups were administered clonidine and versed. This study showed that intravenous ketamine administered in an outpatient setting resulted in statistically significant ($p < 0.05$) reductions in many pain parameters. It also showed that subjects in our placebo group demonstrated no treatment effect in any parameter.

TABLE 5.—Percent Change Between Baseline Values and Mean Values for Weeks 1–4 Post-treatment

Parameter	Placebo	Ketamine
McGill affective component	14.3	−50.3
Twenty gram monofilament on affected limb	0.7	−36.0
Brush allodynia of affected limb	−7.1	−34.2
Burning pain	−4.5	−33.0
McGill Sensory component	5.1	−29.7
Pain when touched or brushed lightly	−10.9	−25.3
Pain score (activity watch)	−3.1	−21.4
Pain in the most affected area	−2.3	−20.5
Degree your pain interferes with your general activity	−6.5	−18.4
Overall pain level	0.0	−18.1
Joint pain	−4.0	−16.9
Pain when deep pressure or squeezing is applied	−5.6	−16.1
Average	−2.0	−26.7

The table entries are gives as percent. Negative values show decreases (improvement) and positive values increases (worsening) from the pre-treatment score. Parameters are listed in decreasing order (most improvement in the ketamine group listed first). The activity watch entries evaluate the percent change between baseline values and mean values for weeks 1–2 post-treatment.

The results of this study warrant a larger randomized placebo controlled trial using higher doses of ketamine and a longer follow-up period (Table 5).

▶ This article provides further evidence that ketamine can improve symptoms of complex regional pain syndrome (CRPS) that outlasts the duration of the drug's analgesic effect (Fig 1 in the original article, Table 5). Most previous studies have been case reports or case series, and it is encouraging to see that the symptomatic improvement was statistically superior to that of a placebo. It is not clear whether the persistent benefit is related to the N-methyl-D-aspartate (NMDA) antagonist effects. The benefits of other NMDA antagonists such as dextromethorphan and memantine in chronic neuropathic conditions have not been very substantial. There are a number of potential therapeutic regimens for ketamine administration, including daily oral administration.

S. E. Abram, MD

Motor cortex electrical stimulation applied to patients with complex regional pain syndrome

Velasco F, Carrillo-Ruiz JD, Castro G, et al (General Hosp of Mexico)
Pain 147:91-98, 2009

Motor cortex stimulation (MCS) is useful to treat patients with neuropathic pain syndromes, unresponsive to medical treatment. Complex regional pain syndrome (CRPS) is a segmentary disease treated successfully by spinal cord stimulation (SCS). However, CRPS often affects large body segments difficult to cover by SCS. This study analyzed the MCS efficacy in patients with CRPS affecting them. Five patients with CRPS of different etiologies underwent a small craniotomy for unilateral 20-grid-contact implantation on MC, guided by craniometric landmarks. Neurophysiological and clinical tests were performed to identify the contacts position and the best analgesic responses to MCS. The grid was replaced by a definitive 4-contacts-electrode connected to an internalized system. Pain was evaluated by international scales. Changes in sympathetic symptoms, including temperature, perspiration, color and swelling were evaluated. Pre-operative and post-operative monthly evaluations were performed during one year. A double-blind maneuver was introduced assigning two groups. One had stimulators turned OFF from day 30–60 and the other from day 60–90. Four patients showed important decrease in pain, sensory and sympathetic changes during the therapeutic trial, while one patient did not have any improvement and was rejected for implantation. VAS and McGill pain scales diminished significantly ($p < 0.01$) throughout the follow-up, accompanied by disappearance of the sensory (allodynea and hyperalgesia) and sympathetic signs. MCS is effective not only to treat pain, but also improve the sympathetic changes in CPRS. Mechanism of action is actually unclear, but seems to involve sensory input at the level of the spinal cord.

▶ While it is not feasible or ethical to do randomized controlled trials of therapies such as motor cortex stimulation (MCS), this study does compare extended blinded trials of stimulation versus no stimulation, and showed significant symptomatic benefit during the trial in 4 of 5 patients. The proposed mechanisms of action include activation of centers controlling sensory input in the thalamus, activation of neurons in the cingulate gyrus, and initiation of descending control to the spinal dorsal horn. The patient who failed MCS had a brachial plexus avulsion injury with extensive upper extremity denervation. Larger studies will be needed to determine the characteristics of patients most likely to respond (eg, presence of allodynia, warm versus cold skin, response to sympathetic blocks, etc).

S. E. Abram, MD

Experimental Pain Management

Immune cell–derived opioids protect against neuropathic pain in mice

Labuz D, Schmidt Y, Schreiter A, et al (Freie Universität Berlin, Germany)

J Clin Invest 119:278-286, 2009

The analgesic effects of leukocyte-derived opioids have been exclusively demonstrated for somatic inflammatory pain, for example, the pain associated with surgery and arthritis. Neuropathic pain results from injury to nerves, is often resistant to current treatments, and can seriously impair a patient's quality of life. Although it has been recognized that neuronal damage can involve inflammation, it is generally assumed that immune cells act predominately as generators of neuropathic pain. However, in this study we have demonstrated that leukocytes containing opioids are essential regulators of pain in a mouse model of neuropathy. About 30%–40% of immune cells that accumulated at injured nerves expressed opioid peptides such as β-endorphin, Met-enkephalin, and dynorphin A. Selective stimulation of these cells by local application of corticotropin-releasing factor led to opioid peptide–mediated activation of opioid receptors in damaged nerves. This ultimately abolished tactile allodynia, a highly debilitating heightened response to normally innocuous mechanical stimuli, which is symptomatic of neuropathy. Our findings suggest that selective targeting of opioid-containing immune cells promotes endogenous pain control and offers novel opportunities for management of painful neuropathies.

▶ Peripheral opioid receptors are upregulated during inflammation, a phenomenon that has prompted studies of the effects of intra-articular opioids for knee surgery. This receptor upregulation appears to be associated with the appearance of opioids derived from immune cells that accumulate in regions of tissue injury. This study indicates that opioids – namely β-endorphin, Met-enkephalin, and dynorphin A – are released from immune cells in the vicinity of nerve injury, and that they may be important in reducing allodynia following nerve injury. Future therapies for the management of acute nerve injury may therefore involve suppressing the release or blocking the effects of proinflammatory cytokines and chemokines, which augment pain perception and enhance the effect of locally released opioid peptides.

S. E. Abram, MD

Axotomy Depletes Intracellular Calcium Stores in Primary Sensory Neurons

Rigaud M, Gemes G, Weyker PD, et al (Med College of Wisconsin, Milwaukee; Univ of Wisconsin, Madison; et al)

Anesthesiology 111:381-392, 2009

Background.—The cellular mechanisms of neuropathic pain are inadequately understood. Previous investigations have revealed disrupted Ca^{2+} signaling in primary sensory neurons after injury. The authors examined the effect of injury on intracellular Ca^{2+} stores of the endoplasmic reticulum, which critically regulate the Ca^{2+} signal and neuronal function.

Methods.—Intracellular Ca^{2+} levels were measured with Fura-2 or mag-Fura-2 microfluorometry in axotomized fifth lumbar (L5) dorsal root ganglion neurons and adjacent L4 neurons isolated from hyperalgesic rats after L5 spinal nerve ligation, compared to neurons from control animals.

Results.—Endoplasmic reticulum Ca^{2+} stores released by the ryanodine-receptor agonist caffeine decreased by 46% in axotomized small neurons. This effect persisted in Ca^{2+}-free bath solution, which removes the contribution of store-operated membrane Ca^{2+} channels, and after blockade of the mitochondrial, sarco-endoplasmic Ca^{2+}-ATPase and the plasma membrane Ca^{2+} ATPase pathways. Ca^{2+} released by the sarco-endoplasmic Ca^{2+}-ATPase blocker thapsigargin and by the Ca^{2+}-ionophore ionomycin was also diminished by 25% and 41%, respectively. In contrast to control neurons, Ca^{2+} stores in axotomized neurons were not expanded by neuronal activation by K^+ depolarization, and the proportionate rate of refilling by sarco-endoplasmic Ca^{2+}-ATPase was normal. Luminal Ca^{2+} concentration was also reduced by 38% in axotomized neurons in permeabilized neurons. The adjacent neurons of the L4 dorsal root ganglia showed modest and inconsistent changes after L5 spinal nerve ligation.

Conclusions.—Painful nerve injury leads to diminished releasable endoplasmic reticulum Ca^{2+} stores and a reduced luminal Ca^{2+} concentration. Depletion of Ca^{2+} stores may contribute to the pathogenesis of neuropathic pain.

▶ For many years much of the research on the pathophysiological changes accompanying tissue injury and inflammation and nerve injury have focused on changes in the spinal dorsal horn. *N*-methyl D-aspartate (NMDA) receptor activation and glial activation in the spinal cord are clearly important changes in mediating hyperalgesia. Recent research has identified a cascade of events that take place in the dorsal root ganglia (DRGs). The identification of reduced calcium stores consistently seen following spinal nerve ligation injury may lead to more specific therapies for patients with radiculopathy or mononeuropathies. Targeting the DRG with transforaminal steroid injections is an example of a therapy directed toward this neural structure. Direct injection of therapeutic substances at this site makes sense, as the DRG is outside of the blood-brain/blood-nerve barriers, and a variety of drugs that do not cross these tight junction barriers can gain access to the DRG.

S. E. Abram, MD

Differential mediation of descending pain facilitation and inhibition by spinal 5HT-3 and 5HT-7 receptors

Dogrul A, Ossipov MH, Porreca F (Gulhane Military Academy of Medicine, Ankara, Turkiye; Univ of Arizona College of Medicine, Tucson)

Brain Res 1280:52-59, 2009

The rostroventromedial medulla (RVM) is an important source of descending modulatory systems that both inhibit and facilitate pain at the level of the spinal cord. Noxious stimuli can activate serotonergic neurons in the RVM and accelerate the turnover of 5-HT in the spinal cord. While numerous studies suggest a bidirectional role for serotonergic transmission at the spinal level, the subtypes of the 5-HT receptors that are associated with descending facilitation or inhibition have not been clearly determined. Here, we explore the relative contribution of spinal 5-HT7 and 5-HT3 receptors to antinociception or hyperalgesia associated with states of enhanced net descending inhibition or facilitation from the RVM. In uninjured rats, RVM microinjection of morphine produced dose-dependent antinociception in the noxious thermal paw flick test while RVM microinjection of CCK produced thermal hyperalgesia and tactile allodynia. Spinal administration of the 5-HT7 antagonist SB-269970, but not of the 5-HT3 antagonist ondansetron, blocked the antinociceptive effects of RVM morphine. In contrast, hyperalgesia induced by RVM-CCK was blocked by spinal ondansetron, but not by SB-269970. The antinociceptive effects of systemic morphine were also blocked by spinal SB-269970 but not ondansetron while hyperalgesia and allodynia resulting from SNL injury were blocked by spinal ondansetron, but not SB-269970. These studies suggest that descending pain inhibitory or facilitatory pathways from RVM act ultimately in the spinal cord in acute and chronic pain states through activation of 5-HT7 and 5-HT3 receptors, respectively.

▶ For more than 2 decades, the role of serotonin in modulating pain perception through descending fibers from the rostroventromedial medulla (RVM) has been recognized. Early discussions focused on descending inhibitory effects, but efforts to increase central serotonergic effects, such as through the use of SSRIs, have not proven effective. It is now clear that some serotonin-containing descending pathways are pain-inhibitory while others are facilitatory. Dopaminergic and noradrenergic pathways also play a significant role in descending modulation of nociceptive inputs. The complexity of these modulatory systems is well documented in an extensive review published by Millan in 2002.[1] This study by Dogrul et al suggests that there is a net pain inhibitory effect mediated by 5-HT7 receptors and a facilitatory effect of 5-HT3 receptors in the spinal cord. The importance of this finding may be minimized by the possibility that this is a species-specific finding. Nevertheless, trials of appropriate agonists and antagonists in other animal models and eventually in humans may be promising.

S. E. Abram, MD

Reference

1. Millan MJ. Descending control of pain. *Prog Neurobiol.* 2002;66:355-474.

Cancer Pain Management

Morphine-Methadone Opioid Rotation in Cancer Patients: Analysis of Dose Ratio Predicting Factors

Benítez-Rosario MA, Salinas-Martín A, Aguirre-Jaime A, et al (NS Candelaria Univ Hosp, Tenerife, Spain; et al)

J Pain Symptom Manage 37:1061-1068, 2009

The dose ratio that is effective when switching opioid therapy from morphine to methadone in cancer patients varies widely. There are no conclusive data explaining the source of this variability. We analyzed 54 cancer patients undergoing opioid rotation to clarify those factors that influenced the morphine/methadone dose ratio (MMEDR) at Day 10 after the switch. Reasons for switching were uncontrolled pain (10 patients) or side effects (with or without pain, 44 patients). Initial MMEDR was 5:1 or 10:1 (82% or 18% of patients, respectively). Multivariate regression analysis was used to identify the demographic, cancer-related, and treatment-related variables that were potential predictors of MMEDR. Median previous morphine dose for the entire sample was 220 mg/day (range: 30–1000 mg/day). The stable MMEDR median was 5:1 (range: 2:1–15:1). In the univariate analysis, reasons for opioid rotation, age, and previous morphine doses were associated with MMEDR. Multiple linear regression analysis showed that only the reason for switching (pain vs. side effects; $P < 0.001$) and previous morphine doses (lower vs. upper to 300 mg/day; $P < 0.001$) were associated with MMEDR. From this analysis, the MMEDRs for patients rotated for side effects at 300 mg/day or more or less than 300 mg/day of morphine were 9.1:1 or 5.6:1, respectively, and the MMEDRs for those switched for pain at 300 mg/day or more or less than 300 mg/day of morphine were 4.9:1 or 3:1, respectively. Both the reasons for opioid rotation and previous morphine doses are predictive factors and should be used to select the MMEDR more accurately (Table 6).

▶ Switching from morphine to methadone can be difficult, primarily because it takes several days for the initial methadone dose to become evident. This study

TABLE 6.—MMEDR Predicted from Multivariate Linear Regression Analysis According to Predicting Factors[a]

Reason for Rotation and Previous Morphine Doses	MMEDR	95% CI
Side effects and >300 mg/day	9.1:1	22.9:1, 3.6:1
Pain and >300 mg/day	4.9:1	9.5:1, 2.5:1
Side effects and ≤300 mg/day	5.6:1	11.5:1, 2.8:1
Pain and ≤300 mg/day	3:1	4.8:1, 1.9:1

CI = confidence interval.
[a]Results are expressed in the habitual MMEDR scale after the antilogarithmic transformation of the final adjusted model.

indicated that the usual morphine to methadone daily dose ratio was 5:1, but high- versus low-dose morphine and the reason for switching (uncontrolled pain vs side effects) were independently predictive of different dose ratios (Table 6).

S. E. Abram, MD

Outpatient Continuous Interscalene Brachial Plexus Block in Cancer-Related Pain

Buchanan D, Brown E, Millar F, et al (Ninewells Hosp, Scotland, UK)

J Pain Symptom Manage 38:629-634, 2009

This case outlines the use of a continuous interscalene brachial plexus block to treat cancer-related pain. Using an elastomeric device, the patient's previously intractable pain was controlled and he was able to return home. Furthermore, the patient developed a pragmatic and effective method of balancing loss of power and sensation against pain control using the flow restrictor. This case illustrates the potential of an integrated approach to cancer pain management to obtain rapid pain relief in the acute hospital setting.

▶ Continuous regional analgesic techniques can be extremely effective at providing pain control during radiation therapy. These techniques are particularly helpful for patients who are unable to remain still in positions required for radiation sessions. In addition, such infusions provide excellent end-of-life analgesia. Many practitioners underestimate the duration that epidural or perineural catheters can remain effective. I was able to manage a single epidural catheter taken from a standard epidural tray for nearly 3 years in a patient with a slow-growing multiple myeloma involving the lumbar spine. Tunneled epidurals can easily be maintained for many months. There are definite advantages to externalized infusion systems over intrathecal pumps. In addition to the lower cost, the benefits of relatively high volumes of local anesthetics are substantial. The authors of this study added an adjustable clamp to the infusion tubing to allow the patient to adjust the flow from the elastomeric pump – an excellent cost-cutting measure.

S. E. Abram, MD

12 Geriatric Medicine Issue

Educational attainment and cognitive decline in old age

Wilson RS, Hebert LE, Scherr PA, et al (Rush Univ Med Ctr, Chicago, IL; Ctrs for Disease Control and Prevention, Atlanta, GA)

Neurology 72:460-465, 2009

Background.—Level of education is a well-established risk factor for Alzheimer disease but its relation to cognitive decline, the principal clinical manifestation of the disease, is uncertain.

Methods.—More than 6,000 older residents of a community on the south side of Chicago were interviewed at approximately 3-year intervals for up to 14 years. The interview included administration of four brief tests of cognitive function from which a previously established composite measure of global cognition was derived. We estimated the associations of education with baseline level of cognition and rate of cognitive change in a series of mixed-effects models.

Results.—In an initial analysis, higher level of education was related to higher level of cognition at baseline, but there was no linear association between education and rate of change in cognitive function. In a subsequent analysis with terms to allow for nonlinearity in education and its relation to cognitive decline, rate of cognitive decline at average or high levels of education was slightly increased during earlier years of follow-up but slightly decreased in later years in comparison to low levels of education. Findings were similar among black and white participants. Cognitive performance improved with repeated test administration, but there was no evidence that retest effects were related to education or attenuated education's association with cognitive change.

Conclusions.—The results suggest that education is robustly associated with level of cognitive function but not with rate of cognitive decline and that the former association primarily accounts for education's correlation with risk of dementia in old age.

▶ Boy is this disappointing. I thought that when I got a higher degree it would not only give me better cognitive function when I had the degree, but it would help prevent the decline in cognitive function when I got older. What a disappointment. I guess that means we have to keep learning and attaining.

M. F. Roizen, MD

Ageing populations: the challenges ahead

Christensen K, Doblhammer G, Rau R, et al (Univ of Southern Denmark, Odense; Univ of Rostock, Germany; et al)

Lancet 374:1196-1208, 2009

If the pace of increase in life expectancy in developed countries over the past two centuries continues through the 21st century, most babies born since 2000 in France, Germany, Italy, the UK, the USA, Canada, Japan, and other countries with long life expectancies will celebrate their 100th birthdays. Although trends differ between countries, populations of nearly all such countries are ageing as a result of low fertility, low immigration, and long lives. A key question is: are increases in life expectancy accompanied by a concurrent postponement of functional limitations and disability? The answer is still open, but research suggests that ageing processes are modifiable and that people are living longer without severe disability. This finding, together with technological and medical development and redistribution of work, will be important for our chances to meet the challenges of ageing populations.

▶ Why comment on this article? Because our populations of patients are getting older, and also because of what it says about the future for us. The article suggests that aging processes are modifiable and that people are living longer without severe disability. Its implication for us is that a second residency, and maybe a third after the age of 120, is well within view. No, I haven't been smoking tonight; that is what the data look like. This is one article to read for your personal and professional benefit.

M. F. Roizen, MD

13 Medical Education and Simulation

Gender difference in mask ventilation training of anesthesia residents
Koga T, Kawamoto M (Hiroshima Univ, Japan)
J Clin Anesth 21:178-182, 2009

Study Objective.—To investigate whether gender difference has an effect on an anesthesia resident's ability to perform successful mask ventilation.

Design.—Cohort study.

Setting.—Surgical operation theater of a university-affiliated hospital.

Patients.—839 ASA physical status I, II, and III patients undergoing general anesthesia performed by residents.

Intervention.—Mask ventilation was performed by 21 different anesthesia residents.

Measurements.—Difficult mask ventilation was defined as the inability of an unassisted resident to maintain oxygen saturation, significant gas flow leakage beneath the face mask, need to increase gas flow, no perceptible chest movement, assistance required using a two-handed mask ventilation technique, or use of the oxygen flush valve more than twice.

Main Results.—Instances of difficult mask ventilation were observed in 210 patients (25.0%), though all were adequately ventilated with a face mask. Difficult mask ventilation was observed significantly more often with female (29.8%) than male (20.0%) residents. Residents' gender was shown to be an independent risk factor for difficult mask ventilation.

Conclusions.—Gender difference has an effect on the mask ventilation learning process, as it was more difficult for female residents to provide a tight air seal in the early stage of training.

▶ Male and female residents are inevitably treated differently by different faculty over the course of their residency training. I was surprised to learn that, in this study, women required 10 cases more than men to master the skills of airway management. Whether the observed differences in ease of mastery of airway skills speak to a relative lack of muscle strength in female residents or something else is not known. That the women were able to learn to manage pediatric airways over the same time course as men would speak to the former. However, one has to wonder whether instructors more readily assisted their female residents rather than expecting that with a couple more attempts to ventilate a patient they would just get it.

Most anesthesiologists in academic programs do not undergo formal training in resident education. Certainly, though, residents of both genders satisfactorily complete their residency training programs and are able to appropriately manage adult airways. As the focus on resident education increases, however, training may become more standardized. As simulation begins to play an increasingly important role in resident education, teaching can, in fact, be tailored to an individual's needs. With ventilating a mannequin rather than a patient, early education will be less pressured and skills more easily mastered. Subsequent experience in the operating room will reinforce these early educational experiences.

C. A. Lien, MD

14 Anesthesia Outside the Operating Room

Overnight Observation in Stand-Alone Surgicenters: Is The Practice Safe?
Otterburn DM, Paredes A, Hester RT (Emory Univ, Atlanta, GA)
Ann Plast Surg 62:502-504, 2009

The safety of performing operations in surgery centers that require overnight stays has not been established. To determine whether this practice is safe we performed a retrospective chart review of all cases performed at Paces over a 12-year period. There were 12,072 total cases and 11,147 general anesthesia (GA) or monitored anesthesia care (MAC) cases. Four thousand eight hundred ten patients stayed overnight. The hospital admission rate for patients undergoing either GA or MAC was 0.12% and for local anesthesia it was 0%. Overnight stay patients had a rate of 0.15%, while same day discharge patients had a rate of 0.08%. Excluding local anesthesia cases, the rate increased to 0.10%. For the GA and MAC patients, there was no statistical difference in hospitalization rates between the same day and the overnight stay groups. All patients had good outcomes after hospitalization. Performing operations that require an overnight stay in a surgery center can be a safe practice.

▶ That this study found overnight observation in stand-alone surgicenters is safe is more a testament to the way that the surgicenter in Atlanta is staffed and run than a general commentary on freestanding ambulatory surgery clinics. There is too much information missing to draw sweeping conclusions.

The rate on unanticipated admissions over 12 years was 0.11%. While patients undergo what seems to be a thorough preoperative evaluation to determine their suitability for a procedure in an ambulatory setting, it is not apparent for specifically which procedures a period of overnight observation was scheduled. Was the need for overnight observation based on the surgical procedure, the duration of the surgery, intraoperative complications, comorbidities, or some other factor? While the admission rate for patients being observed overnight was 0.05% greater than those discharged home after their procedures, this difference did not achieve statistical significance. Additionally, the reasons for admission included bronchospasm or laryngospasm, oversedation, psychosis, hyponatremia, pulmonary embolus, deep vein thrombosis, and most commonly, hemorrhage. Interestingly, at least 6 of the patients requiring hospitalization had undergone abdominoplasties. The surgical procedures that the 3 patients with bronchospasm, the 1 with psychosis, and the 1 with hyponatremia had were not specifically mentioned. However, it appears that patients having abdominoplasties are more prone to require hospitalization than patients having other plastic surgical procedures in this surgicenter.

It would have been interesting and important to know how admission rates had changed over the course of the 12 years. Anesthesia (general and that provided for monitored anesthesia care) has changed over that period of time, and whether or not the admission rate had changed as well would have been important to know. Additionally, admission rates were not quantified based on whether a patient had received a general anesthetic or a monitored anesthetic. With over 12 000 cases, a comment on the specifics of the anesthetics patients requiring admission had received would have been warranted.

If patients are to be monitored overnight in a free-standing surgicenter, even after prolonged plastic surgical procedures, the center must be adequately staffed and located within a short distance from the hospital to which patients will be transferred should they need more acute care. Any surgical procedure, though, no matter how minor, as seen in this report, carries with it risks that, even with thoughtful preoperative evaluation, cannot be completely avoided.

C. A. Lien, MD

Article Index

Chapter 1: Studies of Outcomes, Risks, Costs, and Benefits

Chapter 2: Anesthesia-Related Pharmacology and Toxicology

Chapter 3: Anesthesia Techniques and Monitors

Chapter 4: Cardiothoracic and Vascular Anesthesia

Chapter 5: Pediatric Anesthesia

Chapter 6: Head Injury and Neuroanesthesia

Chapter 7: Critical Care Medicine

Chapter 8: Other Perioperative Patient Care Issues

Chapter 9: Patient Safety, Complications, and Mishaps in Anesthesia

Chapter 10: Obstetric Anesthesia

Chapter 11: Pain Management

Author Index

N

O

P

Q

R

S

T

U

V

W

X

Y

Z